Ambient Assisted Living (AAL) Technologies

Ambient assisted living (AAL) utilizes information and communication technology to empower individuals to maintain an active and independent lifestyle for as long as possible. The concept of AAL has been around for decades, but with the evolution of the healthcare sector, we have seen significant advancements in AAL technologies. In recent years, there has been a growing trend towards living alone, and AAL plays a crucial role in supporting individuals to live independently. *Ambient Assisted Living (AAL) Technologies: Transitioning from Healthcare 4.0 to Healthcare 5.0* is divided into four comprehensive sections that explore the shift from Healthcare 4.0 to Healthcare 5.0.

It covers AAL technology in the context of Healthcare 4.0 and the Internet of Things (IoT) and fog computing frameworks for real-time applications of natural language processing (NLP) in AAL. The text also delves into advanced artificial intelligence methods for data analytics in AAL, focusing on real-time applications and data analysis for practical use. Additionally, the book covers advanced enabling technologies like blockchain, big data, fog computing and cutting-edge AI techniques for assisted living in Healthcare 5.0. The integration of these technologies and perspectives is crucial for advancing assisted living in the realm of Healthcare 5.0. This book is perfect for students and researchers specializing in AAL and NLP. Professionals working on products for assisted living can also benefit from the valuable insights provided by recent research to improve the efficiency and advancement of their products.

The topic of AAL is already a part of the curriculum in many universities and institutes, and this book will help students explore the various applications of NLP within this field. In addition, individuals looking to engage in innovative projects can find inspiration from the latest advancements in AAL.

Innovations in Health Informatics and Healthcare: Using Artificial Intelligence and Smart Computing

Ambient Assisted Living (AAL) Technologies:
Transitioning from Healthcare 4.0 to Healthcare 5.0
Edited by Rashmi Gupta, Xiomara Patricia Blanco Valencia, Lalit Mohan Goyal and Jeetendra Kumar

Ambient Assisted Living (AAL) Technologies

Transitioning from Healthcare 4.0 to Healthcare 5.0

Edited by
Rashmi Gupta, Xiomara Patricia Blanco Valencia,
Lalit Mohan Goyal and Jeetendra Kumar

CRC Press
Taylor & Francis Group
Boca Raton London New York

CRC Press is an imprint of the
Taylor & Francis Group, an **informa** business

Designed cover image: Stock-Asso/Shutterstock

First edition published 2025
by CRC Press
2385 NW Executive Center Drive, Suite 320, Boca Raton FL 33431

and by CRC Press
4 Park Square, Milton Park, Abingdon, Oxon, OX14 4RN

CRC Press is an imprint of Taylor & Francis Group, LLC

ISBN: 978-1-032-85859-3 (hbk)
ISBN: 978-1-032-85860-9 (pbk)
ISBN: 978-1-003-52018-4 (ebk)

DOI: 10.1201/9781003520184

Typeset in Times
by Newgen Publishing UK

Contents

SECTION III Artificial Intelligence (AI) for Data Analysis for Assisted Living in Healthcare 5.0

Preface

Ambient assistant living (AAL) is the use of information and communication technology to enable individuals to stay active and live independently as long as possible. The concept of AAL came into existence in previous decades but along with the evolvement of the healthcare sector from Healthcare 1.0 to Healthcare 4.0, advancement is also seen in ambient assisted living technologies. In previous years, the trend of living alone has increased and AAL helps people to live independently.

This book explores the current advancements in ambient assisted living technology in the healthcare field, specifically in the context of Healthcare 5.0. It also examines the significant shift from Healthcare 4.0 towards Healthcare 5.0. The book is divided into four unique sections, providing a full exploration of this revolutionary topic. The introductory section offers readers a comprehensive overview and introduction to ambient assisted living. The text delves into the changing societal living patterns and the role of ambient assisted living technologies in enabling increased autonomy for individuals. Transitioning to the second section, the book explores a diverse range of subjects including wearable and ambient sensors, communication modules, assistive technologies, IoT/fog computing for AAL and blockchain for privacy and security in AAL. The third section explores the utilization of artificial intelligence methods in healthcare analytics, encompassing topics such as fall prediction, prediction of clinical drug response, diet and diabetes management, drug dispenser systems, telemedicine, remote health monitoring etc. The last section of the book examines the practical implementations of natural language processing (NLP) in the context of ambient assisted living. This includes NLP techniques for AAL, speech emotion recognition for AAL and text analytics of health records using various natural language processing techniques.

This book provides a comprehensive review of technological advancements in ambient assisted living technologies in Healthcare 4.0 as well as in forthcoming Healthcare 5.0. The major benefit of this book is that along with the fundamental and technological advances in AAL, it also elaborates on applications of natural language processing techniques for AAL. In recent years, major advancements have been seen in natural language processing techniques and it is also becoming an integrated part of ambient assisted living. Along with NLP, many advanced technologies for Healthcare 5.0 like IoT/fog infrastructure, blockchain, advanced AI techniques for AAL, remote patient monitoring, etc., for assisted living are also discussed in the book.

Features

- Readers will obtain knowledge of the latest AAL technologies developed to solve the toughest business challenges in sectors such as healthcare and medicine assistance, smart cities and smart homes, IoT, fog computing and more.
- The professional contributions will provide readers with clear insights into how the most recent exciting advancements may be expected to aid in meeting the desired requirements of people living alone.

- This book will be helpful for the reader to get insights into advancements in AAL, its enabling technologies and the application of NLP in AAL in one place.
- This book will also help to get an insight into various state-of-the-art research in the area of AAL that have been performed in the last two to three years and are not covered in other books, thus encouraging future research work.
- This book also discusses advanced enabling technologies like 5G, big data, blockchain, edge computing and advanced AI methods for assisted living in forthcoming Healthcare 5.0.

Acknowledgments

We would like to express our sincere gratitude to everyone who contributed to the development and publication of this book.

First and foremost, we extend our deepest gratitude to Dr. Mamta Mittal, series editor of *Innovations in Health Informatics and Healthcare: Using Artificial Intelligence and Smart Computing* for her precious guidance, encouragement and unwavering support during the entire content preparation and publication process. Her insights and direction were essential in shaping the structure and scope of this book. We are very grateful for all the contributors who provided high-quality chapters and shared their expertise. Their dedication and hard work have significantly enhanced the depth and breadth of the content. We would like to extend our sincere gratitude to CRC PRESS (A Taylor & Francis Company) for accepting our book and offering a platform for its publication. Their professionalism and support have been vital throughout the process.

Our thanks also go out to all of our colleagues, whose constant help, advice and encouragement were helpful during the preparation of this book. Their support and collaboration were essential in making this project a success. We are deeply grateful for our families for their constant support, patience and encouragement during this journey. Without their love and understanding, the completion of this work would not have been possible.

Lastly, we offer our heartfelt thanks to God for giving us the strength, inspiration and determination to make this book project complete.

— The Editors

About the Editors

Rashmi Gupta holds a Ph.D. degree in Computer Applications from the NIT, Raipur. Currently, she serves as an Assistant Professor in the Department of Computer Science and Application at Atal Bihari Vajpayee University Bilaspur, Chhattisgarh. With over 11 years of teaching experience, her research interests encompass natural language processing, EEG signal processing and human activity recognition. She has published more than 20 research papers, conference papers and book chapters. She has been awarded grants by AICTE to organize the ATAL Faculty Development Program and by the Science and Engineering Research Board, DST for conducting high-end workshops and internships. Demonstrating her commitment to mentorship, Dr. Gupta has guided over 30 PG and 20 UG students in their research-related major projects.

Xiomara Patricia Blanco Valencia, a Ph.D. holder in Computer Science and Automation with a Master's in Intelligent Systems, is a faculty member at Universidad International de la Rioja since 2019. She excels as a teacher and researcher in artificial intelligence and data governance, notably as Managing Editor at IJIMAI since 2021. Formerly at CYTOGNOS as a Software Analyst-Programmer, her work on the MIDAS project showcased her proficiency in Java programming and AI techniques. With a rich academic journey, including Ph.D. candidacy at the University of Salamanca, Xiomara's expertise spans case-based reasoning, medical diagnosis and AI applications. Her extensive publication record underscores her commitment to advancing computer science and automation, making her a pivotal figure in academia and industry.

Lalit Mohan Goyal, an Assistant Professor in the Department of Computer Engineering at J.C. Bose University of Science and Technology, YMCA, Faridabad, boasts over 19 years of extensive experience in both teaching and research. He has significantly contributed to the academic realm with 29 SCI and SCIE indexed research papers published across esteemed journals such as IEEE, Springer and Elsevier. Additionally, Dr. Goyal holds eight patents and has served as the editor for 5 books and author of 11 book chapters published by renowned publishers like Springer and CRC Press. His leadership further exemplifies his dedication to advancing knowledge in a research project granted by ICMR, New Delhi, and his role as a reviewer for reputable journals including Springer, IEEE and ACM publications. Dr. Goyal's research interests span various domains, including data mining, theory of computation, discrete mathematics and data structures and algorithms. Moreover, he has imparted his expertise by delivering over 20 keynote lectures in numerous workshops and conferences, further establishing himself as a respected person in the field.

Jeetendra Kumar holds Ph.D. degree in Computer Science from GLA University, Mathura, India and has worked as an Assistant Professor in the Department of Computer Science & Application at Atal Bihari Vajpayee University, Bilaspur,

Chhattisgarh, India for the last 11 years. He holds a Master's degree (M.Sc.) and a Master of Technology (M.Tech.) in Computer Science. He has published various research articles in reputed journals and conferences, including topics like sentiment analysis, fall detection using machine-learning techniques, IoT applications, automatic question generation, etc. He has also contributed book chapters on topics related to neuroscience, smartphone applications and fog computing in healthcare. He has completed two research projects sponsored by the State Planning Commission, C.G., and Commonwealth Media Centre for Asia (CEMCA) New Delhi and Atal Bihari Vajpayee University, Bilaspur. He is also a member of prestigious academic societies such as IEEE, the Indian Science Congress, the International Association of Engineers (IAENG), the International Computer Science and Engineering Society (ICSES) and the International Association of Academicians (IAASSE).

Contributors

Francesco Amenta
Telemedicine and Telepharmacy Centre,
School of Medicinal and Health Products Sciences,
University of Camerino, Italy

N. Sharmila Banu
School of CS&AI, SR University, Warangal,
Telangana, India

Gopi Battineni
Telemedicine and Telepharmacy Centre,
School of Medicinal and Health Products Sciences,
University of Camerino,
Italy

Nidhika Chauhan
Chandigarh University,
Punjab, India

Nalini Chintalapudi
Telemedicine and Telepharmacy Centre,
School of Medicinal and Health Products Sciences,
University of Camerino,
Italy

Sharmin Chougule
School of Law, University of Camerino,
Camerino, Italy

Dharmendra Dangi
Indian Institute of Information Technology (IIIT),
Bhopal, India

R. Nancy Deborah
Velammal College of Engineering and Technology,
Madurai, Tamil Nadu, India

K. Deepa
School of CS&AI, SR University,
Warangal, Telangana, India

Rashmi Gupta
Department of Computer Science and Application,
Computer Science and Application,
Atal Bihari Vajpayee University,
Bilaspur, Chhattisgarh, India

P. Harish
Department of ECE,
Annamacharya Institute of Technology and Sciences,
Tirupati, Andhra Pradesh, India

Alan James
Tata Elxsi,
Kerala, India

Jomin Joy
Department of EEE,
Amal Jyothi College of Engineering,
Kanjirappalli, Kerala, India

Inderpreet Kaur
Chitkara University
Institute of Engineering and Technology Chitkara University
Rajpura, Punjab, India

Navneet Kaur
Chandigarh University,
Punjab, India

Atul Kumar
Department of Computer Science,R.G.M.
Govt. College Joginder Nagar,
Himachal Pradesh, India

Jeetendra Kumar
Department of Computer Science and Application,
Computer Science and Application, Atal Bihari Vajpayee University,
Bilaspur, Chhattisgarh, India

S.N. Kumar
Department of EEE, Amal Jyothi College of Engineering,
Kanjirappalli, Kerala, India

Paula Lamo
Universidad Internacional de La Rioja,
La Rioja. Spain

Pattisapu Manikanta Manohar
Department of Computer Science and Engineering,
GITAM School of Technology,
GITAM (Deemed to be University), Visakhapatnam.
Andhra Pradesh, India

Eno Chongs Mantu
Department of Medical Microbiology,
Federal College of Medical Laboratory Science & Technology
Jos, Nigeria

Ujjwal Matoliya
Computer Science and Application, Atal Bihari Vajpayee University,
Bilaspur, Chhattisgarh, India

Shikha Mittal
Chitkara University Institute of Engineering and Technology
Chitkara University
Rajpura, Punjab, India

Chetna Monga
Chitkara University Institute of Engineering and Technology
Chitkara University
Rajpura, Punjab, India

Kashish Mukhija
Chitkara University Institute of Engineering and Technology
Chitkara University
Rajpura, Punjab, India

Seema P. Nehete
Datta Meghe College of Engineering,
Airoli, Maharashtra, India

Nkechinyere Linda Obeta
Department of Legal Services,
Federal College of Medical Laboratory Science and Technology
Jos, Nigeria

Uchejeso Mark Obeta
Department of Medical Laboratory Management,
Federal College of Medical Laboratory Science & Technology
Jos, Nigeria

Dooshima Augustina Orshio
Chemical Pathology Unit, Department of Medical Laboratory Services,
Federal Medical Centre,
Makurdi, Nigeria

P. Pujari
Department of Computer Science & Information Technology,
Guru Ghasidas Vishwavidyalaya, Bilaspur,
Chhattisgarh, India

Nainaru Pushpalatha
Department of ECE, Annamacharya Institute of Technology and Sciences,
Tirupati, Andhra Pradesh, India

J. Javier Rainer
Universidad Internacional de La Rioja,
La Rioja. Spain

Nicole Rakov
Universidade de Averio,
Portugal

Kasarapu Ramani
School of Computing, Mohan Babu University, Tirupati,
Andhra Pradesh, India.

Giovanna Ricci
School of Law, University of Camerino,
Camerino, Italy

Prabu Selvam
Department of CSE, SRM Institute of Science and Technology,
Tamil Nadu, India

Suvarna Sharma
Chitkara University Institute of Engineering and Technology
Chitkara University
Rajpura, Punjab, India

Richa Singh
Department of Psychology, Vasanta College for Women, Rajghat Fort,
Varanasi, India

G. Sivakarthi
Velammal College of Engineering and Technology,
Madurai, Tamil Nadu, India

M. Soundarya
Velammal College of Engineering and Technology,
Madurai, Tamil Nadu, India

Irala Suneetha
Dept. of ECE, Annamacharya Institute of Technology and Sciences,
Tirupati, Andhra Pradesh, India.

Anurag Upadhyay
Department of Psychology, Udai Pratap Autonomous College,
Varanasi, India

A. Vinora
Velammal College of Engineering and Technology,
Madurai, Tamil Nadu, India

Section I

Overview and Recent Advances in Ambient Assisted Living (AAL) Technologies in Healthcare 4.0

1 Overview and Recent Advances in Ambient Assisted Living Technologies Transitioning from Healthcare 4.0 to Healthcare 5.0

Pattisapu Manikanta Manohar

1.1 INTRODUCTION

Ambient assisted living (AAL) pertains to information technology (IT) solutions and systems specifically developed to aid the elderly. The goal is to improve their standard of living and assist with everyday tasks. AAL solutions strive to prevent or defer the transition to long-term care facilities, offering important assistance to elderly individuals in their own surroundings. These solutions integrate modern information and communication technologies (ICTs) with social circumstances, promoting active aging and improving overall well-being throughout the life cycle.

AAL deals with a concept where technology is indispensable when it comes to the independence and safety of elderly citizens in their own homes (Martins et al., 2018). Thus, it is in the interest of aging people to stay in familiar surrounding for as long as possible and receive proper care through smart systems. AAL means technologies that help elderly or disabled persons to go through their daily activities, being protected from potential risks. As a result, the AAL systems are intended to help people to have a healthier and more independent life for more years due to the advancement in the age of the populations. AAL solutions aim to connect digital environments with inherent and profound intelligence to boost the quality of life for older individuals (Martins et al., 2018). The organization of the work is depicted in Figure 1.1.

DOI: 10.1201/9781003520184-2

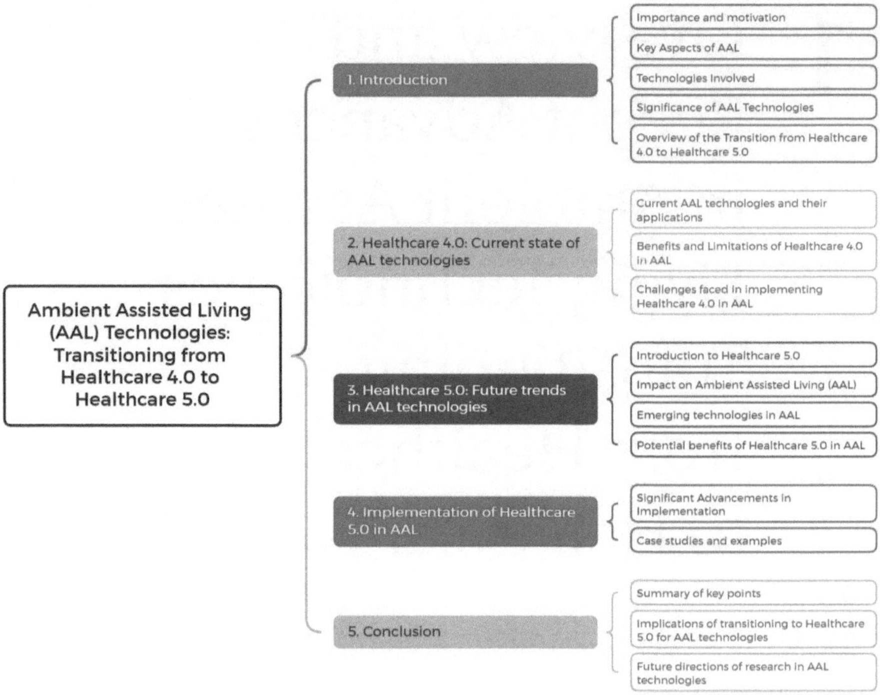

FIGURE 1.1 Overview of recent advances in AAL technologies transitioning from Healthcare 4.0 to Healthcare 5.0.

1.1.1 Key Aspects of AAL

Technological Adoption for Active Aging: In performing an activity or task, the real age matters since it is commonly observed that doing comparative tasks and activities as one gains age has a poorer outcome. However, it is imperative to adopt unique technologies to improve the support services and foster the policy on active aging. Technological applications of AAL solutions assist elderly people and contribute to the enhancement of their quality of life. Such solutions comprise integrated packages of products and services aimed at fulfilling the needs, including disease prevention and health promotion, as well as managing the difficulties of chronic diseases (Blackman et al., 2016).

Safety and Monitoring: With AAL solutions, the security of elderly people is improved by including alarm instruments and remote tracking. Such systems have a way of identifying emergencies or anomalies inherent in daily activities and notifying the caregivers or the appropriate authorities (Martins et al., 2018).

Cost Reduction in Healthcare Services: Applying AAL solutions, various healthcare costs may be hugely saved in the future. Preventing and early management of cases reduce the load on a healthcare system (Martins et al., 2018).

1.1.2 Technologies Involved

They consist of smart equipment, wireless networks, software services, computer systems, and healthcare sensors installed in the living structure. They allow people to continue accessing healthcare, help perform activities, and maintain interaction (Caballero et al., 2023). Figure 1.2 shows the technologies involved in AAL.

Wearable Sensors: In AAL, wearable devices include smart watches and fitness trackers. They always observe older adults' condition, activity rate, and gait. These sensors provide real-time information to control health issues and help take early interventions (Stodczyk, 2020; Cicirelli et al., 2021)

Smart Objects and Devices: The innovative applications and products become integrated into the context of the living space to enhance security and life experience. Some of the current smart devices are intelligent thermostats, smart lighting

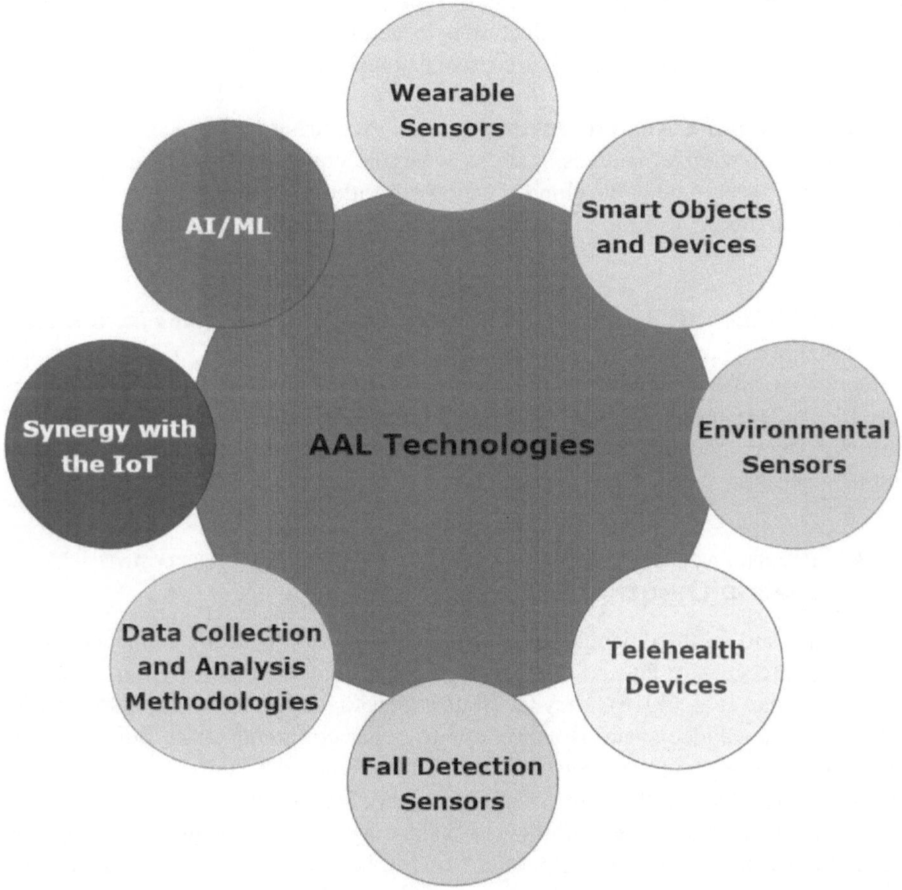

FIGURE 1.2 Technologies involved in ambient assisted living.

controls, voice control assistants, and smart appliances. These devices enable older adults to manage their environment effectively and modify it if need be (Stodczyk, 2020; Jovanovic et al., 2022; Wilton, 2023).

Environmental Sensors: Sensors feel the environment, including temperature, humidity, and air quality, among other things. They assist in safety by creating alarms for the caregivers or the emergency services once there are signs that something is wrong (e.g., gas leakage or fire) and make sure that the client's living condition is comfortable (Stodczyk, 2020; Cicirelli et al., 2021).

Telehealth Devices: Telehealth technologies are useful tools for remote health checks and communication between the oldest people and doctors. Under this, we are talking about video consultation, medicine reminders, and the sharing of health information. Telehealth encourages self-sufficiency and limits the number of hospital visits the patient needs (Stodczyk, 2020; Wilton, 2023).

Fall Detection Sensors: Fall detection sensors employ accelerometers and gyroscopes to detect falls that occur suddenly. Such sensors call for the attention of the caregivers or the emergency services if a fall has been registered (Stodczyk, 2020; Wilton, 2023).

Data Collection and Analysis Methodologies: Acquiring and processing big and small data from various sources, such as wearable equipment and sensors, is crucial for AAL development. Machine-learning algorithms, as well as statistic models, are widely used to analyze the data that has been collected (Aumayr, 2016; Cicirelli et al., 2021).

Synergy with the IoT: The IoT plays a significant role in developing an intelligent environment that supports AAL systems (Caballero et al., 2023). IoT facilitates the interaction of different applications and objects, hence making the AAL solutions more transparent and intelligent. Thus, integrating AAL and IoT will enable the creation of systems that support the elderly, raise their quality of life, and provide them with the necessary care while staying at home (Caballero et al., 2023).

1.1.3 Significance of AAL Technologies in Improving Elderly and Disabled Quality of Life

Most elderly and disabled people enhance their quality of life through enhanced independence, safety, warmth, and comfort through AAL technologies (Martins et al., 2018; Blackman et al., 2016). They facilitate access to medical services, help perform daily tasks, and reduce social isolation due to better communication. Subsequently, the expansion of AAL in the context of the IoT has promoted the development of smart spaces that promote healthy aging (Caballero et al., 2023; Blackman et al., 2016).

The significance of AAL technology in enhancing the well-being of elderly and disabled individuals has been emphasized as follows: *improving independence and autonomy.* AAL systems assist elderly people and individuals with impairments to maintain independent living for longer durations. Smart objects, wearable sensors, and environmental monitoring contribute to safety and autonomy within their living spaces (Cicirelli et al., 2021; Jovanovic et al., 2022).

Health Monitoring and Early Detection: Wearable sensors continuously monitor vital signs, activity levels, and movement patterns. Early identification of ailments allows for prompt interventions, which reduce hospital visits and improve general well-being (Cicirelli et al., 2021).

Enhancing Social Connectivity: AAL technologies foster social interaction by enabling communication through smart devices. Smartphones, tablets, and video conferencing tools connect older adults with family, friends, and support networks (Cynthia S Y LAU et al., 2021).

Supporting Caregivers and Medical Staff: AAL systems provide real-time data to caregivers and medical professionals. Remote monitoring and alerts help caregivers respond promptly to emergencies or changes in health status (Cicirelli et al., 2021)

Quality of Life Enhancement: By promoting independence, safety, and well-being, AAL technologies significantly enhance the overall standard of life for elderly and disabled individuals (Benetazzo et al., 2015).

1.1.4 Overview of the Transition from Healthcare 4.0 to Healthcare 5.0

The transition from Healthcare 4.0 to Healthcare 5.0 signifies combining human abilities with new technologies to establish a healthcare ecosystem that prioritizes the patient, operates efficiently, and demonstrates empathy (Aumayr, 2016). Healthcare 5.0 emphasizes personalization and customer focus, leveraging expertise like AI and cloud computing to boost patient care and the overall healthcare experience (Aumayr, 2016).

Healthcare 5.0: A human-centered approach known as Healthcare 5.0 seeks to reconcile the economy's progress with resolving societal issues. It aims to create a society where technological innovation eliminates disparities and provides services tailored to individual needs. In this society, AAL technologies will be pivotal in delivering personalized, efficient, and inclusive healthcare solutions (Martins et al., 2018). The transition from Healthcare 4.0 to Healthcare 5.0 represents the many stages of growth in the healthcare sector, where advanced technology are integrated to enhance patient care and overall health.

Healthcare 4.0: The Fourth Industrial Revolution (4IR) marked the beginning of digital transformation in healthcare. Notable aspects encompassed Health 4.0, an approach prioritizing interoperability, personalized medicine, and decision-making based on data. By employing advanced technologies such as machine learning, IoT, and big data analytics, healthcare delivery was enhanced (Coile, 2024).

TABLE 1.1
Some Main Aspects of Healthcare 4.0 and Healthcare 5.0

Aspect	Healthcare 4.0	Healthcare 5.0
Focus	Process optimization for healthcare professionals	Patient-oriented care
Technologies	AI, machine learning, IoT, big data	AI, IoT, blockchain, virtual & augmented reality, digital twin
Patient Involvement	Limited patient involvement	Active patient involvement
Communication	Traditional doctor–patient interactions	Transparent communication for effective relationships
Benefits	Improved efficiency, informed decisions	Personalized care, holistic treatment
Limitations	digital literacy, context, digital transformation, privacy and security	Patient acceptance, customization complexity, standardization

Healthcare 5.0: Industry 5.0 (I5.0) redefines healthcare by expanding the symbiotic relationship between human capabilities and technological advancements. It prioritizes an environment that is expeditious, empathetic, and patient-centred. It leverages emerging technologies such as IoT, AI, and digital twins to transform patient care and services. Increased collaboration exists between physicians, patients, and devices (Basulo-Ribeiro & Teixeira, 2024).

Digital Wellness and Personalization: Healthcare 5.0 focuses on customer-centricity, well-being, and quality of life. Personalized healthcare solutions empower patients and enhance their experience (Byrne, 2023).

Policy Guidelines and Strategic Integration: I5.0 strategic integration in healthcare necessitates a shift in policy. This integration benefits the healthcare sector significantly (Basulo-Ribeiro & Teixeira, 2024).

Healthcare 5.0 represents a transformative shift where technology augments human competence, leading to a more holistic and practical healthcare ecosystem. Some of the main aspects of Healthcare 4.0 and Healthcare 5.0 are shown in Table 1.1.

1.2 HEALTHCARE 4.0: CURRENT STATE OF AAL TECHNOLOGIES

The current state of AAL technologies showcases a blend of AI, IoT, and other digital advances. These technologies are designed to assist with daily activities, monitor health parameters, and provide emergency assistance. The focus is on creating intuitive systems that users can easily adopt without technical expertise (Cicirelli et al., 2021). Including AAL in IoT has further progressed the development of intelligent environments for healthy aging.

Healthcare 4.0 and AAL Technologies: Healthcare 4.0 is distinguished by the attempt to include technology in the healthcare approaches to improve the delivery of services, enhance patients' experiences, and give attention to individual needs. On this basis, there have been improvements in AAL technologies. They are becoming more intelligent, sophisticated, and functional, making the elderly and disabled persons self-reliant (Cicirelli et al., 2021).

1.2.1 Artificial Intelligence (AI) in AAL

The application of AI is critical for AAL as it contributes to the smart decision-making process, personalization, and automation. The application of AI in AAL is the following:

Health Monitoring: AI models utilize vital physiological indicators, like pulse rate, blood pressure, and breathing rate, through intelligent sensors and IoT devices. Listed below are the usual key techniques employed in the field, such as deep learning, natural language processing, and clustering (Jovanovic et al., 2022). These models help to identify errors and future health conditions and to care for the patient on time.

Activity Assistance and Recognition: AI-based systems identify daily tasks (for example, walking, eating, and taking a shower) with the help of data collected by wearable gadgets and sensors. The availability of contextual data and the introduction of machine-learning methods improve the detection accuracy and make the methods more flexible (Cicirelli et al., 2021).

Personalization: AI technologies help personalize services with recommendations based on patients' choices, routines, and state of health. AI includes features like reminders according to the user's preference, medication doses, and the light's changing colors.

1.2.2 Internet of Things (IoT) in AAL

IoT is the enabling technology that supports the connectivity of the devices, services, and applications in AAL environments. IoT has the capacity to enhance the well-being for elderly individuals by utilizing sophisticated AAL environments. These environments utilize IoT technologies to establish smart residences that promote self-sufficient safe living for elderly citizens. Key aspects of IoT in AAL includes the following:

Ambient Sensing: IoT-enabled sensors collect data on temperature, humidity, light, and movement. This data informs decisions related to comfort, safety, and energy efficiency.

Mobile Technology: Wearable devices (smart watches, fitness trackers) connect seamlessly to AAL systems. Real-time monitoring and emergency alerts are facilitated through mobile apps.

Robotic Devices: Robots assist with medication reminders, companionship, and mobility support. They enhance independence and reduce caregiver burden.

1.2.3 Benefits of Healthcare 4.0 in AAL

The advancements of Healthcare 4.0 in the context of AAL have the capacity to greatly influence the quality of life for old and disabled individuals.

Enhanced Care and Support: Healthcare 4.0 leverages smart technologies, including IoT and AI, for comprehensive care and support. AAL systems are equipped with wearable sensors, environmental sensors, and intelligent algorithms to monitor daily activities and health conditions. Early detection of anomalies, fall prevention, and personalized assistance have become possible (Cicirelli et al., 2021).

Independence and Autonomy: AAL solutions extend the time individuals can live independently. Smart devices assist with daily routines, enabling elderly and differently abled individuals to maintain autonomy. Personalized support enhances their overall well-being and standard of life.

Reduced Healthcare Costs: By integrating Healthcare 4.0 into AAL, we can reduce the reliance on human resources in healthcare. Smart monitoring and preventive measures minimize emergencies and hospital visits.

1.2.4 Limitations of Healthcare 4.0 in AAL

Digital Literacy Challenges: The elderly population, especially those who lack digital skills, may struggle to benefit fully from AAL technologies. Bridging the digital literacy gap is essential to ensure equitable access.

Context Constraints: The application environment (both indoor and outdoor, private or public) limits technological choices. Balancing invasiveness, range distance, and usability is crucial (Cicirelli et al., 2021).

Privacy and Security Concerns: Gathering information through health sensors is invasive of the individual's privacy. The secure transmission and storage of data are critical.

In AAL, Healthcare 4.0 is a signalling value that can potentially enhance people's lives. Still, working through specific issues concerning digital literacy, context, and privacy is crucial to success.

1.2.5 Challenges Faced in Implementing Healthcare 4.0 in AAL

In the case of Healthcare 4. 0 and AAL, there exist numerous research challenges and gaps that require attention and resolution:

Digital Literacy: In the past, Healthcare 4.0 emerged for patients, allowing customization services. The first service that differentiated from competitors was providing highly individualized services to patients, increasing the use of IoT, and smart technologies, thus highlighting the need to improve elders' digital competency. The lack of proper digital competencies may result in the exclusion of information and elderly persons not benefiting from AAL technologies (Digital Literacy, n.d., 1998).

Technological Barriers: It is necessary to remove the technological barriers to enhance the existing and future demand for digital health, especially for seniors. Applying AAL technologies to seniors with special health requirements for upgrades and security (Márquez & Taramasco, 2023).

Usability and Accessibility: In Cicirelli et al. (2021), the issue of developing AAL systems that are easy to use and that, in addition to providing services to the users, can support disabled ones, is described, and it is a complex issue, which includes ergonomy, human-computer interaction, and information organization.

Personalization: AAL systems should be able to adapt to a person's care needs according to the profile and conditions of that person. Therefore, it is necessary to have an efficient analysis of the data and an integration of context-aware technologies (Marques et al., 2020).

Integration with Healthcare Services: AAL e-services need to be seamlessly integrated with existing healthcare services to improve quality and access to care, reduce labour costs, and engage the elderly in their health and well-being decisions (Marques et al., 2020). Addressing these challenges will be vital to advancing AAL systems and ensuring they meet the needs of an aging population within the framework of Healthcare 4.0.

Staffing and Cost Constraints: Solutions for elderly care often require medical personnel and specialists. However, cost constraints and limited staff availability pose challenges in providing comprehensive care to the elderly (Cicirelli et al., 2021).

1.2.6 Challenges and Opportunities

AAL technology has advanced, but issues remain to be resolved, like protecting privacy and data security as well as ethical and legal concerns, skill development for healthcare professionals, improving device interoperability, and making these solutions affordable and accessible to a broader population. Integrating human intelligence with cutting-edge technology is central to advancing AAL technologies, aiming to improve healthcare delivery and patient outcomes. However, the opportunities for enhancing the standard of life for the elderly and disabled are vast, with continuous research and development paving the way for more sophisticated and integrated AAL solutions in the future (Denecke, 2021).

1.3 HEALTHCARE 5.0: FUTURE TRENDS IN AAL TECHNOLOGIES

Expanding upon the previous phases of healthcare development (ranging from Healthcare 1.0 to 4.0), Healthcare 5.0 represents a major revolution in the healthcare field. The patient-centred approach emphasizes individualized care, proactive health management, and patient participation. Key features of Healthcare 5.0 include the following:

(1) *Integration of Cutting-Edge Technologies:* Healthcare 5.0 integrates technologies like IoT, AI, and digital twin.
(2) *Empowerment and Precision:* Patients become empowered, and medicine becomes more precise.
(3) *Anticipatory Healthcare:* Access to healthcare services at any time has revolutionized care delivery.
(4) *Democratization of Healthcare:* AI algorithms provide evidence-based medical information to the general population, often bypassing conventional healthcare systems (Digital Transformation in Healthcare 5.0, n.d.).

1.3.1 Impact on AAL

The objective of AAL is to facilitate the ability of elderly individuals to maintain their independence in their own homes for an extended time. It achieves this through intelligent systems that enhance their quality of life.

IoT and AAL Synergy: IoT allows devices to communicate with each other wirelessly. When combined with AAL, it creates intelligent environments that support independent living.

Intelligent Systems: IoT enables transparent and intelligent AAL systems, ensuring care and attention for older adults.

Virtual Reality (VR): Simulators enhance examinations and diagnoses, improving healthcare outcomes.

Data-Driven Healthcare: IoT and AI improve diagnostic accuracy and patient care.

Customized Computational Models: Patients can have personalized models, aiding doctors in anticipating illness, guiding therapy, and improving diagnosis and prognosis.

Challenges: Accessibility of data and energy/resource constraints remain challenges, especially in resource-limited countries (Naureen et al., 2023; Digital Transformation in Healthcare 5.0, n.d.).

Healthcare 5.0 is the latest stage of development in the healthcare industry, and it addresses the research gaps in Healthcare 4.0 concerning AAL. Healthcare 5.0 represents the blend of enhanced technologies into healthcare, focusing on personalization and efficiency. It emphasizes using AI, IoT, and robotics to tailor treatments, enhance diagnostics, and facilitate remote healthcare services. Ambient assisted living technologies will play a crucial role, with smart devices monitoring health, managing treatments, and ensuring medication adherence. The objective is to establish a cohesive healthcare ecosystem that enhances patient outcomes while addressing challenges like data security and cost-effectiveness. This evolution aims to harmonize technological advancement with human-centric care, shaping the future of healthcare delivery.

Healthcare 5.0's maximum potential can only be realized by addressing obstacles, including privacy and security of data, ethical and legal concerns, healthcare professional skill development, and cost-effectiveness (Denecke, 2021). Consequently, combining human intelligence with technological solutions, which constitutes the fundamental aspect of enhancing AAL technologies, targets the optimization of healthcare services and, by extension, the health of patients (Caballero et al., 2023).

1.3.2 Emerging Technologies in AAL

These technologies are AI, IoT, and robotics in AAL; they significantly improve the well-being of elderly people with specific needs (Garg, 2022).

Artificial Intelligence (AI) in AAL: Far from its static implementation, AI offers a dynamic means of addressing AAL's necessities, considering a more individualized approach. Here is how it impacts AAL:

- *Health Monitoring:* Smart sensors measure the physiological parameters, including pulse rate and the patient's blood pressure, and AI algorithms are used to process such information.
- *Activity Recognition:* AI models identify daily activities from sensor data regarding assistance with preventing falls and care, such as walking and cooking.
- *Personalization:* AI specifically adapts management strategies to the client's choice, habits, or medical state.
- *Predictive Analytics:* AI anticipates health incidents such as falls, deterioration, and so on so that appropriate action can be taken promptly.
- *Natural Language Processing (NLP):* AI-supported virtual assistants or chatbots provide communication and provide support.

IoT in AAL: IoT links smart devices and sensors and develops smart surroundings. The following shows how IoT transforms AAL:

- *Smart Homes*: Smart devices or intelligent things (e.g., smart thermostats, smart lighting) improve comfort and accessibility of the environment.
- *Wearable Sensors:* Smart clothes in IoT keep track of healthiness, alert the user of danger, and monitor their daily physical activity.
- *Ambient Sensing:* It may be about IoT sensors that pick up environmental changes, such as temperature or humidity, and respond accordingly.

- *Data Sharing:* IoT enables data exchange between devices, caregivers, and healthcare practitioners.
- *Remote Monitoring:* This uses IoT-based systems to monitor some health status and compliance with medication.

Robotics in AAL: Challenges in implementing robotic systems in AAL, user acceptance, safety, and applicable ethical issues are prerequisites.

- *Socially Assistive Robots:* Such robots offer social interaction, proactively call patients to take drugs, and help complete tasks. Telepresence robots facilitate interaction between the patients, caregivers, and health authorities. Robotic exoskeletons help to ambulate and regain strength and function.
- *Fall Detection and Assistance:* Robots can identify the moments when a person has fallen and assist them quickly.

1.3.3 Digital Twins in Healthcare 5. 0 and AAL

Digital twins can be a real-time, dynamic definition of a physical object or a process. It allows simulation, monitoring, and optimization of the system's performance. Digital twins present healthcare with prospects to identify emerging frailties, detect risk situations, and automate scenarios according to individual routines and behaviors (Cicirelli et al., 2021; Denecke, 2021). The main roles and benefits of digital twins in AAL are the following:

Cognitive Buildings: The combination of digital twin models and AAL seeks to develop cognitive buildings that can learn, reason, and seamlessly collaborate with humans.

AI-Driven Recognition: Digital twins use AI models and sensors to recognize behaviors, detect anomalies, and support elderly individuals living alone, especially those with cognitive disorders (Cynthia S Y LAU et al., 2021; Benetazzo et al., 2015).

Scenario Awareness: Digital twins attain situational awareness by independently acquiring advanced knowledge. They can identify irregularities in domestic environmental situations and assist consumers (Cynthia S Y LAU et al., 2021).

Personalization: Digital twins allow customized monitoring and intervention based on individual needs.

Risk Detection: They help identify risks early, improving safety and well-being.

Efficiency: Real-time monitoring and optimization enhance efficiency in care delivery.

User Support: Two-way interaction and AI agents assist users through speech-to-text and text-to-speech capabilities (Cynthia S Y LAU et al., 2021).

1.3.4 Potential Benefits of Healthcare 5.0 in AAL

Healthcare 5.0, closely linked to Society 5.0, involves merging cutting-edge technologies with healthcare to enhance our quality of life and tackle existing issues. Here are some key points:

Improved Access to Medical Advancements: Healthcare 5.0 seeks to provide affordable access to cutting-edge medical innovations. Advancements in medical research and technology enable patients to engage in real-time communication with clinicians at any time and from any location. VR surgical simulators facilitate more sophisticated examinations and diagnosis (Basulo-Ribeiro & Teixeira, 2024; Dlamini et al., 2023).

IoT and AI for Diagnostic Accuracy: The IoT, a network of wireless and networked devices, plays a crucial part in Healthcare 5.0. IoT, combined with AI, improves diagnostic accuracy. These technologies possess the capacity to significantly enhance healthcare and patient care (Coile, 2024; Dlamini et al., 2023).

Precision Medicine and Empowered Patients: Medicine becomes more precise in Healthcare 5.0. Patients are empowered with customized computational models of themselves. Doctors can anticipate illnesses, guide therapy, and improve diagnosis and prognosis.

Anticipatory Healthcare and Democratization: Healthcare becomes anticipatory, available anytime, and transforms care delivery. A "democratisation of healthcare" is achieved when AI algorithms provide the general public with personalized access to evidence-based medical information (Sofiat Makanjuola-Akinola, 2022).

However, there are the following challenges:

Data Accessibility and Misuse*:* The accessibility of IoT data has the potential to be exploited, resulting in a breach of human rights and privacy. Some nations, particularly those with limited resources, encounter energy and resource obstacles that affect the sustainability of the Internet of Things (Gomathi et al., 2023).

1.4 IMPLEMENTATION OF HEALTHCARE 5.0 IN AAL

Implementing Healthcare 5.0 in AAL technologies is poised to revolutionize the healthcare industry by providing tailored healthcare services, enhancing the quality of life, and ensuring that healthcare is proactive, personalized, and accessible. Healthcare is being transformed by technology with five key advancements: Democratization of healthcare, where IoT and AI make medical care more accessible and anticipatory; cyber-physical systems, merging digital and physical realms to enhance diagnostics and preventive care; digital twins and precision medicine, using AI for accurate patient modelling and tailored treatments; smart energy management, integrating smart grids for sustainable healthcare operations; and legal and ethical considerations, ensuring data is managed responsibly amidst new privacy challenges. The implementation of Healthcare 5.0 in AAL is expected to bring about significant changes:

The democratization of Healthcare: IoT and AI in Society 5.0 aims to make medical advancements more accessible and cost-effective, allowing available healthcare anytime and anticipatory (Demetriou et al., 2023).

Cyber-Physical Systems: Merging cyberspace with physical space through IoT devices and AI analysis will improve diagnostics and patient care, focusing on preventive medicine (Demetriou et al., 2023).

Digital Twins and Precision Medicine: AI and machine learning will facilitate the development of digital twins for patients, enabling more precise simulation in healthcare situations and adopting precision medicine (Cicirelli et al., 2021).

Smart Energy Management: To guarantee the sustainability of healthcare technologies, smart grids and novel energy sources will be implemented in response to the energy crisis.

Legal and Ethical Considerations: The implementation will also navigate new legal and ethical challenges, ensuring responsible data management and addressing privacy concerns (Cicirelli et al., 2021).

1.4.1 Case Studies or Examples of Successful Healthcare 5.0 Implementations in AAL

Healthcare 5.0 implementation examples in the context of AAL demonstrate how advanced technologies enhance healthcare and improve individuals' quality of life.

Cervical Cancer Screening/Management: In a low- and middle-income country (LMIC) healthcare setting, Society 5.0 principles were applied to cervical cancer screening, prevention, and management. The blend of AI, cloud computing, and the IoT allowed for efficient data gathering, analysis, and personalized interventions. By leveraging digital twins of patients and populations, healthcare professionals could model and predict outcomes more accurately (Byrne, 2023).

Enhanced Living Environments (ELE) for Health: ELE is a paradigm that focuses on improving well-being, social inclusion, and autonomy. It integrates ambient intelligence (AmI), IoT, and cyber-physical systems to create smart spaces. In healthcare, ELE aims to personalize systems and services for patients, especially the elderly or those with disabilities. The goal is to enhance living conditions and independence (Digital Literacy, n.d., 1998).

Advancements in Ambient Assisted Systems for Independent Living: Ambient assisted living systems (AALS) are essential for cost-effective care of the elderly. These systems continuously monitor the environment and occupant behavior using intelligent event-driven systems. However, challenges remain, such as integrating environmental factors for long-term care and addressing privacy and security concerns (Márquez & Taramasco, 2023).

Use Case – The Ambient Assisted Living Joint Programme (AALJP): The European Commission has put out the Action Plan Ageing Well in the Information Society to develop ICTs for older people. In 2007, 14 EU member states established the AAL JP, aiming to improve older adults' quality of life, prolong working life, promote social activity, and reduce health and social care costs (Cicirelli et al., 2021; Anzola & Moreno, 2021).

These examples highlight the transformative potential of Healthcare 5.0 in AAL, emphasizing personalized care, predictive modelling, and improved quality of life. As we move toward a human-centred society, these technological advancements promise healthier, longer, and more productive lives for individuals.

1.5 CONCLUSIONS

AAL is a system that uses AI and IoT to assist the elderly and disabled in their daily lives. It enables remote healthcare, reduced isolation, and improved efficiency. However, challenges include digital literacy, accessibility, and integration. Healthcare 5.0 aims to address these issues and improve care and cost efficiency by integrating advanced technologies like AI and cloud computing. This human-centred approach eliminates disparities and enhances healthcare delivery and patient outcomes. Healthcare 5.0 integrates economic advancement with social problem resolution, utilizing AAL technologies for personalized, efficient, and inclusive healthcare. It will be possible to accommodate the increased convergence of cyberspace with the physical space and improve the management of health, reducing the cost of healthcare systems. Research within technologies for AAL under the domain of Healthcare 5.0. It lacks any specific proposal, and its target is to enhance the quality of life of disabled individuals and cope with the problem of demographic aging. Possible directions for future research are personal and contextualized systems, wearable devices and smart things, prognostics, interfaces and interactions, ethical and privacy aspects, and interactions with medical environments. Some issues that need to be addressed are the satisfaction, security, and privacy of users and the ability to fit more users into a system since the population of aging individuals is increasing. Future studies need to be directed to improving user interfaces, ethical issues, and data protection and security.

REFERENCES

Anzola, E. W. C., & Moreno, M. N. M. (2021). Enhanced Living Environments (ELE): A Paradigm Based on Integration of Industry 4.0 and Society 5.0 Contexts with Ambient Assisted Living (AAL). In José García-Alonso & César Fonseca (Eds.), *Lecture notes in bioengineering* (pp. 121–132). Springer, Cham. https://doi.org/10.1007/978-3-030-72567-9_12

Aumayr, G. (2016). From Ambient Assisted Living to Active and Assisted Living: A Practical Perspective on Experiences and Approaches. In Ewa Piętka, Pawel Badura, Jacek Kawa, & Wojciech Wieclawek (Eds.), *Advances in intelligent systems and computing* (pp. 3–13). Springer, Cham. https://doi.org/10.1007/978-3-319-39904-1_1

Basulo-Ribeiro, J., & Teixeira, L. (2024). The Future of Healthcare with Industry 5.0: Preliminary Interview-Based Qualitative Analysis. *Future Internet*, *16*(3), 68. https://doi.org/10.3390/fi16030068

Benetazzo, F., Ferracuti, F., Freddi, A., Giantomassi, A., Iarlori, S., Longhi, S., Monteriù, A., & Ortenzi, D. (2015). AAL Technologies for Independent Life of Elderly People. In Bruno Andò, Pietro Siciliano, Vincenzo Marletta, & Andrea Monteriù (Eds.), *Biosystems & biorobotics* (pp. 329–343). Springer, Cham. https://doi.org/10.1007/978-3-319-18374-9_31

Blackman, S., Matlo, C., Bobrovitskiy, C., Waldoch, A., Fang, M. L., Jackson, P., Mihailidis, A., Nygård, L., Astell, A., & Sixsmith, A. (2016). Ambient Assisted Living Technologies for Aging Well: A Scoping Review. *Journal of Intelligent Systems*, *25*(1), 55–69. https://doi.org/10.1515/jisys-2014-0136

Byrne, C. (2023, May 9). *Healthcare 5.0: Digital wellness through transformative shifts - digital CxO*. Retrieved May 25, 2024, from https://digitalcxo.com/article/healthcare-5-0-digital-wellness-through-transformative-shifts/

Caballero, P., Ortiz, G., & Medina-Bulo, I. (2023). Systematic Literature Review of Ambient Assisted Living Systems Supported by the Internet of Things. *Universal Access in the Information Society*. https://doi.org/10.1007/s10209-023-01022-w

Cicirelli, G., Marani, R., Petitti, A., Milella, A., & D'Orazio, T. (2021). Ambient Assisted Living: A Review of Technologies, Methodologies and Future Perspectives for Healthy Aging of Population. *Sensors*, *21*(10), 3549. https://doi.org/10.3390/s21103549

Coile, R. C. (2024). Digital Transformation in Healthcare 5.0. *De Gruyter eBooks*. https://doi.org/10.1515/9783111327853

Cynthia S Y LAU, & Ben Y F FONG. (2021, March). *Technology adoption among the elderly – smart older adults in the new decades*. Retrieved September 11, 2024, from https://hklaureateforum.org/en/technology-adoption-among-the-elderly-smart-older-adults-in-the-new-decades

Demetriou, D., Mathabe, K., Lolas, G., & Dlamini, Z. (2023). *Internet of Things in Society 5.0 and the Democratization of Healthcare* (pp. 111–130). Springer, Cham. https://doi.org/10.1007/978-3-031-36461-7_5

Denecke, K. (2021). What Characterizes Safety of Ambient Assisted Living Technologies? *Studies in Health Technology and Informatics*. https://doi.org/10.3233/shti210263

Dlamini, Z., Miya, T. V., Hull, R., Molefi, T., Khanyile, R., & De Vasconcellos, J. F. (2023). *Society 5.0: Realizing Next-Generation Healthcare* (pp. 1–30). Springer, Cham. https://doi.org/10.1007/978-3-031-36461-7_1

Digital Literacy. (n.d.). Google Books. https://books.google.ie/books?id=ppVx7pHr07kC

Digital Transformation in Healthcare 5.0. (n.d.). Google Books. https://books.google.com/books/about/Digital_Transformation_in_Healthcare_5_0.html?id=j2EDEQAAQBAJ

Garg, P. K. (2022). The Future Healthcare Technologies: A Roadmap to Society 5.0. In Pradeep Kumar Garg, Nitin K. Tripathi, Martin Kappas & Loveleen Gaur (Eds.), *Disruptive technologies and digital transformations for society 5.0* (pp. 305–318). Springer, Singapore. https://doi.org/10.1007/978-981-16-9476-9_14

Gilster, P. 1998. *Digital Literacy*. Wiley.

Gomathi, L., Mishra, A. K., & Tyagi, A. K. (2023). Industry 5.0 for Healthcare 5.0: Opportunities, Challenges and Future Research Possibilities. *2022 6th International Conference on Trends in Electronics and Informatics (ICOEI)*, pp. 204–213. https://doi.org/10.1109/icoei56765.2023.10125660

Jovanovic, M., Mitrov, G., Zdravevski, E., Lameski, P., Colantonio, S., Kampel, M., & Florez-Revuelta, F. (2022). Ambient Assisted Living: Scoping Review of Artificial Intelligence Models, Domains, Technology, and Concerns. *Journal of Medical Internet Research*, *24*(11), e36553.

Marques, G., Saini, J., Pires, I. M., Miranda, N., & Pitarma, R. (2020). Internet of Things for Enhanced Living Environments, Health and Well-Being: Technologies, Architectures and Systems. In Pradeep Kumar Singh, Bharat K. Bhargava, Marcin Paprzycki, Narottam Chand Kaushal, & Wei-Chiang Hong (Eds.), *Advances in intelligent systems and computing* (pp. 616–631). Springer, Cham. https://doi.org/10.1007/978-3-030-40305-8_29

Márquez, G., & Taramasco, C. (2023). Barriers and Facilitators of Ambient Assisted Living Systems: A Systematic Literature Review. *International Journal of Environmental Research and Public Health*, *20*(6), 5020. https://doi.org/10.3390/ijerph20065020

Martins, A. I., Queirós, A., & Da Rocha, N. P. (2018). Ambient Assisted Living: Introduction and Overview. In Alexandra Queirós & Nelson Pacheco da Rocha (Eds.), *Human-computer interaction series* (pp. 1–12). Springer, Cham. https://doi.org/10.1007/978-3-319-91226-4_1

Naureen, A., Vamshi, K., Krishna, K. C., & Hussain, M. M. (2023). Healthcare 5.0 Fundamentals. In A. Hassan, V. Prasad, P. Bhattacharya, P. Dutta, & R. Damaševičius (Eds.), *Advances in healthcare information systems and administration book series* (pp. 1–25). IGI Global Scientific Publishing. https://doi.org/10.4018/979-8-3693-1082-3.ch001

Sofiat Makanjuola-Akinola. (2021, March 30). *What is the biggest benefit technology will have on ageing and longevity?* World Economic Forum. Retrieved May 25, 2024, from www.weforum.org/agenda/2021/03/what-is-the-biggest-benefit-technology-ageing-longevity-global-future-council-tech-for-good/

Stodczyk, R. (2020). Ambient Assisted Living an Overview of Current Applications, End-Users and Acceptance. *Biomedical Journal of Scientific & Technical Research*, *30*(3). https://doi.org/10.26717/bjstr.2020.30.004949

Wilton, M. (2023, April 26). *What is ambient assisted living?* Retrieved May 26, 2024, from www.resilientlife.tech/what-is-ambient-assisted-living

Section II

Advances in Enabling Technologies for Assisted Living in Healthcare 5.0

2 Wearable and Ambient Sensors Applicable in the Medical Laboratory and Diagnostic Services in Healthcare

Eno Chongs Mantu, Dooshima Augustina Orshio and Uchejeso Mark Obeta

2.1 INTRODUCTION

A sensor is any device that can measure or record the physicality, physiology, and activity of a human body while a wearable is anything that can be worn by the body, and internet-network-enabled devices are capable of monitoring activities like physical and physiological signals about personal well-being and are capable of delivering feedback (Devine et al., 2022). In active or assisted ambient leaving (AAL), there has been a serious increase in the use of sensors, most of which are wearable in nature. AAL technologies were mostly employed among disabled and old people.

The post COVID-19 era saw a surge in healthcare technologies, of which wearable devices are numerous among them. The target for such technologies is not only disabled and aged people but is for everybody who needs healthcare no matter where the patient is located. The medical laboratory and other diagnostic services were commonly carried out with the patient present in the healthcare facility. Most of the procedures involve sample collection, imaging, and use of big healthcare equipment.

Wearable ambient sensors means "something that can be worn" and the study and development of such devices has astronomically increased recently (Kageyama et al., 2022). Wearable and ambient sensor technologies are providing an opportunity to remain at a distance and allow some tests and appropriate monitoring to be carried out to sustain the lives of individuals. The aim of this chapter is to isolate those wearable and ambient sensors that can be deployed in the medical laboratory and other diagnostic units of healthcare.

DOI: 10.1201/9781003520184-4

2.2 HEALTHCARE SERVICES

Healthcare is the provision of medical care services to individuals (clients) or to a community in general as it is applicable in an organized set up. This is in a bid to provide, maintain, or restore the mental, physical, or emotional well-being of the patient. The healthcare provision in an organized set up may be by the government or private sector. In various nations, healthcare may be stratified into primary, secondary, or tertiary healthcare as the case may be (Obeta et al., 2024).

The services in healthcare may include hospital and outpatient services, medical laboratory and diagnostic services, dental services, nursing services, etc. Figure 2.1 describes the basic section of healthcare while others represent other sections like works, accounts, laundry, cleaners, etc. With the advent in technology, telehealthcare, digital health blood and cord blood banking services, and other advanced diagnosis are practiced in healthcare.

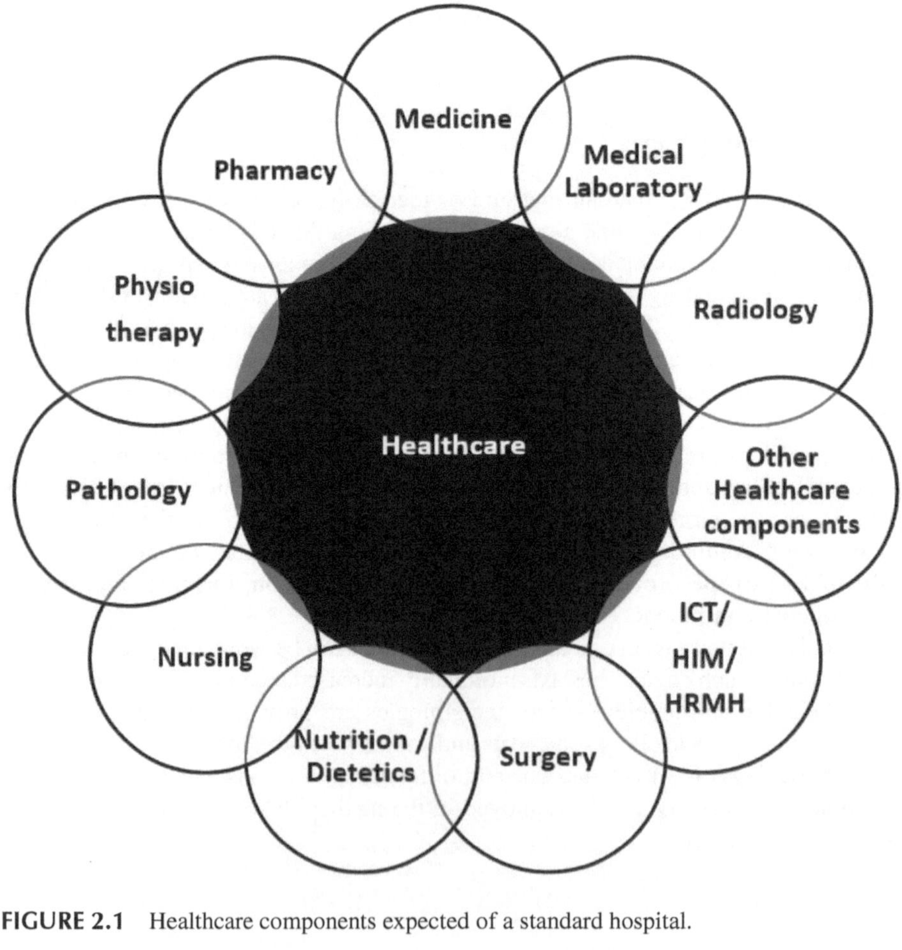

FIGURE 2.1 Healthcare components expected of a standard hospital.

There are several healthcare practitioners including specialists who make the healthcare institutions and services viable. They include physicians/doctors, pharmacists, nurses, medical laboratory scientists, physiotherapists, imaging scientists/radiologists, health information management officers, public health officers, community health officers, nutritionists, information technology officers, and several others whom participate in the healthcare industry.

Healthcare services cannot be exhausted especially with the advancement in technologies in healthcare services. In the healthcare sector, aside from healthcare professionals, hospitals, clinics, and other healthcare facilities exist, which are laced with various health insurance plans at various levels depending on the national healthcare packages. Some of the healthcare services maybe for profit or non-profit entities. In healthcare, the regulation and support of government in various capacities are key. Healthcare is a social and political undertaking by various governments. In various ways, it is like the DOD (Department of Defense); FEHBP (Federal Employees Health Benefits Program); IHS (Indian Health Service); NHIA (National Health Insurance Authority); and VHA (Veterans Health Administration) as the case may be including hospital administration packages (IOM, 2002).

2.3 MEDICAL LABORATORY AND DIAGNOSTIC SERVICES

Medical laboratory services are an aspect of healthcare diagnostics that involve the use of various human and animal samples, such as blood, stools, urine, and other fluids, for the accurate diagnosis and testing of patients and issuing of quality results to clients for effective treatments (Obeta et al., 2022). The medical laboratory as a diagnostic service provides not less than 70% of clinical decisions based on the results towards healthcare management. It also contributes to the high income of healthcare organizations (Obeta et al., 2019). Although the medical laboratory diagnostic areas have distorted nomenclature across the globe, their services worldwide are the same (Obeta et al., 2020).

There are other diagnostic components in healthcare especially the non-invasive aspect of diagnosis, in particular, imaging diagnostics. Figure 2.2 presents the medical laboratory and diagnostic segments of healthcare depending on the size and status of healthcare. Medical laboratory and diagnostic services are essential components of healthcare, providing some vital health data and information for diagnosis, treatment, and management of diseases. These diagnostic services are as follows:

Chemical Pathology or Clinical Chemistry: This involves analysis of chemical components of the body from blood, urine, and other body fluids. Some tests in this laboratory are electrolytes, enzymes, kidney and liver function parameters and hormones.

Hematology and Blood Transfusion Science: This involves analysis of blood to detect blood abnormalities such as cell count, blood typing, transfusion transmissible infections tests, cross-matching, and coagulation studies. In some cases, immunological studies are carried out.

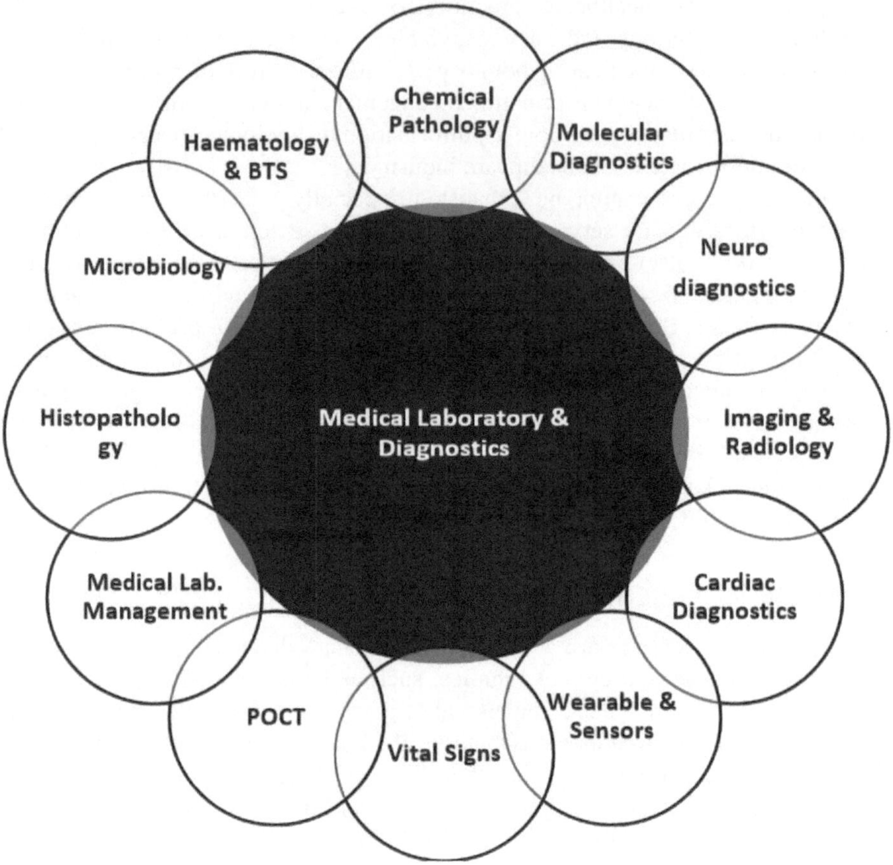

FIGURE 2.2 Medical laboratory and diagnostics in healthcare.

Histopathology and Cytopathology: This involves the microscopic examination of tissues and cells including cells from fluids and tissues.

Microbiology: This area may be subdivided into bacteriology for identification of bacteria and susceptibility testing; virology for detection and identification of viruses; mycology for fungal identification and susceptibility testing; parasitology for parasites' identification and in some cases some immunological studies.

Molecular Diagnostics: This is the DNA and RNA testing for genetic disorders and infectious diseases. This may involve other advanced technical laboratory studies.

Medical Laboratory Management: This is the area that organizes and manages the laboratory components. It is also involved with the quality management, research, and new technologies in diagnostics.

Point of Care Testing (POCT): This is the use of mobile/movable measuring equipment towards the position of the patient to carry out some levels of test. It encompasses *wearable and ambient sensors.*

Imaging and Radiology Diagnostics: This involves use of machines that show features or images of organs and tissues of interest. It includes x-rays, CT scans, MRI, ultrasound, and radioisotope imaging for organ function and disease detection.

Cardiac Diagnostics: This involves diagnosis in relation to heart diseases such as electrocardiography (ECG) for heart rhythm and function testing, and echocardiography for ultrasound examination of the heart.

Neurodiagnostics: This is for studies of neurons and transmitters as in electroencephalography (EEG) for brain activity testing and nerve conduction studies (NCS) for nerve function tests.

Vital Signs: This is majorly the measuring of some vital signs like blood pressure, pulse rate, weight, temperature, and oxygen saturation.

There is no doubt that the medical laboratory and diagnostic services for those mentioned and many more provide essential information to healthcare professionals and care givers to diagnose, treat, and manage various medical conditions, thereby improving patients' care and outcomes.

2.4 HEALTHCARE SERVICES IN THE AGE OF THE INTERNET OF THINGS AND NEW TECHNOLOGIES

Healthcare services in every country has its peculiarity. The government and private entities provide healthcare services according to their standard and governing regulations. In Nigeria, for instance, the healthcare indices of WHO rating for Nigeria is very low to the extent that out of 160 countries assessed, Nigeria is at 157th position (Folinas et al., 2021). This has lingered to the extent that healthcare tourism and capital flight continues to increase starting from political leaders who have the capacity to improve the healthcare system. The malaria situation worsens by the year (WHO, 2023) and the available option for consideration for improvement is the internet of healthcare.

Healthcare systems are challenged across the globe and in developing countries, in particular, by non-unified patients' data, poor teamwork of healthcare professionals, security and privacy matters, poor patients' consent and authorization documentation, uncoordinated hospital workflow, and poor/unavailable system capacities (Dauwed & Meri, 2019); of which the internet of healthcare would greatly change the narrative.

The healthcare in the age of the internet may be characterized by connectivity with the aid of network, hardware and sensors; dynamic changes as time changes in services and operation; safety and security end-to-end; heterogeneity based on devices and applications with networks requiring extensibility, modularity, scalabilities, and interoperability; enormous scale of communication via the internet; interconnectivity of healthcare devices for connecting healthcare clients and all the Internet of Things related services (Obeta et al., 2024).

2.5 NON-INVASIVE TECHNIQUES IN HEALTHCARE

Non-invasive techniques in healthcare refer to methods that do not penetrate the body or require insertion of instruments or devices into the body. Most laboratory and diagnostic procedures are invasive except with the latest technologies that encourage non-invasive techniques. The level of the invasive nature of some technologies applied in diagnostics are highlighted in Table 2.1 in accordance with Smith et al., (2023).

TABLE 2.1
Wearable Sensor Technologies with their Level of Invasiveness

S. No.	Nature of Ambient Sensors	Activity Description	Level of Invasiveness
1	Accelerometer	The acceleration and force measurement sensed on the body where fixed	Low
2	Ambient temperature	This measures the ambient environmental temperature	Low
3	Ambient light	The measurement surrounding light level	Low
4	Gyroscope	Measures a device's rate of rotation around each of the three physical (x, y, and z) axes	Low
5	Magnetometer	Measures the geomagnetic field strength	Low
6	Pressure	Measures the surrounding air pressure	Low
7	Proximity	Measures an object distance from the sensor	Low
8	Electrocardiogram	The measure of heart rate or cardiac activity	Medium
9	Galvanic Skin Response	Measuring the electrical conductivity of the skin	Medium
10	Screen state	Recording the turning on or off of the screen always	Medium
11	Touch state	This records the body movement, pressure, and level of screen touch interactions	Medium
12	Bluetooth	Detects nearby Bluetooth capable devices	High
13	Cell towers	Provides information about the nearby cellphone towers	High
14	GPS	Provides user location direction and coordinates	High
15	Video	Captures video and pictures of user activities	High
16	Wi-Fi	Providing data needed to the nearby Wi-Fi access points based on the signal strength and connectivity	High

These techniques are used for diagnosis, monitoring, and treatment, and are often preferred over invasive methods by clients to minimize risk, discomfort, and recovery time. Some examples of non-invasive techniques applied in healthcare include the following:

Medical Imaging such as x-rays, computed tomography (CT) scans, magnetic resonance imaging (MRI), ultrasound, and mammography; diagnostic tests such as electrocardiogram (ECG), electroencephalogram (EEG), electromyogram (EMG), and nerve conduction studies (NCS).

Monitoring Techniques such as blood pressure monitoring, pulse oximetry (oxygen saturation), heart rate monitoring, and respiratory rate monitoring.

Therapeutic Techniques such as physical therapy (e.g., exercise, massage), occupational therapy, speech therapy, and acupuncture.

Ventilation such as oxygen therapy, continuous positive airway pressure (CPAP), and bi-level positive airway pressure (BiPAP).

Cardiac Output Monitoring such as echocardiography and impedance cardiography.

Glucose Monitoring such as infrared spectroscopy and optical coherence tomography.

Brain Stimulation such as transcranial magnetic stimulation (TMS), and transcranial direct current stimulation (tDCS).

Wound Healing such as low-level laser therapy and ultrasound therapy.

Telemedicine and Remote Monitoring such as virtual consultations, wearable devices, and mobile apps for monitoring vital signs and other health metrics especially for very ill patients, elderly and disabled subjects.

It is very clear that these non-invasive techniques have revolutionized healthcare by providing accurate and timely diagnoses, improving patient comfort and outcomes, and reducing healthcare costs without penetrating the patients or causing pains. This is what wearables and sensors are doing in healthcare and it is spreading very fast for all interested subjects.

2.6 WEARABLE AND AMBIENT SENSORS

Wearable sensors are those devices that are fixed on the body parts which are designed to collect health data using electrical, biochemical, and electrophysiological methods. Wearable sensors are made in such a way that they have a reagent layer, sensing layer, and readout/packaging layer (Janghorban et al., 2022).

The European Union Medical Device Regulation (EUMDR) described wearables and sensors as "medical devices" meaning

> *"any instrument, apparatus, appliance, software, implant, reagent, material, or other article intended by the manufacturer to be used, alone or in combination, for human beings for one or more of the following specific medical purposes:*
>
> - *diagnosis, prevention, monitoring, prediction, prognosis, treatment, or alleviation of disease;*
> - *diagnosis, monitoring, treatment, alleviation of, or compensation for, an injury or disability;*
> - *investigation, replacement, or modification of the anatomy or of a physiological or pathological process or state;*
> - *providing information by means of in vitro examination of specimens derived from the human body, including organ, blood, and tissue donations;*
>
> *and which does not achieve its principal intended action by pharmacological, immunological, or metabolic means, in or on the human body, but which may be assisted in its function by such means".*

This era stimulates all to pursue a better healthy and high-quality living but is challenged by paying attention to maintaining a very reasonable and healthy life and lifestyle. This challenge presents the opportunity to use wearables and sensors. Wearables and sensors are non-invasive devices that can measure some medical parameters, physiological biomarkers, and environmental changes to notify the person wearing it or in some cases the care giver. Walter et al. (2024) described it as "potentially disruptive and powerful tools to promote health equity at scale". No wonder Loucks et al. (2022) stated that "Smartwatches and wearable medical devices help people monitor their health 24/7. Their impact could increase if doctors trust their utility and people feel their data is secure". Wearable devices in healthcare can be said to have adopted "4P medical model" of healthcare practice representing that wearable devices should not deviate from being preventive, predictive, personalized, and participatory in the healthcare environment and practice (Lin, 2019).

Lu et al. (2020) describe the historical origin of wearables in healthcare, which, as corroborated by Smith et al. (2023), was traced to the year 1960 in relation to Jeffrey and Parsonnet's study on a pacemaker that was implanted in a 40-year-old patient in 1958 due to the effort of a thoracic surgeon Dr Erik Senning of Karolinska Hospital in Stockholm. There is no doubt that such pacemakers are being implanted day-in day-out but improved versions including wearables, sensors, and patches/stickers.

2.7 NATURE AND FORM OF WEARABLES AND AMBIENT SENSORS

Since 1960, there has been more developments and improvements going on in wearable sensors. This effort has to be multiplied by the Internet of Things, intelligent hardware/AI, big data dynamics, in the presence of security and privacy. So many sectors are attuned to wearables and sensors not leaving healthcare, culture, education, social networking, security, and military interventions (Smith et al., 2023; Lu et al., 2020). Initially, wearables and sensors were meant for the disabled, aged, and seriously ill individuals, however, the technologies have become part and parcel of

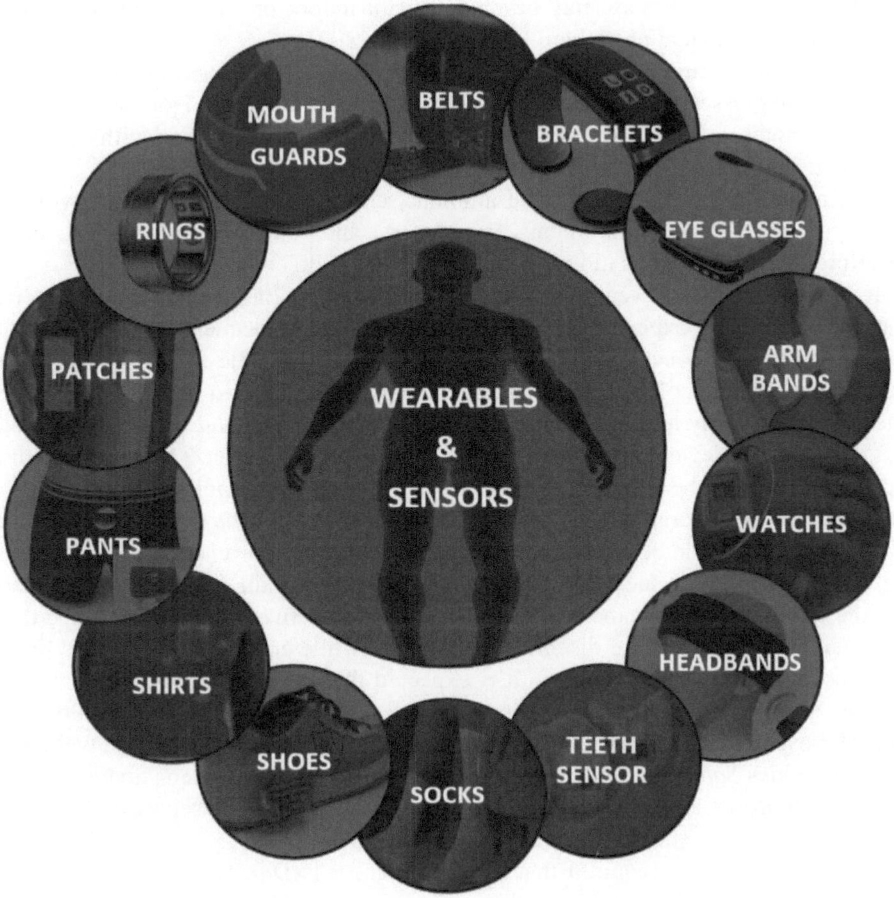

FIGURE 2.3 Some wearables at different parts of the body.

everyday lives among all that are interested in the form of armbands, belts, bracelets, eye glasses, head bands, mouth guards, patches, pants, rings, shoes, socks, watches, and lots more (Figure 2.3). Guk et al. (2019) presented wearable sensors to be piezoelectric, resistive and capacitive sensors in nature. Wearable sensors can be portable devices in the form of wrist-mounted devices, head-mounted devices, e-textiles, and several others while some are attachable devices like wearable skin patches and contact lens. It can also be implantable and ingestible devices and several of them are displayed in Figure 2.3.

The wearable sensor devices are portable and mostly are directly worn on the body and are able to analyze, perceive, regulate, record, and intervene to maintain, monitor and raise health alarms or even treat diseases. These wearables are in different shapes and categories depending on the vendors and vendees. Various technologies with the aid of the internet and other network connections laced with AI have helped to identify, sense, connect several data to the cloud for possible storage. It is also important to note that those technologies may be made to suit indoor or outdoor environmental needs of the people that need them (Cicirelli et al., 2021).

Some of the wearables can achieve multi-parameter assays and monitoring like wearable eye glasses or integrated sensor arrays can test lactate and glucose, respectively. It is notable that some wearables perform real-time and on-line with accuracy while carrying out self-diagnosis and self-monitoring.

The nature and form of wearable ambient sensors cannot be complete without looking at the design requirements, parameters, and roles of each one and their descriptions with functions in line with Francés-Morcillo et al. (2020).

It is required that a wearable sensor gives *Comfort*. Based on the parameters, namely, *Shape*, it is expected that the wearable has an adjustment to suit the body part it is meant for, ensuring that the device is well attachable to the user without any danger and fear of losing it. The device should be able to fit the body shape intended and be easy to fix and remove the instrument. *Breathability* – it is expected that the wearable device is breathable without sweat accumulation. The device should have some space to be able to circulate air without any compromise. *Hygiene* – it is expected that the wearable is washable or cleanable. *Temperature* – the temperature of the wearable should be maintained as recommended by the vendors/producers and that the maintenance of such temperature should not cause pain. *Sizing* – it is expected that the wearable adapts to the targeted users' size. *Obtrusiveness* – it is expected that the wearable does not cause discomfort or fatigue while enabling all expected body movements of the wearer. *Weight* – it is expected that the wearable is very light for ease of carriage. *Movement* – the wearable device should be very flexible to allow the natural movement of the body where attached. Also, it is required that the wearable sensor provides *Safety*. Parameters, like *Harmless*, ensure that there is no pain to the wearer with proper attachment and the heat-dissipating wearable separated from the skin. *Anxiety* – there should be no anxiety among users.

To add to that, it is required that wearable sensor is *Durable*. The parameter is *Resistance*, showing how the wearable is resisting any identified damaging factor protected from external elements. More so, it is required that the wearable sensor has adequate *Usability*. Parameters, like *Intuitiveness*, show how the wearer understands the device and the *Simplicity* shows how easy and simple the wearer uses it. In addition, it is required that the wearable sensor has adequate *Reliability* based on *Precision* and accuracy with adequate *Effectiveness* in terms of function and result. It is required that the wearable is *Aesthetic* thereby providing the expected *Fashion* as defined, with the presence of *Form Language* in a coherent manner and the ability to be *Customizable* to suit the purpose. It is also required that the wearable follows the rule and purpose of *Engagement* in terms of *Long-Term Use* and being *Appealing* for the user all the time. *Wearable Privacy* is highly required for confidentiality to prohibit the exchange of information from unauthorized users and nearby devices. Finally, wearable *Functionality* should be very high with *Satisfaction***.** Some of the wearable biosensors are made specifically for skin, sweat, saliva, tears, and environmental biosensor adaptations with specific principles and mechanisms. Canali et al. (2022) present the function of various forms of wearable to include the following: monitoring of pulse, telehealth, COVID-19 symptoms and long-term effects; screening of atrial fibrillation, sleep apnea, cardiovascular disease; detection of physical activity levels, pre-symptoms of COVID-19 infections, seasonal influenza; prediction of mortality and clinical risk, COVID-19 infections, and exacerbations of chronic obstructive pulmonary diseases.

2.8 WEARABLES AND AMBIENT SENSORS APPLICABLE IN MEDICAL LABORATORIES

So many before now see the medical laboratory as a section of healthcare where there must be blood, urine, stools, and other body fluids to be able to carry out various tests. As medical laboratory scientists, we can confirm that many tests cannot be carried out by wearables and sensors but this section of the chapter shall enumerate some of the parameters that can be tested with the aid of wearables especially where such wearables are standardized and quality managed. Table 2.2 presents some wearables and parameters tested by them.

Looking more closely at the wearables/sensors available, it seem that glucose has the highest number of wearable devices. It would be important to highlight some of the principles and techniques of operation of the devices, using glucose as an example. Some of the techniques employed by wearable sensors for glucose includes dual iontophoresesis, epidermal, interstitial fluids, subcutaneous, electromagnetic, ion electronic, HEAM lens, radiofrequency, and machine learning.

The glucose assay using biosensors and wearables can be traced back to the 1960s and several companies have produced a lot of the wearables and sensors for use such as

TABLE 2.2
Wearable Ambient Sensors and Tested Parameters in the Medical Laboratory Services

S. No.	Wearable and Ambient Sensors	Parameter Tested
1	Armbands	Glucose
2	Belt	Cholesterol
3	Bracelets	Glucose, bilirubin
4	Eye glasses/contact lens	Glucose, cholesterol and lactate
5	Head bands	Glucose, bilirubin
6	Implantable sensor	Glucose
7	Mouth guard	Uric acid
8	Patches	Glucose, haemoglobin and lactate
9	Pants	Glucose
10	Rings	Cholesterol, glucose
11	Shoes	Glucose and diabetic ulcers
12	Shirts	Glucose
13	Socks	Glucose, bilirubin, lactate,
14	Tooth sensor	Bacteria
15	Watches	Glucose

Note: Some of the wearables for particular parameters are not yet approved by appropriate authorities.

the following: FreeStyle Freedom Lite (Abbott), WaveSense KeyNote (AgaMatrix), Glucocard X-meter (Arkray), Ascensia Contour (Bayer), Rightest GM300 (Bionime), Advocate Redi-Code (Diabestic Supply of Suncoast), Prodigy Autocode (Diagnostic Devices), Nova Max (Nova Biomedical) OneTouch UltraLink (LifeScan), and Accu-Chek Aviva (Roche) (Yoo & Lee, 2010)

2.9 WEARABLES AND AMBIENT SENSORS APPLICABLE IN OTHER DIAGNOSTICS

The diagnostic components outside the medical laboratory includes vital signs carried out at nursing stations, diagnostics and monitoring in physiotherapy sections, services rendered in radiology and imaging clinics and investigations at the nutritional clinics. With the healthcare improved technologies and wearable sensors, Table 2.3 provides such sensors and their roles in the other diagnostic areas of healthcare.

It is noteworthy that in addition to diagnostic purposes for human health, there are diagnosis of the environment that take place for the benefits of health of the occupants of such environment especially the elderly, disabled, and critically ill. Such environmental diagnosis and monitoring are useful for stroke-affected patients, the blind, the lame, the deaf and numerous others who are in sports programmes. These wearables are contributing meaningfully to ambient and assisted living of all who are interested in such technological services.

TABLE 2.3
Wearable Ambient Sensors and Tested Parameters with Activities in other Healthcare Diagnostic Services

S. No.	Wearable and Ambient Sensors	Parameter/Activities Tested and Monitored
1	Armbands	Pulse rate, blood pressure, ECG
2	Belt	Positions, heart monitoring
3	Bracelets	ECG, positions
4	Eye glasses	Sight obstruction, stroke assessment
5	Head bands	EEG, brain monitoring, disease tracking
6	Implantable sensor	Movement, environmental conditions
7	Jewelry	Temperature, sweat patterns
8	Mouth guard	Eating and drinking habit
9	Patches	Pulse, ECG, temperature
10	Pants	Physical activities, falls
11	Rings	Blood pressure, mood monitoring, sleep monitoring, infection detection
12	Shoes	Sports activity; weight, gait, and fall monitoring, Stroke management
13	Shirts	Physical activity monitoring
14	Socks	Walking and gaits, dementia care, sports activity tracking
15	Tooth sensor	Eating and drinking habit
16	Watches	Oxygen saturation, blood pressure, ECG

2.10 THE ADVANTAGES, DISADVANTAGES, AND LIMITATIONS OF WEARABLES AND AMBIENT SENSORS

This area shall be discussed from the perspective of earlier researchers (Xing et al., 2023; Kang & Exworthy, 2022) and (Jovanovic et al., 2022; Canali et al., 2022; Vijayan et al., 2021).

The advantages of wearable sensors include accurate monitoring of human body laboratory parameters, diagnostic parameters and other body activities and indicators in real-time. Notably, the wearables provide comfort based on the design to the wearer. It is mostly admired because of the portability thereby allowing the wearer to move around freely. The wearables have enormous convenience that provide a convenient and timely solution for urgency especially in motion detection. The health monitoring capacity of wearable sensors can monitor various physiological signals and body movements. These advantages in health monitoring goes ahead to provide real-time feedback thereby encouraging the wearer or care provider to take immediate action. Because of the hereditary and chronic diseases, wearables provide the opportunity of long-term monitoring of health conditions over a long period, providing valuable insights into the wearer's health. In addition, the wearable sensors are mostly non-invasive making them a more comfortable and convenient option compared to traditional medical devices. They are also cost-effective compared to traditional medical devices and hospital visits. Most of the wearables are very easy to use because they are designed to be user-friendly, making them easy to use and interpret.

The ability of wearables to help in remote patient monitoring especially in pandemic and endemic diseases in the context of reducing the demand for healthcare systems is an advantage. Also, wearables are an aspect of patient empowerment in personal healthcare. Furthermore, the wearable devices is helpful in ambient assisted living especially with the disabled, elderly, and children.

The possible disadvantages and limitations of wearable sensors may include accuracy issues due to their limited storage and computing capabilities. There is also difficulty in data transmission of captured data to a powerful remote computer or a cloud implementation, where the sensor information is deciphered, deconstructed, and results are meaningfully generated, interpreted and presented to the user or healthcare provider. In some cases, there may be data loss as a result of the vulnerability of wireless communication channels that can result in data loss during transmission, as well as errors in data analysis and prediction. Also, sensor-wearer error may unintentionally cause errors throughout a lengthy time of use.

To add to the disadvantages are the complexity and high cost of wearable technologies involved. There could be possible contaminations of wearables by oils and proteins. This could be reduced by adequate cleaning and blocking of contaminant inlet routes.

The challenges of wearable sensors to healthcare is about the standards for data quality and access to wearable devices for health equity; whereas the wearable users are concerned about their privacy, limited digital literacy, and limited socioeconomic resources available but the vendors are trying to ensure clinical validity, address translational gaps, balance technology readiness with clinical validation and real-world viability assessments, and establish strategic partnerships between technical and clinical stakeholders.

2.11 ECONOMIC IMPLICATIONS OF WEARABLE AND AMBIENT SENSORS

Wearable devices have significant economic implications on the healthcare industry, including health equity for all, data quality for reliable and trustworthy healthcare services, interoperability and integration with other health data, to enable the comparison and balancing of results collected by different devices, sensors, and approaches.

The economic benefits are numerous to healthcare, users and vendors. Wearable devices can reduce healthcare costs by enabling remote monitoring and early detection of health issues. The vendors and users' economic consideration shall border on manufacturing costs, selling cost, and purchase cost. This will definitely affect the perceived "market for the sensor information and the perceived impact of the sensor on the market price" (Devine et al., 2022).

2.12 FUTURE PERSPECTIVES OF WEARABLE AND AMBIENT SENSORS

At the moment, the need and production of wearable sensors are on the increase. More attention has been on data accuracy as most of them are at the infancy and with less accuracy of data. Few and single or double data collection is ongoing such as temperature, oxygen saturation, respiration rate, heart rate and heart rhythm and there is the need to upscale the collection of complex data and more laboratory parameters. The personal privacy security of wearable sensor devices may not be enough leading to risk, leakage, and tampering of data. This calls for more security measures. Also there is single function and poor compatibility of wearables. The wearables should improve from the level of health monitoring to integrate multiple functions more. The industrial standardization and technological improvements in the various wearable software with new regulatory standards are required (Lu et al., 2020).

There is an urgent need to strengthen the wearable device industry for stronger security features for adequate privacy. The weak wearable should be strengthened to withstand environmental factors, have a long duration of rechargeable battery life, and possess processing efficiency.

The future of wearables would be bastardized if there are no strong guiding principles and regulation worldwide. The regulation should not be only national regulations as cross-border services shall be very high. This would include inspection, monitoring, and evaluation systems for wearable sensor devices. The wearable sensors should be expanded to combine big data, involve cloud computing, and the Internet of Health Things to build a robust healthy database. In consideration of elders' care, wearable devices should be incorporated with healthcare insurance and pension care services for effective use.

2.13 WEARABLE AND BIO-SENSORS, THE BANE OF AMBIENT ASSISTED LIVING (AAL)

Wearables are employed in domiciliary care (patient's home), hospital care (in the hospital), or in wearable health monitoring (anywhere). The use of the wearables are applicable for all clients though mostly used in the past for the elderly, disabled, and critically ill patients. The use of wearables because of their portability, robustness, and ease of use shall advance among the elderly and the disabled for the sake of environmental monitoring and activities (Vijayan et al., 2021). Such wearables employ deep learning (DL) or machine learning (ML) for motion monitoring and capture in the form of biometrics goniometers, data gloves, head sensors, smart shoes, pressure mats, sensors attached to legs, smart watches, and Torsiometers on toes and arms. The healthcare and environmental monitoring is moving up to the wearable technology supported by the internet and latest technologies of this century. All healthcare service workers, various interested subjects and vendors of such wearable sensors are to be very much informed the extent of use of wearables and especially for the sake of ambient and assisted living across the globe.

2.14 CONCLUSION

Wearable and ambient sensors are currently used in healthcare. The use expands to the elderly care, disabled, critically ill, children and sports lovers. The future of healthcare may be seeing wearables and sensors taking the lead when the standard and confidence of the people are greatly improved because of the numerous advantages following the wearables including cost effectiveness.

The healthcare providers should improve in their technological acceptability, usage, and knowledge so that the challenges associated with the latest technologies would not take them unaware with the current push for wearable technologies. The wearable manufacturers and vendors should, as a matter of urgency, address the associated privacy and security challenges with improvement of durability and contamination levels so that the future use would have little or no challenge for longer usage in healthcare.

The mindset that human samples especially in medical laboratory science, should be the best sample for running healthcare tests in healthcare practice should be addressed as new technologies can use sensors to carry out adequate diagnosis that can address health issues and save lives.

REFERENCES

Canali, S., Schiaffonati, V., Aliverti, A. (2022). Challenges and Recommendations for Wearable Devices in Digital Health: Data Quality, Interoperability, Health Equity, Fairness. *PLOS Digit Health,* 1(10), e0000104. https://doi.org/10.1371/journal.pdig.0000104

Cicirelli, G., Marani, R., Petitti, A., Milella, A., D'Orazio, T. (2021). Ambient Assisted Living: A Review of Technologies, Methodologies and Future Perspectives for Healthy Aging of Population. *Sensors*, 21, 3549. https://doi.org/10.3390/s21103549

Dauwed, M., Meri, A. (2019). IOT Service Utilisation in Healthcare. (In) Internet of Things (IoT) for Automated and Smart Applications. IntechOpen. http://dx.doi.org/10.5772/intechopen.86014

Devine, J.K., Schwartz, L.P., Hursh, S.R. (2022). Technical, Regulatory, Economic, and Trust Issues Preventing Successful Integration of Sensors into the Mainstream Consumer Wearables Market. *Sensors*, 22, 2731. https://doi.org/10.3390/s22072731

Folinas, S., Obeta, M.U., Etim, G.B., Etukudoh, N.S. (2021). COVID-19 Pandemic: The Medical Tourism and its Attendant Outcome for Nigeria. *IOSR Journal of Business and Management*, 23(7), VI, 26–35.

Francés-Morcillo, L., Morer-Camo, P., Rodríguez-Ferradas, M.I., Cazón-Martín, A. (2020). Wearable Design Requirements Identification and Evaluation. *Sensors*, 20, 2599. http://dx.doi.org/10.3390/s20092599

Guk, K., Han, G., Lim, J., Jeong, K., Kang, T., Lim, E.K., Juyeon Jung, J. (2019). Evolution of Wearable Devices with Real-Time Disease Monitoring for Personalized Healthcare. *Nanomaterials*, 9, 813. http://dx.doi.org/10.3390/nano9060813

IOM. (2002). The Future of the Public's Health in the 21st Century. / Committee on Assuring the Health of the Public in the 21st Century, Board on Health Promotion and Disease Prevention. National Academy of Sciences. www.nap.edu/catalog/10548.html

Janghorban, M., Aradanas, I., Kazemi, S., Ngaju, P., Pandey, R. (2022). Recent Advances, Opportunities, and Challenges in Developing Nucleic Acid Integrated Wearable Biosensors for Expanding the Capabilities of Wearable Technologies in Health Monitoring. *Biosensors*, 12, 986. https://doi.org/10.3390/bios12110986

Kageyama, I., Kurata, K., Miyashita, S., Lim, Y., Sengoku, S., Kodama, K.A. (2022). Bibliometric Analysis of Wearable Device Research Trends 2001–2022—A Study on the Reversal of Number of Publications and Research Trends in China and the USA. *International Journal of Environmental Research and Public Health*, 19, 16427. https://doi.org/10.3390/ijerph192416427

Kang, H.S., Exworthy, M. (2022). Wearing the Future—Wearables to Empower Users to Take Greater Responsibility for Their Health and Care: Scoping Review. *JMIR Mhealth Uhealth*, 10(7), e35684. http://dx.doi.org/10.2196/35684

Lin, B. (2019). Wearable Smart Devices for P4 Medicine in Heart Disease: Ready for Medical Cyber Physical Systems. *Omics,* 23, 291–2. https://doi.org/10.1089/omi.2019.0059

Loucks, J., Stewart, D., Bucaille, A., Crossan, G. (2022). Wearable technology in Health Care: Getting Better all the time. In J. Kaji et al. (Eds.), *Technology, Media and Telecommunication Predictions*; 64–68. Deloitte Insights.

Lu, L., Zhang, J., Xie, Y., Gao, F., Xu, S., Wu, X., Zhewei Ye, Z. (2020). Application and investigation of wearable devices in the field of health care. *JMIR mHealth and uHealth.* https://doi.org/10.2196/preprints.18907

Obeta, M.U., Ejinaka, O.R., Etukudoh, N.S. (2022). Data Mining in Medical Laboratory Service Improves Disease Surveillance and Quality Healthcare. In T. Saba et al. (Eds.), *Prognostic Models in Healthcare: AI and Statistical Approaches, Studies in Big Data;* 109. Springer.

Obeta, M.U., Maduka, M.K. Ejinaka, O.R. (2020). Medical Laboratory Science; the Distortion of Nomenclature across the Globe. *New Zealand Journal of Medical Laboratory Science,* 74, 52–53.

Obeta, M.U., Maduka, K.M., Ofor, I.B., Ofojekwu, N.M. (2019). Improving Quality and Cost Diminution in Modern Healthcare Delivery: The Role of the Medical Laboratory Scientists in Nigeria. *International Journal of Business and Management Invention (IJBMI)*, 08(03), 08–19.

Obeta, U.M,, Lawrence, A,. Etukudoh, N.S., Ejinaka, O.R., Ibanga, I. (2024). Internet of Medical Laboratory Things (IoMLTs) in the High-Tech Healthcare Industry. In Chapter 14 Alex Khang (Ed.), *Driving Medical Diagnostics through AI-Powered Technologies and Applications*; 222–237. IGI Global Press. https://doi.org/10.4018/979-8-3693-3679-3.ch014

Smith, A.A., Li, R., Tse, Z.T.H. (2023) Reshaping Healthcare with Wearable Biosensors. *Scientific Reports*, 13, 4998. https://doi.org/10.1038/s41598-022-26951-z

Vijayan, V., Connolly, J.P., Condell, J., McKelvey, N., Gardiner, P. (2021). Review of Wearable Devices and Data Collection Considerations for Connected Health. *Sensors*, 21, 5589. https://doi.org/10.3390/s21165589

Walter, J.R., Xu, S., Rogers, J.A. (2024). From Lab to Life: How Wearable Devices can Improve Health Equity. *Nature Communications*, 15, 123. https://doi.org/10.1038/s41467-023-44634-9

WHO. (2023). WHO's 2023 World malaria report downloaded on 12th May, 2024 from www.who.int/publications/i/item/9789240086173

Xing, Z., Hui, J., Lin, B., Wu, Z., Mao, H. (2023). Recent Advances in Wearable Sensors for the Monitoring of Sweat: A Comprehensive Tendency Summary. *Chemosensors*, 11, 470. https://doi.org/10.3390/chemosensors11090470

Yoo, E.H., Lee, S.Y. (2010). Glucose Biosensors: An Overview of Use in Clinical Practice. *Sensors*, 10, 4558–4576; https://doi.org/10.3390/s100504558

3 GuardianMeds

Empowering Elderly Care with IoT Medication Monitoring

Kasarapu Ramani, Irala Suneetha, Nainaru Pushpalatha and P. Harish

3.1 INTRODUCTION

Alzheimer patients and elderly people struggle to remember the schedules of medications as per doctor's prescription. Sometimes, they may be confused as to whether medicines were taken or not leading to missed doses or double doses leading to adverse effects on health. Even distinguishing between different medications, managing numerous medications with different dosages, may increase the likelihood of medication errors or non-adherence (IoT in Healthcare: Applications, Benefits, and Challenges in 2023 | Stfalcon, n.d.). They may need caregiver's assistance to follow proper medication schedules. The Internet of Things (IoT) is a revolutionary technology leading to many sophisticated interactive medical devices and applications. It caters to the needs of individual stakeholders and is healthcare specific for patients, physicians, hospitals, and insurance companies, etc. (Acharya & Patil, 2020).

An automated medicine reminder system avoids the dependency on care givers. In traditional systems, patients used to engage with doctors during physical visits or telecommunication. Therefore, continuous monitoring of the patient's health and subsequent treatment-based recommendations by doctors is not feasible (Sawand et al., 2014). With the advancements of IoT-enabled remote monitoring by doctors, the well-being of patients can be taken care of, and readmissions and expenditures can be reduced. IoT enables the real-time acquisition of patient's health data, early disease detection, tracking of vital signs and emergency response, which enhances the patient's care (Singh et al., 2023). Wearable devices empower patients' self-care management. Mobile apps facilitate an efficient healthcare ecosystem (Li et al., 2024).

3.2 IOT DEVICES IN HEALTHCARE

Prior to the advent of the IoT, most healthcare technology consisted of independent devices necessitating human intervention. However, with the introduction of IoT, a digitally interconnected healthcare ecosystem has been enabled. Figure 3.1 illustrates various healthcare applications of IoT (Rathee et al., 2018).

DOI: 10.1201/9781003520184-5

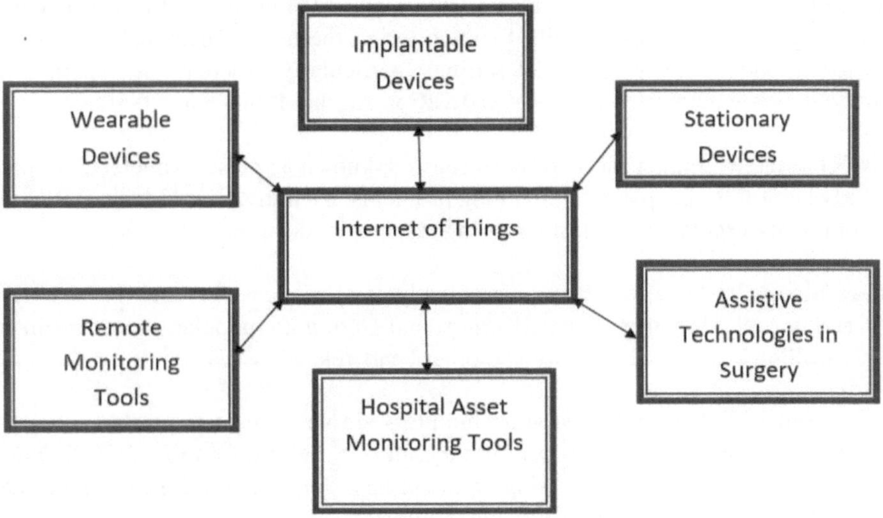

FIGURE 3.1 Applications of IoT in the healthcare sector.

3.2.1 Wearable Devices

Wearable devices encompass a wide range of gadgets that focus specifically on monitoring health metrics like oxygen levels, blood pressure, heart rate, or even electrocardiograms (ECGs). These can be useful for people with specific health concerns or for general wellness monitoring. These gadgets are mainly crafted to consistently monitor essential stats, activity levels, and overall health metrics. Within healthcare, they fulfil two intertwined yet separate functions: monitoring patients outside clinical settings and enabling individuals to track their personal health.

Medical-grade wearables are utilized for monitoring patients outside clinical environments. These devices collect real-time data crucial for tracking ongoing health conditions, aiding post-surgical recovery, or supporting elderly care. In contrast, consumer-grade wearables, designed more for tracking general well-being metrics than diagnosing or treating medical conditions, form the basis of personal health tracking (Rathee et al., 2018)

Fitness Trackers: These devices that track various health metrics like steps taken, calories expended, and sleep quality, making them extremely beneficial for individual use. Fitbit and Garmin are useful devices for monitoring the physical activity of patients during rehabilitation.

Smart Watches: Besides showing the time, these devices can track heart rate, sense falls, and occasionally conduct ECGs. Wearable devices like the Apple Watch and Samsung Galaxy Watch are beneficial for tracking patients in non-hospital environments, especially those dealing with heart issues, as well as for personal use.

Wearable ECG Monitors: Wearable ECG monitors, often in the form of patches or straps, are designed specifically for monitoring the heart. Their main use is for monitoring patients in non-hospital settings, particularly in situations that involve heart care. Some notable examples are AliveCor, KardiaMobile, and QardioCore.

Pulse Oximeters: Finger blood oxygen sensors, known as pulse oximeters, are particularly helpful for people with breathing problems. iHealth Air and Masimo Rad-5v are commonly used devices for monitoring respiratory disorders.

Smart Blood Pressure Monitors: These gadgets offer measurements for both systolic and diastolic blood pressure. *Withings* and *Omron* are popular gadgets utilized for controlling high blood pressure and other heart-related issues.

Temperature Monitors: Temperature monitors are wristbands or patches worn by patients for continuous body temperature monitoring, helpful for monitoring infants, the elderly, or individuals recovering from surgery. TempTraq and Fever Scout are widely utilized tools for monitoring temperature.

Glucose Monitors: These often involve pricking fingers with a needle to monitor glucose levels, which is an invasive process. Glucose levels in diabetic individuals can be assessed using non-invasive techniques that involve electromagnetic fields, ultrasonic waves, or radio waves. Glucowise and Gluco Track are both devices commonly employed for monitoring glucose levels.

Neurological Monitors: These devices, typically headbands or caps, track brain waves for diagnostic or monitoring purposes related to neurological conditions like epilepsy and sleep disorders. Some gadgets are made for use in homes, whereas others are suitable for clinical environments.

In clinical settings, examples include the Emotiv EPOC+ and B-Alert X-Series. For at-home use, options like Muse and NeuroSky provide accessible solutions for individuals to monitor their brain activity and potentially gain insights into their cognitive health.

3.2.2 Implantable Devices

A type of medical technology uniquely capable of providing ongoing monitoring and, in certain cases, treatment for various ailments. These devices, typically surgically implanted into the body, are engineered to function autonomously for extended durations.

Cardiac Pacemakers: These devices are mostly used in clinical settings to treat problems like bradycardia and heart failure. They are specifically designed to monitor heart rate and rhythm. Prominent instances comprise Boston Scientific's ACCOLADE MRI pacemakers and Medtronic's Azure pacemaker, which incorporates BlueSync technology and is well-known for its sophisticated features and effectiveness in heart care.

Neurostimulators: These gadgets measure the electrical activity in specific nerves or brain regions to provide a high level of specialized treatment, typically in clinical settings. They are employed in treating disorders such as epilepsy and chronic pain by administering electrical stimulation to targeted nerves or brain areas. Two notable examples are the Vercise DBS system from Boston Scientific and Medtronic's InterStim Therapy, both renowned for their effectiveness in delivering customized neuromodulation therapy.

Continuous Gluclose Monitors: By eliminating the need for regular finger pricking, these devices monitor blood glucose levels, enhancing the convenience and effectiveness of diabetes management. Two notable products in this category are Abbott's FreeStyleLibre and Dexcom's G6 (IoT in Healthcare 2023: IoT Medical Devices & Companies, n.d.).

Spinal Cord Stimulators: By intercepting pain signals before they reach the brain, spinal cord stimulators, primarily utilized in clinical settings for chronic pain management, effectively mitigate the perception of pain. Prominent examples in this field include Nevro's Senza System and Boston Scientific's Spectra WaveWriter.

Cochlear Monitors: Innovative devices known as cochlear implants are surgically implanted into the inner ear to assist individuals with profound hearing loss. Typically configured in clinical settings, these implants significantly improve hearing capacity.

Top companies such as Cochlear and MEDEL have developed advanced cochlear implants such as the Nucleus 7 and SYNCHRONY2, advancing the development of hearing implant technology.

Intraocular Pressure Sensors: Sensors implanted in the eye continuously monitor intraocular pressure to help treat glaucoma. These products have features for tracking at home and in clinical settings, giving important information on how the condition is developing. Sensimed's Triggerfish is a noteworthy technology that streamlines the process of monitoring and treating glaucoma.

Implantable Drug Delivery Systems: These systems are mainly used in medical settings to deliver drugs in a controlled and targeted manner for a wide range of conditions, including cancer and chronic pain. The Medtronic SynchroMed II pump is a well-known example that provides various delivery rates to customize treatment based on the specific requirements of each patient and improve its effectiveness.

3.2.3 Stationary Devices

These devices are essential to conventional healthcare settings, covering a wide range of treatment from diagnosis to surgical syringes. With the application of IoT technology, stationary devices are evolving towards unparalleled connectivity. Although they are immobile, they will be more powerful on remote monitoring, transmitting and integrating data, for providing better health services.

Smart Beds: Hospital beds are now smart beds, which are able to position the patient, for their comfort and to increase the efficacy of the treatments being delivered. These beds often have monitoring functions for weight, temperature and movement metrics. Interestingly, some of the smartest beds, such as The ProCuity Bed made by the company Stryker and the Centrella Smart+ Bed made by Hill-Rom, improve care by creating real-time data that can inform a healthcare provider's decisions (Acharya & Patil, 2020).

Automatic Dispensing Systems: These are sophisticated vending machines programmed to dispense medication, when authorized, to the right patient and ensure the right medicines are stocked in the right way at all times in a healthcare facility to control pharmaceutical errors and automate stock inventory control in the health institution. For instance, a PYXIS MedStation, which is an automatic programmed medication dispensing system, guarantees medication reconciliations and reduced pharmaceutical errors; and aids medications management process and protecting patients from being exposed to serious errors from medications in the healthcare setting.

EKG Machines: Modern EKG (electrocardiogram) machines have been augmented to be IoT-enabled, allowing them to supply 'live' data to doctors and expedite the diagnosis and treatment of the patient's heart problem. The best EKG machines are available from GE Healthcare, Philips, among other top manufacturers. They are primarily used in hospitals for advanced monitoring and analysis of heart function.

Ventilators: Internet-connected ventilators have transformed the field of critical care by allowing remote control and real-time monitoring of data. Ventilators like the Draeger Evita Infinity V500 and the Hamilton Medical G5 demonstrate this progress and are widely used in ICUs. These ventilators improve patient care by giving clinicians instant access to crucial information and the option to remotely adjust settings, resulting in better treatment effectiveness and patient results.

MRI and CT Scanners: The incorporation of IoT technology has transformed diagnostic instruments like CT and MRI scanners, enhancing communication and information sharing among healthcare providers. Siemens and General Electric are leading the way in this progress by providing some of the most advanced interconnected scanners on the market. These scanners with IoT capabilities improve diagnostic precision and productivity while also facilitating smooth collaboration and communication in healthcare, ultimately leading to better patient care (What Is the Internet of Medical Things (IoMT)? | Definition from TechTarget, n.d.).

Dialysis Machines: These gadgets have evolved to become IoT capable, providing enhanced data-tracking features and the ability to make changes remotely. Fresenius Health Care, Inc. and Baxter are leading providers of these smart dialysis machines, which are primarily utilized in specialized clinics. By incorporating IoT technology, these machines enhance the efficiency and effectiveness of dialysis treatments while enabling healthcare providers to monitor patient data more closely and make timely adjustments as needed.

3.2.4 Remote Monitoring Tools

Functioning as IoT devices, these technologies are engineered to sustain a continuous exchange of health data between patients and medical professionals, especially in scenarios where in-person consultations are impractical. While wearable technology and remote monitoring tools may share some similarities, remote monitoring solutions typically concentrate on specific, targeted health metrics. They enhance the remote monitoring and supervision of patients' health conditions and find extensive application in home settings, long-term care facilities, and transitional care units (Al-Haider et al., 2020).

Blood Pressure Monitors: Blood pressure measurements obtained from IoT-enabled devices, such as Omron Platinum BP5450 or Withings BPM Connect can be sent directly to the care providers or stored on the cloud for further evaluation. They are often used at home to assist hypertensive patients with routine surveillance. With its convenient use, precision, and seamless data transmission, it assists in better managing hypertension and understanding its causes towards promoting patient outcomes.

Smart Scales: Some models of smart scales like Fitbit Aria 2 and Withings Body+ measure not only weight but also other parameters such as body fat percentage, BMI, muscle mass among others. Such gadgets are most popularly used at homes for overall health or as part of targeted weight loss programs. Therefore, these smart scales offer complete body composition information that allows users to make accurate assessments of their progress and choose the right paths concerning their fitness goals.

Specialized Cameras: Certain specialized cameras enable remote examination of skin disorders remotely through sending clear high-resolution images for diagnosis by doctors. This is why there are many wound care products such as MolecuLight i:X, which can be useful in both home and clinical settings. These devices can provide detailed images of wounds that serve as a useful reference in assessing progress of healing, preventions of complications and in making better decisions on how to best treat the wound. This service would help improve patient care and save resources.

Glucose Monitoring Systems: Continuous glucose monitoring that can be made possible by remote monitoring devices such as Freestyle Libre system that sends data to patients and healthcare professionals. Although mostly for easy continuous glucose monitoring at home these devices can also be used in clinical settings where more specialized treatment is required, for instance, in the management of diabetic cases. For faster decision-making to facilitate timely interventions and finally improve diabetes management, these systems provide real-time information concerning the blood sugar.

Home EKG Monitors: Patients can easily measure their EKG tests from home with items like AliveCor's KardiaMobile, and immediately convey the same results to their medical attendants. These gadgets come in handy especially among heart patients who need constant surveillance because they allow on-time identification of arrhythmias among other cardiac abnormality disorders. Apart from reducing the needs for frequent clinic visits, remote monitoring through such gadgets as KardiaMobile enhances cardiological care, improves patient's conditions and allows early intervention.

Pulse Oximeters: Patients who have chronic respiratory conditions such as cystic fibrosis find the iHealth Air or Masimo's MightySat device very helpful in monitoring their blood oxygen levels while at home. In addition to clinics, these devices also perform well in other patient care settings. By providing constant monitoring of the level of oxygen in blood, these machines enable patients and medical professionals to manage lung health more effectively by catching any possible defects earlier enough and give appropriate interventions when needed. This translates into improved patient outcomes and better quality of life (Singh et al., 2023).

3.2.5 Hospital Operation Tools

They play a vital role in assisting healthcare facilities to run efficiently, even if they do not directly interact with patients. Leveraging IoT technology, these devices facilitate various functions such as asset tracking and environmental control. By enhancing efficiency and safety within the healthcare environment, these tools indirectly impact patient care by ensuring that resources are effectively managed and that the facility operates optimally to meet patient needs (IoT in the Healthcare Industry: Applications, Benefits and Challenges | Cloud Credential Council, n.d.).

Asset Tracking Systems: Medical equipment and staff members are among the precious assets whose locations can be tracked in real-time using real-time location systems (RTLS), such as the Stanley Healthcare AeroScout or CenTrak's offerings. By providing accurate and up-to-date information on the whereabouts of assets, RTLS ensures that resources are always optimally utilized within healthcare facilities. This not only enhances operational efficiency but also contributes to better patient care by ensuring that necessary equipment and personnel are readily available when needed.

Environmental Monitoring: Devices like the ElproEcologNet system are essential in critical healthcare environments, such as operating rooms and sensitive material storage areas, to monitor factors like temperature, humidity, and air quality. By continuously monitoring these environmental factors, these devices ensure compliance with safety guidelines and regulations and improve patient health. Ensuring ideal conditions in healthcare facilities is critical to stopping the spread of infection, ensuring the quality of medical equipment, and creating a comfortable and safe space for patients and staff (Gillespie et al., 2020).

Hand Hygiene Monitoring: Tools like Ecolab's Hand Hygiene Compliance Monitoring System and GOJO's SMARTLINK are essential for infection control because they can automatically identify healthcare workers' handwashing habits. Hand hygiene is critical to preventing the spread of infection in healthcare settings. These protocols help ensure healthcare workers follow proper handwashing procedures. Through instant monitoring and feedback, these systems promote adherence to hand-hygiene guidelines, ultimately improving patient safety and reducing the likelihood of healthcare-associated infections (IoT in Healthcare, n.d.).

Waste Management System: Intelligent waste disposal systems, such as the Enevo solution, utilize sensors to detect when garbage containers are nearing their maximum capacity. These systems use real-time data to improve the waste collection process, making sure that waste is only collected as needed. This helps cut down on unnecessary pickups and enhances operational efficiency, ultimately reducing costs. Furthermore, through the optimization of waste management procedures, these systems aid in environmental sustainability initiatives by cutting down on unnecessary waste transportation and lessening the carbon footprint linked to waste collection operations.

3.2.6 Assistive Technologies in Surgery

Organ-on-Chip: Emulate Inc. and CN Bio are replicating microfluidic cell culture chips used by companies such as Whole Organ Functions and Reactions. These advanced chips provide more advanced laboratory organ models, revolutionizing drug testing and disease modeling. By accurately replicating the environment and function of real organs, these chips allow researchers to more effectively study drug responses and disease mechanisms, accelerating the development of new therapies and improving patient outcomes (IoT in Healthcare: Applications, Benefits, and Challenges in 2023 | Stfalcon, n.d.).

Robot-Assisted Surgery Systems: The da Vinci Surgical System, which is among other surgical devices, assists surgeons in complicated procedures. In fact, such modern robot-assisted surgical systems offer improved precision, dexterity as well as visualization leading to minimally invasive surgeries, which are more accurate and controllable. They also empower the surgeons with increased accuracy of incision through which he can operate on different parts of the body that are hard to reach thus reducing trauma, resulting in quicker recovery rates for patients and better results (Li et al., 2024).

3.3 THE NEED OF SMART MEDICATION PILL REMINDER

There are countless people, some of them old, and some of them who have special needs, who need constant help, due to their being in constant need. Conforming to a medication regimen is especially important in the older population, as it contributes greatly to the success of the therapy. Nonetheless, problems related to age, such as vision reductions and memory loss can be the reason why patients have difficulty remembering and adhering to medication schedules. Persons with dementia, the likes of alzheimer's, show that this gap is even more noticeable. Provided an initial proposal to this type of situation, we must come up with an accurate and easy-to-use way so that we have less need for 24/7 nurse attendance and, thus, a decreasing chance of missing the drug doses.

3.4 SMART MEDICATION MONITORING SYSTEM THROUGH IOT

One of the key elements for effective medication monitoring technology is the sending of timely reminders. The said reminders are critical to prompt the patients to take their medicine. Also it can be sent using different kinds of methods, such as SMS, mobile applications, and voice-based assistants are also used. The adaptation of the reminders to the medicament schedule of each individual is important, wherein the changeable frequencies allow for the possibility of the individual deciding the amount of repetition necessary for them. They play a large part in keeping the patients on track by mitigating the possibilities of the patients taking an incorrect dose or even skipping a dose.

Modern drug monitoring technology has several advantages for both patients and medical professionals. It improves medication compliance first and foremost, which improves health outcomes. It also lowers medical costs related to hospital stays and ER visits that result from non-compliance with drug guidelines. Thirdly, it makes it possible for medical professionals to keep a closer eye on patients' adherence, which leads to better drug-management strategies. Ultimately, it fosters a sense of control and accountability by empowering people to take control of their health and encouraging patient involvement.

The intelligent pill container is a specially made tool intended to help people, particularly the elderly, manage their prescription schedules efficiently. With the use of this innovative technology, which integrates several features including GPS monitoring, smartphone connectivity, and provides medication reminders. Block diagram of the smart medication remainder system through IoT is shown Figure 3.2.

3.4.1 Components of Smart Medication Remainder System Through IoT

Heart Rate Sensor: Carrying out a heart rate monitor in a smart pill organizer system has a number of advantages, especially for people, who need to consider their heart rates frequently or people, who have a number of existing health conditions. This sensor opens up another level of security and convenience in terms of use of the pill box system for the user and their caregivers. Based on the effectiveness and ease of use created by this feature, it augments the heart rate monitoring capabilities to help the user manage their health and respond quickly to any irregularities in their heart rate.

Temperature Sensor: Besides using a data recorder with a GPS device, integrating a temperature sensor in the smart pill box system has its advantages, particularly

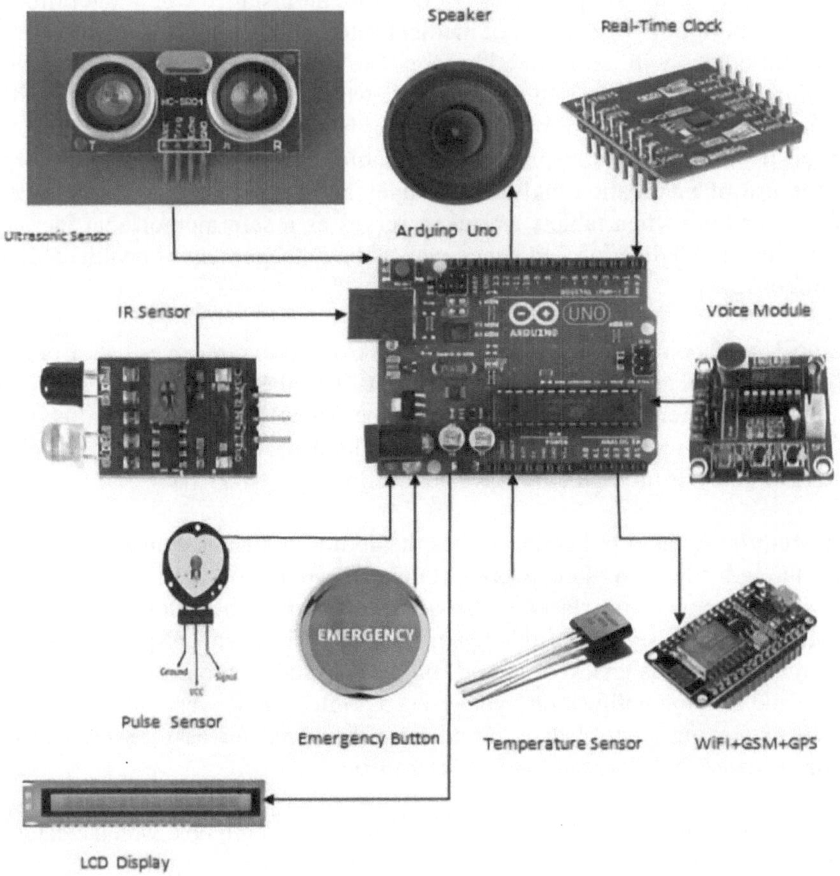

FIGURE 3.2 Block diagram of the smart medication remainder system through IoT (SMRSI).

to drugs that chemical or physical properties require a certain temperature storage range. This sensor when incorporated in the pill box system means that the temperature is monitored at all times.

Ultrasonic Sensor: An easy way to monitor the pill quantities is to blend an ultrasonic sensor with medical IoT into the smart medication box. Distance measuring ideas are applied to identify the number of pills that are available within the container with the help of the sensor. To compute the distance and pill level that the system determines, the time taken by the ultrasonic signal to travel and reflect off the tablets is measured. The pill level has not changed if the received signal and the broadcast signal are the same and if the distance change is minimal. These include the possibility to contemplate the dosages of pills continuously to ensure that patients use medicines religiously, and to order the next stock immediately.

IR Sensor: One of the simplest ways of defining an instance where the pillbox is opened is by adopting the concept of medical Internet of Things to develop a smart pillbox that comes with an infrared sensor. The sensor is also highly effective in discriminating between the state of the box; whether it is open or closed. Thus, the smart medication system might recognize that a tablet is being used for consumption if the cover is transparent. This feature enhances the aspect of correct real-time use of medication and also includes an extra layer of review. In other words, confirming when tablets are taken serves as a safe method that increases the adherence to medication and hence makes the management of health safer and more effective.

Arduino-Uno: The main ingredient here is an Arduino that receives data from several sensors as well as stores the data and outputs it on the LCD display. Each sensor transmits information in the proportion with the patient's utilization. Furthermore, UART is also utilized since the Arduino transmits data to the IoT device to obtain oversight or analysis through the UART connection.

Wi-Fi Module: A smart pill container has the ability to make a connection with the internet through a local Wi-Fi network through the use of a Wi-Fi module. Data from the pill box can now be interfaced with a diverse system such as cloud-based servers or smartphone apps because of this hyperlink. The Wi-Fi module provides options for the real-time status check of the pill box, easy modification of the prescription schedule and sending notification to the users as well as caregivers. Also, it provides a connection for the flow of data to and from the cloud for easy retrieval of data regarding medication adherence and its performance.

GSM Module: This is incorporated in the intelligent smart pill box, which creates the opportunity of linking up with the cellular network. Implementing this function, the persons or caretakers can call and (or) send messages through this pill container even if Wi-Fi connection is unavailable. Furthermore, the GSM module also plays a role in alerting the user and making the medication schedule recent so that timely alerts are received irrespective of the internet connection. This characteristic enhances the reliability and usability of the intelligent pill container and enhances confidence and medication management to the users and their care givers as well.

GPS Module: The smart pill container is equipped with the Wi-Fi and GSM modules and thus, the GPS integration-enabled accurate monitoring of the user location. With this capability, the smartphone may know the exact location of the user and using the GSM module may be able to send notifications in the instances of emergencies or any other special occasion. GPS, Wi-Fi, and GSM connectivity make the smart pill container easy to monitor and help the consumers to get the required help and action wherever they are.

Voice Module and Speaker: Using the Internet of Things to combine a speech module/speaker with a smart pill box, the signal is given through speaking instructions and notifications. Thus, translating important data into the audio format and making sure that alarms or instructions are heard and comprehensible, including for the visually impaired or users, who prefer audio, this feature improves usability and accessibility. Further, the smart pill box gives the caregivers an option that they can offer vocal support and reminders of the need to take the medicine to the patient from a distance enhancing the medicine adherence.

Real-Time Clock (RTC): For accurate delivery of medication at a certain time the IoT smart pill box necessarily requires the RTC, real-time clock. Since real time is synchronized within the device, the RTC enables the administration of the drug at the right time in the user's timetable. Thus, by synchronizing its time with the RTC, the smart pill box can be very specific in terms of time and can provide medicine events as demanded by the RM. This trait denotes that doses can be taken as scheduled and therefore promotes drug adherence in people to support effective healthcare.

Emergency Button: The incorporation of an emergency button in a smart pill box helps the users to notify their caregivers in any dire situations. The emergency button activates itself to send a massage to the caretaker informing them about the patient emergency; these details are very essential to the caretaker. This alert could include information about the current location as a result of a possibility of the patient being in need of assistance, which caretakers can address immediately. This function enhances the security of the users and provides an additional level of comfort to both patients and caretakers since it is ensured that help can be summoned for whenever the need arises. This alert could hold the location of the patient at the moment and since caregivers always monitor him or her, they can be able to assist where necessary. It increases user security and provides comfort to patients and caregivers, ensuring that help can be called at any time of the day or night.

3.4.2 Working Model of the Smart Medication Reminder System Through IoT

Several portions discussed in previous sections make up the intelligent medication container, which is filled with various pills according to the doctor's prescription. Based on the distance measure, an ultrasonic sensor determines whether or not there are any pharmaceuticals in the box. When the box is empty, an LCD display not only notifies the caregiver to replenish the medication but also shows the message. An IR sensor detects when the box is opened, indicating medication consumption by the patient. The RTC module ensures accurate timekeeping for scheduling medication reminders and updating sensor data. Arduino communicates with the IoT module via a Wi-Fi module and GSM module. This allows for data transmission to cloud servers and mobile apps. GPS module monitors the location of the medication box and alerts the caretaker in case of emergencies.

When the box is opened and the patient does not take the medication, the sensor will detect for a little while. If the medication is not taken within the recommended amount of time, an audio alert to take the medication will be played. It will communicate with the RTC, IoT module, and Arduino in addition to sending data to them. This will update every entry in the cloud database. When the sensor detects data, the

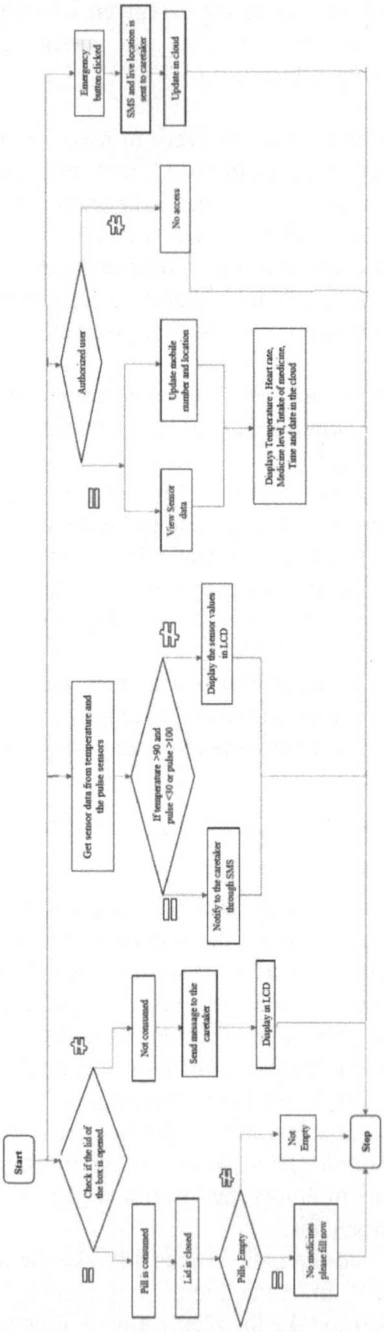

FIGURE 3.3 The process of the IoT-based smart medication remainder system.

messages will appear on the LCD panel. The speech module is utilized to receive the voice output of the alert notice, which is transmitted from the Arduino to the speaker. The voice playback module's memory card houses the message, and sensor data is stored in the cloud server, along with medication intake records and timestamps. The flow of the smart medication system is shown in Figure 3.3.

Figure 3.3 depicts the pill consumption status by the patients and checks the medication level of the pill box, the process of collecting data from diverse sensors, storing it within an Arduino, and transmitting it to the cloud via an IoT device. The Arduino gathers and stores data in its allocated memory space, then transmits it to the Wi-Fi device for upload to the cloud. This data is subsequently mirrored in the mobile application, and SMS generation is done when the emergency button is clicked.

3.5 CONCLUSIONS AND FUTURE WORK

IoT provides an excellent foundation for developing creative solutions such as a smart pill dispenser. An intelligent medication box helps patients take their medication on schedule, decreases the chances of skipped doses, and improves adherence to treatment regimens. Sensors that are integrated track important indicators such as heart rate and temperature, providing proactive healthcare and early identification of health problems. IoT gathers and combines information from different sensors to provide a comprehensive overview of patient well-being and medicine consumption. Data can be stored, analyzed, and accessed from anywhere by uploading it to the cloud. If there is an emergency or if medication is missed, the system can notify authorized caregivers through SMS with the patient's location for immediate help. A smart medication box reduces medication misuse and enhances patient safety by promoting medication adherence and proactive health monitoring. In essence, the intelligent medication box employs Internet of Things technology to oversee medication, promote patient health, and provide reassurance to caregivers. It has the capability to connect with various sensor devices and cloud platforms, making it a valuable asset in contemporary healthcare systems. This mechanism utilizes an ultrasonic sensor to gauge the amount of medicine by distance measurement, with the potential addition of a counter for monitoring pill quantity in the future.

REFERENCES

Acharya, A. D., & Patil, S. N. (2020). IoT based Health Care Monitoring Kit. 2020 Fourth International Conference on Computing Methodologies and Communication (ICCMC), 363–368. https://doi.org/10.1109/ICCMC48092.2020.ICCMC-00068

Al-Haider, A. J., Al-Sharshani, S. M., Al-Sheraim, H. S., Subramanian, N., Al-Maadeed, S., & Zied Chaari, M. (2020). Smart Medicine Planner for Visually Impaired People. 2020 IEEE International Conference on Informatics, IoT, and Enabling Technologies (ICIoT), 361–366. https://doi.org/10.1109/ICIoT48696.2020.9089536

Gillespie, C.W., Morin, P.E., Tucker, J. M., & Purvis, L. (2020). Medication Adherence, Health Care Utilization, and Spending Among Privately Insured Adults With Chronic Conditions in the United States, 2010–2016. *The American Journal of Medicine, 133*(6), 690–704.e19. https://doi.org/10.1016/j.amjmed.2019.12.021

IoT in Healthcare 2023: IoT Medical Devices & Companies. (n.d.). Retrieved September 14, 2024, from www.emarketer.com/insights/iot-healthcare/

IoT in Healthcare: Applications, benefits & Challenges. (n.d.). Peerbits. Retrieved September 14, 2024, from www.peerbits.com/blog/internet-of-things-healthcare-applications-benefits-and-challenges.html

IoT in healthcare: Applications, benefits, and challenges in 2023 | Stfalcon. (n.d.). Retrieved September 14, 2024, from https://stfalcon.com/en/blog/post/iot-in-healthcare-benefits-challenges

IoT in the healthcare industry: Applications, benefits and challenges | Cloud Credential Council. (n.d.). Retrieved September 14, 2024, from www.cloudcredential.org/blog/iot-in-the-healthcare-industry-applications-benefits-and-challenges/

Li, C., Wang, J., Wang, S., & Zhang, Y. (2024). A Review of IoT Applications in Healthcare. *Neurocomputing*, *565*, 127017. https://doi.org/10.1016/j.neucom.2023.127017

Rathee, A., Poongodi, T., Yadav, M., & Balusamy, B. (2018). Internet of Things in Healthcare Wearable and Implantable Body Sensor Network (WIBSNs). In H. Thi Thanh Binh, & N. Dey (Eds.), *Soft Computing in Wireless Sensor Networks*. Chapman and Hall/CRC.

Sawand, A., Djahel, S., Zhang, Z., & Naït-Abdesselam, F. (2014). Multidisciplinary approaches to achieving efficient and trustworthy eHealth monitoring systems. 2014 IEEE/CIC International Conference on Communications in China (ICCC), 187–192. https://doi.org/10.1109/ICCChina.2014.7008269

Singh, S., Sharma, S., Bhadula, S., & Mohan, S. (2023). Industry 4.0 Internet of Medical Things Enabled Cost Effective Secure Smart Patient Care Medicine Pouch. In A. Nayyar, M. Naved, & R. Rameshwar (Eds.), *New Horizons for Industry 4.0 in Modern Business* (pp. 149–170). Springer International Publishing. https://doi.org/10.1007/978-3-031-20443-2_7

What Is the Internet of Medical Things (IoMT)? | Definition from TechTarget. (n.d.). Retrieved September 14, 2024, from www.techtarget.com/iotagenda/definition/IoMT-Internet-of-Medical-Things

4 Internet of Things (IoT), Fog Computing, and Communication Infrastructures for Assisted Living

Paula Lamo and J. Javier Rainer

4.1 INTRODUCTION

The technological advance of the Internet of Things (IoT) has facilitated significant transformations in various sectors, such as industrial and manufacturing. But its impact is revolutionary in the field of healthcare and support for individuals with special needs, particularly in ambient assisted living (AAL) (Basulo-Ribeiro & Teixeira, 2024), where it has contributed to the creation of adaptive environments that improve the quality of life of their users substantially.

Since its initial industrial application, IoT has matured into the concept of the "Internet of the Future" (Kumar, 2017; Maity et al., 2023), where information is considered extremely valuable. In the context of AAL, optimizing medical interventions and personalizing care based on individual patient needs highly depend on the system's ability to collect real-time data and process and analyze it quickly. Therefore, processing data at the network's edge with fog computing is a significant advancement. Fog computing acts as an intermediary between edge IoT devices and the cloud (Pareek et al., 2021; Sundas et al., 2024), facilitating the management of vast volumes of data and allowing for reduced latency and improved operational efficiency. This is critical because fast decisions can be vital.

On the other hand, modern sensors, which have enabled the expansion of IoT in AAL, collect environmental and physiological data and interact with actuator systems to modify environmental conditions in response to automatically detected needs. An example of applications that can be developed using this technology is those that allow lighting and temperature to be adjusted in smart homes or to activate medical alerts by monitoring patients' vital signs and detecting anomalies. If new developments in low-consumption and high-efficiency microprocessors are incorporated, such as those based on the ARM architecture used in many IoT devices, portable and embedded devices are obtained. These proliferate in the market because

DOI: 10.1201/9781003520184-6

they offer the processing power to analyze sensor data in situ, facilitating rapid and localized decision-making.

Despite the above, the privacy, security, and ethics associated with developing IoT systems in AAL are challenges. The exposure or misuse of personal and health data can seriously affect the people affected. Therefore, systems developed in this field must be accompanied by robust regulatory frameworks and demanding security practices to protect sensitive information and ensure the reliability and security of the systems.

4.2 IOT IN ASSISTED LIVING

Using IoT devices in home care improves patients' quality of life. Figure 4.1 shows a non-exhaustive classification of the types of IoT wearables that can be placed in a

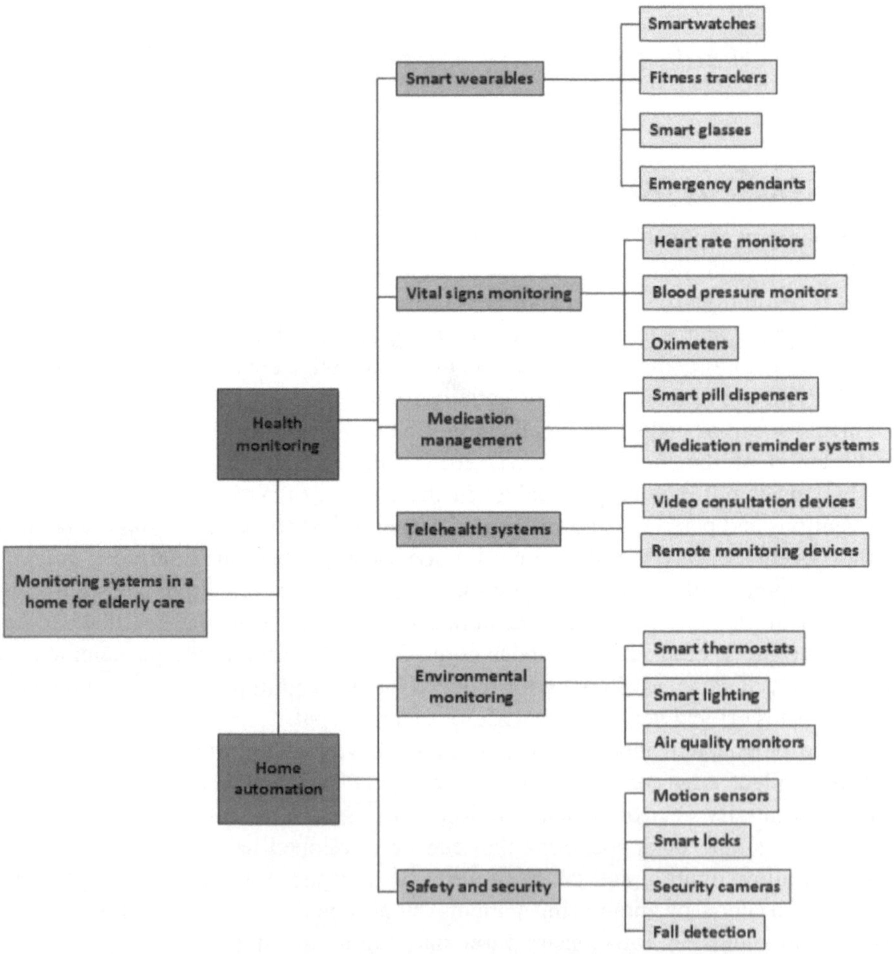
Monitoring systems in a home for elderly care
Health monitoring
Home automation
Smart wearables
Vital signs monitoring
Medication management
Telehealth systems
Environmental monitoring
Safety and security
Smartwatches
Fitness trackers
Smart glasses
Emergency pendants
Heart rate monitors
Blood pressure monitors
Oximeters
Smart pill dispensers
Medication reminder systems
Video consultation devices
Remote monitoring devices
Smart thermostats
Smart lighting
Air quality monitors
Motion sensors
Smart locks
Security cameras
Fall detection

FIGURE 4.1 Classification of monitoring systems in home for elderly care. Photograph by the author.

home. There are devices on the market ranging from wearables to fixed items in the home. Solutions of all kinds can already be found on the market. The IoT has made it possible to connect virtually anything to the Internet. The limit of this technology is the imagination, or it even has no limit. These things or devices are equipped with sensors that allow information to be collected through different stimuli. For example, they can monitor light, heat, movement, humidity, and pressure. To do so, they are exposed to a physical stimulus and convert their physical signal into digital data. The physical stimulus cannot be analyzed directly. However, the digital data generated from it can be monitored and analyzed. Some data that can be parameterized in a person are, among others, heart rate, blood pressure, and physical activity levels (Stavropoulos et al., 2020). An example of possible monitoring of an elderly person using IoT wearable devices are shown in Figure 4.2.

Making "things" or devices connected to the Internet and transmitting the information of interest is just one of the many verticals of the IoT. Moreover, as in other areas, it requires the development of a robust infrastructure that guarantees compatibility, continuous communication, and high security in the transmission and storage of personal and medical data. However, not only the technical aspects must be taken into account. The associated ethical issues must also be considered. The legislation of many countries, to a greater or lesser extent, already requires that people's data be encrypted. Its management must use demanding safety standards (Cicirelli et al., 2021).

Once analyzed, the information collected by sensors gives rise to the need to carry out specific actions. To execute an action, the device must have an actuator. These elements are responsible for converting control signals they receive from the device into physical actions. For example, an actuator can activate an alarm,

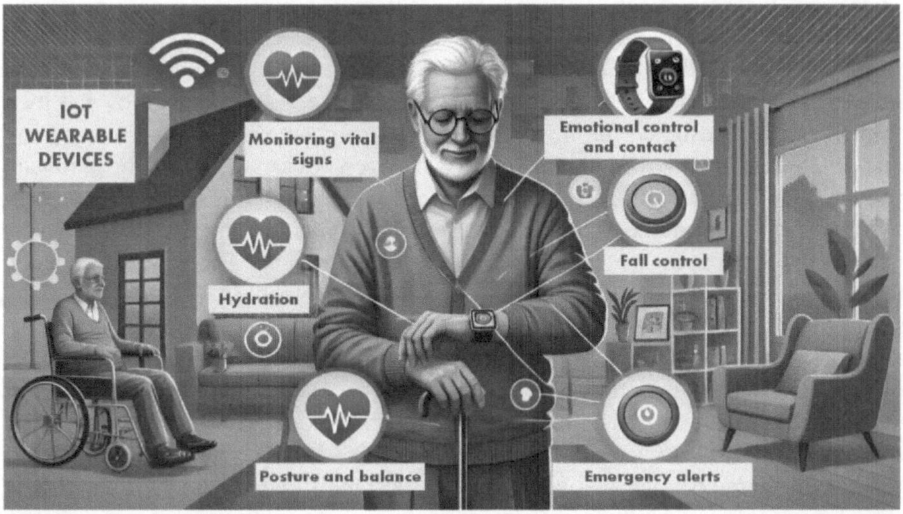

FIGURE 4.2 Example of possible monitoring of an elderly person using IoT wearable devices.

produce a movement or apply pressure at a certain point. With them, it is possible to carry out an automatic response to the needs the system has detected that the patient has. For example, a temperature sensor can trigger an actuator that adjusts the air conditioning in a home to improve patient comfort without human intervention (Erden et al., 2016).

In this context, fog computing, which carries out real-time processing of data collected by sensors, facilitates an immediate and automated response through actuators. This enables critical action in personalized healthcare and automated alert systems, such as medical emergency notifications or medication administration (Dave & Joshi, 2019).

Wilmoth and Sundaravadivel (2021) highlight the importance of a reliable and user-friendly IoT framework for resource management during pandemics is highlighted. It is also highlighted that IoT systems must be designed to be robust and easy to use in times of crisis. Flexible systems for processing multiple data have been booming (Alexandrescu et al., 2022; Ali et al., 2024). The ability to adapt and process information from various sensors ensures the personalization of treatment and care for each patient's specific needs. Another exciting option is telecommunication platforms. Mandalis et al. (2023) discuss working on this architecture, integrating portable IoT devices for real-time data collection and emergency support. All works agree that continuous and personalized medical care allows faster and more efficient medical interventions.

4.3 COMMUNICATION AND DATA

In the field of AAL, machine-to-machine (M2M) technology helps create intelligent environments that provide continuous assistance to people with special needs or the aging population. M2M systems enable seamless interaction between different devices and distributed sensors, facilitating automated monitoring and assistance without constant human intervention.

Protocols are used to communicate between these devices. These fall into two categories: proprietary and open. Proprietary or patented protocols are owned by a company and are designed for closed systems where customization and security are critical. They enable unique communications between devices with specific hardware and software. They facilitate the creation of customized solutions that offer significant competitive advantages for manufacturers seeking to differentiate their products in a saturated market. At the other extreme are open protocols. Examples include the Internet Protocol (IP) or the Constrained Application Protocol (CoAP). No company or entity owns them. The advantage of using them is that they encourage interoperability between heterogeneous devices. Device interoperability is an important aspect of this type of technology because it ensures system scalability and flexibility. This, in turn, means that broader and more diverse integration of devices and systems can be achieved.

When designing devices that work in AAL, designers and engineers try to choose network protocols and communication technologies that are efficient, secure, reliable, and energy-efficient (Qadri et al., 2024). CoAP is a protocol primarily designed for devices with capacity constraints and low power consumption. This protocol is ideal for devices operating on networks with significant bandwidth and power constraints because it is optimized to minimize data overhead and facilitate efficient operations. This makes it very common in AAL applications (Rodrigues et al., 2015).

Network infrastructure is divided into wired and wireless, depending on its use. Wired connections are used where connection stability and speed are a priority because they provide reliable and secure communication paths for high-volume data transfer. Examples of these are Ethernet and Universal Serial Bus (USB).

On the other hand, wireless technologies offer greater flexibility and mobility, which are essential in applications where device portability is a key factor. The most commonly used wireless communications in this area are shown in Table 4.1. Although Bluetooth Low Energy (BLE), ZigBee, and Wi-Fi are among the most chosen, BLE is commonly used in wearable devices, such as those that monitor vital signs or physical

TABLE 4.1
Summary of the Most Common Technologies of Wireless Communications

Technology	Technical Info.	Advantages	Disadvantages	Example AAL Applications
5G	Speeds of up to 10 Gbps, 1 ms latency, high device density per area, improved energy efficiency.	High speed and low latency enable real-time applications, broad coverage and reliability, IoT integration.	High implementation cost, reliance on dense and complex infrastructure.	Remote surgical operations, real-time health monitoring, advanced medical alert systems, autonomous vehicles for transporting the elderly.
LPWAN	Low energy consumption, long range (hundreds of meters to kilometers), low data transfer.	Ideal for applications requiring long battery life and broad coverage, low operational cost.	Limited in data transfer capacity, not suitable for real-time or high-volume data.	Monitoring of environmental conditions in homes, activity-based alert systems for the elderly.
NFC	Short-range communication (a few centimeters), operates at 13.56 MHz, low energy consumption.	Enables simple and secure interactions, widely integrated into mobile devices.	Very limited range, low data transfer capacity.	Personalized access systems to homes or elderly residences, quick exchange of medical information between personal devices and medical staff.

(continued)

TABLE 4.1 (Continued)
Summary of the Most Common Technologies of Wireless Communications

Technology	Technical Info.	Advantages	Disadvantages	Example AAL Applications
RFID	Active and passive tags, frequencies from LF to UHF, variable range depending on tag type.	Widely adopted, passive tags are inexpensive and do not require a battery.	Active tags are more costly, limitations in data transfer and range depending on type.	Patient identification, medication access control, resource tracking in hospitals.
Zigbee Smart Energy	Uses IEEE 802.15.4, supports network topologies such as star and mesh, low power consumption.	Robust and reliable networks, good scalability, low energy consumption.	Complexity in configuring large networks, shorter range compared to other long-range technologies.	Lighting and HVAC control in adapted homes for the elderly, alarm systems and fall detection.
Bluetooth Low Energy	Short range, low power consumption, widely integrated in personal devices.	Low energy use, high market penetration in mobile device platforms.	Limited range, can be susceptible to interference in environments with many devices.	Wearable health monitors, personal medical alerts, mobility assistance devices.
IEEE 802.11ah	Operates in the 900 MHz band, designed for IoT, supports a large number of devices with low power consumption.	Better signal penetration and range than traditional Wi-Fi, optimized for IoT devices.	Not very widespread yet, relies on specific infrastructure.	Health sensor connections in homes, remote monitoring systems for living conditions.
DASH7	ISM band, encryption and IPv6 addressing, designed for light, long-range traffic.	Scalable outdoor coverage, low cost, supports master-slave structure.	Less common compared to other technologies, limited development community.	Real-time tracking systems for location and health status of the elderly in outdoor settings.

activity, because it allows data transmission at low energy. This means the devices can operate for long periods without recharging, thus facilitating continuous monitoring without interruptions. ZigBee connects sensors that monitor the environment, such as motion detectors or door and window opening sensors. It uses a mesh network that improves the coverage and reliability of communication within the home, allowing each device to communicate with the central hub and each other, ensuring that critical information is communicated effectively even in suboptimal conditions.

On the other hand, although Wi-Fi consumes more energy, it is preferred when large volumes of data need to be transferred, such as in devices that require constant connectivity with support services or security cameras (Dzogovic et al., 2020).

On the other hand, the geographic coverage available and required by the project determines the network technology. Personal Area Networks (PANs) allow communication between devices over short distances, which do not exceed the average distance of a room. Bluetooth and ZigBee are typical examples of this technology. When the user needs to cover larger areas, such as an office or an entire building, he must set up a local area network (LAN). Here, Ethernet and Wi-Fi are the most common examples. If this distance is insufficient and the aim is to cover areas as large as an entire city or a country, a wide area network (WAN) is chosen. The best example of a WAN is the Internet, where 4G-LTE, LTE-A, and 5G are technologies that efficiently manage data.

When the designer wants to implement an M2M system, its design is more complex than choosing technologies and protocols. M2M systems include advanced network management to ensure continuous and reliable functionality. Strategies used to accomplish this include, for example, efficient power management and controlling duty cycles so that devices remain idle when not in use. The chosen protocol, for its part, must ensure secure authentication, adequate access management and protection of user privacy by regulations. Meanwhile, the devices must be designed to be able to translate protocols when necessary in order to ensure the integration of systems. In other words, an M2M system must guarantee that all the devices and systems that compose it can work together without any problem.

Another important advance in the area is the development of IoT platforms capable of processing large amounts of data. Using a distributed methodology, two approaches—batch processing and real-time processing—can be differentiated. Batch processing allows for automatically handling large data sets accumulated over long periods. This system facilitates scalability by dynamically adding new processing nodes. A traditional example of the method is used by Apache Hadoop, which integrates resource managers such as YARN and storage systems such as HDFS to manage data at scale efficiently.

On the other hand, real-time processing analyses large amounts of data at the time of their generation. This can be done in milliseconds. The evolution towards "fast data" reflects the need for systems that manage large volumes of information by reducing the time between data reception and use. In addition to processing large volumes of data with minimal latency, these systems must be fault-tolerant and flexible to variations in data volume. In this context, streaming processing has become relevant. This model connects the application layer with the service infrastructure through middleware, allowing data to flow from generation to final analysis in real-time. Applied to AAL, this can translate into the ability to adapt assisted living environments to users' changing behavior and needs in real-time. The actions that can be carried out range from automatically adjusting lighting and temperature to activating emergency alerts for immediate assistance (Nakayama et al., 2022). Fog computing proposes a decentralized architecture where data processing is performed closer to the network's edge, i.e., close to the devices generating the data. This allows for managing network latency and bandwidth, especially in AAL. Fast local processing reduces the dependency on remote data centers' connections, ensuring critical applications run efficiently even with intermittent internet connections.

The market offers numerous options for carrying out data processing tasks. Platforms like Apache Spark and Flink facilitate advanced analytics and offer robust real-time processing capabilities. The former is ideal for processing that requires iterative work and in-memory data analysis. Spark Streaming is part of its ecosystem and handles real-time data stream processing, integrating this capability with batch processing and interactive data analysis. On the other hand, Apache Flink is designed explicitly for stream processing, offering true real-time processing capabilities and handling data streams with very low latencies and high volumes, which is ideal for dynamic and real-time environments. These technologies are complemented by data storage systems such as Apache Cassandra or Redis, which provide fast writes and reads, essential for applications that depend on immediate access to large volumes of operational data.

4.4 USE CASES AND APPLICATIONS

The integration of IoT in smart cities has revolutionized the way health services are connected and made accessible. Featured projects have demonstrated how IoT technology facilitates the creation of integrated healthcare networks, enabling remote patient monitoring and providing real-time data to healthcare providers. Syed (2022) mentions one notable example: holistic IoT applications that incorporate human activity recognition and fall detection, crucial elements for elderly care in urban environments.

Smart homes use IoT technology to improve the management of energy and other home resources, optimizing energy use and ensuring environments that promote the health and well-being of residents. In Chen (2019), intelligent systems can automatically adjust lighting and temperature based on patient needs. The system developed by Almalki et al. (2022) ensures continuous and accurate patient care, alerting caregivers if an essential medical device is disconnected or incorrectly configured.

Syed (2022) studied the incorporation wearable IoT devices that continuously monitor patients, showing how uninterrupted data collection and notifications to caregivers allow for proactive and personalized healthcare. The market allows finding devices that can detect practically everything. This includes subtle changes in sleep patterns or medical emergencies such as falls or critical fluctuations in vital signs. Spoladore et al. (2021) described a smart home that uses IoT and virtual reality systems to anticipate and respond to the needs of inhabitants, addressing the privacy and usability challenges associated with service personalization. Also, Ghorbani et al. (2023) show how the combination of augmented reality and fuzzy decision-making can support older adults with memory impairment by significantly improving their quality of life at home. Gonzalez-Usach et al. (2021) highlight the importance of system interoperability for active and healthy aging, facilitating effective communication between European smart home clusters. This interoperability is crucial for real-time data translation between systems, improving service delivery and device integration within a broader ecosystem, enabling more proactive health management, and improving overall patient safety.

4.5 CHALLENGES AND FUTURE

Creating a generalized IoT framework, with heterogeneous devices and technological support, requires interoperability between products, applications, and services that prevents lock-in between providers. The only solution to this problem is global standardization. In this sense, standardization efforts are not new. Different national and international organizations already work in this aspect today. However, most existing Internet standards do not include IoT, as it is a relatively new concept. Therefore, its scope is insufficient to support this new technology's standardization from a technical and economic point of view. Furthermore, the concept of IoT continues to evolve today, making the homogenization process difficult. Many IoT devices have even been deployed with proprietary protocols, making communication and interoperability between multiple devices very difficult.

Standardization has numerous advantages. It can ensure interoperability across physical communication systems, protocol syntax, data semantics and domain information and across products, applications and services that eliminates vendor lock-in; security and privacy of data and users; economies of scale and reasonable timelines; and space, which allows researchers to take our society to the next level. We are in the midst of the sixth industrial revolution, where researchers, entrepreneurs, interested sellers and buyers work tirelessly to develop new solutions. Government agencies are also trying to bring this technology to their citizens. So, the world needs to agree on a common standard. This means that software and hardware must be standardized, creating standardized programming interfaces and software services to implement future applications in a uniform environment, thus allowing easy migration between systems.

Many companies and organizations, national and multinational, have formed alliances to agree on common standards and technologies for IoT. For example, organizations such as IEEE, IETF, ITU-T, OneM2M, or 3GPP work internationally to develop standardization. However, a universal organization has not yet been formed.

In the context of AAL, standardization can facilitate the adoption of more accessible, effective, and safe technologies that significantly improve the autonomy and quality of life of older people or people with disabilities. For example, IoT devices such as motion sensors that monitor daily activities and detect falls or intelligent systems that control the home environment (temperature, light, access) must be interoperable to work together and provide a better environment that is safe and comfortable. Standardization of these devices ensures that a fall sensor from one manufacturer can effectively communicate with another's medical alarm system, improving responses in emergencies. Additionally, standardization in wearable technology can allow health monitoring devices, such as those that measure blood pressure and heart rates, to integrate with electronic health management systems from various vendors. This facilitates rapid health interventions. Doctors can remotely access and monitor the health of their patients in real-time.

The use of artificial intelligence (AI) has been democratized and extended to all sectors, including AAL. Including AI in any IoT device allows for extending the device's functions, developing new, more advanced functions, and ensuring informed decision-making (Saraswat et al., 2022). To illustrate how this technology can impact, an example is described. The data collected by a sensor can be analyzed by an artificial intelligence algorithm to detect patterns that indicate cognitive and/or physical deterioration of an elderly person and/or a person with a disease. From this information, the algorithm would also allow patient assistance levels to be adjusted as needed. Another clear example is virtual assistants. They can help older people manage their medications and medical appointments. However, although this technology has great potential, its application in healthcare systems is not always easy. AAL is not without its challenges. The most important ones relate to standardization, security, and regularization. If a failure occurs in the AI system used in AAL, the consequences for the patient can be disastrous and affect their health and well-being. This forces regulators to impose rigorous testing frameworks and high-performance standards to ensure that AI systems in AAL are effective and do not compromise users' autonomy or personal rights. In addition, these systems must ensure the confidentiality and security of all data. Future developed standards must address how AI-embedded devices collect, analyze, and use personal data, ensuring the protection of privacy and data integrity. In addition, there must be clear guidelines on the explainability of decisions made by AI so that users and caregivers can understand and trust how these systems operate.

Beyond the above, other multifaceted challenges require attention in healthcare settings. These are interoperability, cybersecurity, adaptability and accessibility (Gomathi et al., 2023). A challenge facing manufacturers and integrators of these devices is to ensure that devices from different manufacturers work consistently and smoothly, creating integrated and efficient systems (Márquez & Taramasco, 2023). As the world's population is aging, AAL systems must scale effectively to safely increase data volumes and services without affecting quality or functionality.

On the other hand, the increase and evolution of cyberattacks manifest a greater need to protect the privacy and security of confidential data collected (Wazid et al., 2022). Protocols must ensure that unauthorized access will not occur, and that the integrity of personal data will be guaranteed. From an ethical point of view, voices are raised calling for informed consent and user autonomy to respect the dignity and rights of the people involved, especially the most vulnerable.

Effective integration of AAL systems with broader healthcare infrastructures ensures coordinated and continuous healthcare. The goal is for AAL devices to communicate seamlessly with electronic medical records and other systems used by patients and healthcare professionals. The flexibility and customizability of the systems play an essential role here, as they must adapt to the changing needs and preferences of users. Finally, it is essential to mention that these types of systems must be accessible and easy to use for people of all ages. The interface design and user experience must be intuitive to ensure that it does not exclude the user due to technical complexity or difficulty of use (Srinivasrao et al., 2024).

4.6 CONCLUSION

This chapter shows the importance of integrating IoT and fog computing in-home care. It highlights how these technologies facilitate transitioning from Healthcare 4.0 to Healthcare 5.0. Thus, combining IoT and fog computing allows efficient and real-time data management at the network's edge, improving the response in critical situations through advanced health monitoring systems, automatic alerts and life support. On the other hand, developing communication technologies, including implementing 5G networks and new satellite networks dedicated to IoT, reinforces the home care infrastructure. They also allow for optimizing energy management and medical monitoring systems in smart cities and homes.

Examples of practical applications have been described that illustrate how these technologies increase patients' efficiency, comfort, independence, and safety. Use cases in smart cities and homes have shown that this new paradigm improves the autonomy and interaction of users, especially those with special needs or belonging to the aging population. Despite the above, there are also challenges associated with standardization and regulation. Addressing these challenges is critical to ensuring an ethical and secure implementation of IoT in-home care while maintaining that personal and health data is handled with the highest standards of security and privacy. The continued development of robust regulatory frameworks and meticulous security practices is essential to protect sensitive information and ensure the reliability and security of AAL systems.

Looking ahead, standardization is presented as a pressing need to facilitate interoperability between heterogeneous devices and systems, essential for effectively implementing IoT technologies on a broader scale. This standardization will allow for broader integration of devices and systems, improving proactive health management and overall patient safety. As technology advances and communication networks expand their coverage, IoT integration into home care is anticipated to become even more prevalent and effective, providing indispensable support for home health management.

ACKNOWLEDGMENTS

This research was funded by Universidad Internacional de La Rioja, grant number JT-2022-04 (Project: "Architecture and communications system for connectivity with low-orbit nanosatellites"). Also, this publication is part of the project "Exploring the Practical Application of Generative Artificial Intelligence in Internet of Things and Connected Industry Educational Environments" (T24-002-I), financed by the Programa Propio de Inversiones Estratégicas para el Desarrollo de Capacidades de Investigación y Transferencia (Programa Incentiva) of the Instituto de Investigación, Transferencia e Innovación (ITEI) of the Vice-Rector's Office for Transfer of the Universidad Internacional de La Rioja.

REFERENCES

Alexandrescu, A., Botezatu, N., & Lupu, R. (2022). Monitoring and Processing of Physiological and Domotics Parameters in an Internet of Things (IoT) Assistive Living Environment. 2022 26th International Conference on System Theory, Control and Computing (ICSTCC), 362–367. https://doi.org/10.1109/ICSTCC55426.2022.9931865

Ali, M. T., Turetta, C., Demrozi, F., & Pravadelli, G. (2024). ICT-Based Solutions for Alzheimer's Disease Care: A Systematic Review. *IEEE Access*, *12*, 13944–13961. https://doi.org/10.1109/ACCESS.2024.3356348

Almalki, M., Alsulami, M. H., Alshdadi, A. A., Almuayqil, S. N., Alsaqer, M. S., Atkins, A. S., & Choukou, M.-A. (2022). Delivering Digital Healthcare for Elderly: A Holistic Framework for the Adoption of Ambient Assisted Living. *International Journal of Environmental Research and Public Health*, *19*(24), Article 24. https://doi.org/10.3390/ijerph192416760

Basulo-Ribeiro, J., & Teixeira, L. (2024). The Future of Healthcare with Industry 5.0: Preliminary Interview-Based Qualitative Analysis. *Future Internet*, *16*(3), Article 3. https://doi.org/10.3390/fi16030068

Chen, F. (2019). *Smart Assisted Living: Toward An Open Smart-Home Infrastructure*. Springer.

Cicirelli, G., Marani, R., Petitti, A., Milella, A., & D'Orazio, T. (2021). Ambient Assisted Living: A Review of Technologies, Methodologies and Future Perspectives for Healthy Aging of Population. *Sensors*, *21*(10), Article 10. https://doi.org/10.3390/s21103549

Dave, V., & Joshi, N. (2019). Fog Computing Enabled Ambient Assisted Healthcare Systems. 2019 IEEE International Conference on Distributed Computing, VLSI, Electrical Circuits and Robotics (DISCOVER), 1–7. https://doi.org/10.1109/DISCOVER47552.2019.9007916

Dzogovic, B., Do, V. T., Santos, B., Jacot, N., Feng, B., & Do, T. V. (2020). Secure Healthcare: 5G-enabled Network Slicing for Elderly Care. 2020 5th International Conference on Computer and Communication Systems (ICCCS), 864–868. https://doi.org/10.1109/ICCCS49078.2020.9118583

Erden, F., Velipasalar, S., Alkar, A. Z., & Cetin, A. E. (2016). Sensors in Assisted Living: A survey of signal and image processing methods. IEEE Signal Processing Magazine, *33*(2), 36–44. https://doi.org/10.1109/MSP.2015.2489978

Ghorbani, F., Ahmadi, A., Kia, M., Rahman, Q., & Delrobaei, M. (2023). A Decision-Aware Ambient Assisted Living System with IoT Embedded Device for In-Home Monitoring of Older Adults. *Sensors*, *23*(5), Article 5. https://doi.org/10.3390/s23052673

Gomathi, L., Mishra, A. K., & Tyagi, A. K. (2023). Industry 5.0 for Healthcare 5.0: Opportunities, Challenges and Future Research Possibilities. 2023 7th International Conference on Trends in Electronics and Informatics (ICOEI), 204–213. https://doi.org/10.1109/ICOEI56765.2023.10125660

Gonzalez-Usach, R., Julian, M., Esteve, M., & Palau, C. E. (2021). IoT Semantic Interoperability for Active and Healthy Ageing. In R. Pandey, M. Paprzycki, N. Srivastava, S. Bhalla, & K. Wasielewska-Michniewska (Eds.), *Semantic IoT: Theory and Applications: Interoperability, Provenance and Beyond* (pp. 323–346). Springer International Publishing. https://doi.org/10.1007/978-3-030-64619-6_14

Kumar, P. (2017). Future Internet & Internet of Things. 2017 International Conference on Innovations in Electrical Engineering and Computational Technologies (ICIEECT), 1–1. https://doi.org/10.1109/ICIEECT.2017.7916594

Maity, P., Sur, K., & Muhopadhyay, I. (2023). The Future of the Internet of Things (IoT) and IoT Authentication. 2023 11th International Conference on Internet of Everything, Microwave Engineering, Communication and Networks (IEMECON), 1–6. https://doi.org/10.1109/IEMECON56962.2023.10092285

Mandalis, K., Pardos, A., Menychtas, A., Gallos, P., Panagopoulos, C., & Maglogiannis, I. (2023). Integrating IoT Wearable Devices in Telemonitoring Platforms for Continuous Assisted Living Services. *Studies in Health Technology and Informatics*, *305*, 612–615. https://doi.org/10.3233/SHTI230572

Márquez, G., & Taramasco, C. (2023). Barriers and Facilitators of Ambient Assisted Living Systems: A Systematic Literature Review. *International Journal of Environmental Research and Public Health*, 20(6), Article 6. https://doi.org/10.3390/ijerph20065020

Nakayama, F., Lenz, P., & Nogueira, M. (2022). A Resilience Management Architecture for Communication on Portable Assisted Living. *IEEE Transactions on Network and Service Management*, *19*(3), 2536–2548. https://doi.org/10.1109/TNSM.2022.3165729

Pareek, K., Tiwari, P. K., & Bhatnagar, V. (2021). Fog Computing in Healthcare: A Review. *IOP Conference Series: Materials Science and Engineering*, *1099*(1), 012025. https://doi.org/10.1088/1757-899X/1099/1/012025

Qadri, Y. A., Jung, H., & Niyato, D. (2024). Towards the Internet of Medical Things for Real-Time Health Monitoring over Wi-Fi. *IEEE Network*, 1–1. https://doi.org/10.1109/MNET.2024.3352598

Rodrigues, J. J. P. C., Misra, S., Wang, H., & Zhu, Z. (2015). Ambient Assisted Living Communications [Guest Editorial]. *IEEE Communications Magazine*, *53*(1), 24–25. https://doi.org/10.1109/MCOM.2015.7010511

Saraswat, D., Bhattacharya, P., Verma, A., Prasad, V. K., Tanwar, S., Sharma, G., Bokoro, P. N., & Sharma, R. (2022). Explainable AI for Healthcare 5.0: Opportunities and Challenges. *IEEE Access*, *10*, 84486–84517. https://doi.org/10.1109/ACCESS.2022.3197671

Spoladore, D., Arlati, S., Colombo, V., Modoni, G., & Sacco, M. (2021). A Semantic-Enabled Smart Home for AAL and Continuity of Care. In G. Marques, A. K. Bhoi, V. H. C. de Albuquerque, & K.S. Hareesha (Eds.), *IoT in Healthcare and Ambient Assisted Living* (pp. 343–371). Springer. https://doi.org/10.1007/978-981-15-9897-5_17

Srinivasrao, K., Joga, S. R. K., Kumar, A. P., Hemanth, O. P., Lavanya, K. L. V., & Yaswanth, D. (2024). User Experience design for IoT-Driven Smart Home Automation interfaces. 2024 3rd International Conference on Artificial Intelligence For Internet of Things (AIIoT), 1–6. https://doi.org/10.1109/AIIoT58432.2024.10574764

Stavropoulos, T. G., Papastergiou, A., Mpaltadoros, L., Nikolopoulos, S., & Kompatsiaris, I. (2020). IoT Wearable Sensors and Devices in Elderly Care: A Literature Review. *Sensors*, *20*(10), Article 10. https://doi.org/10.3390/s20102826

Sundas, A., Badotra, S., Shahi, G. S., Verma, A., Bharany, S., Ibrahim, A. O., Abulfaraj, A. W., & Binzagr, F. (2024). Smart Patient Monitoring and Recommendation (SPMR) Using Cloud Analytics and Deep Learning. *IEEE Access*, *12*, 54238–54255. https://doi.org/10.1109/ACCESS.2024.3383533

Syed, M. Z. A. S. (2022). IoT in smart communities, technologies and applications. *Electronic Theses and Dissertations*. https://doi.org/10.18297/etd/4029

Wazid, M., Das, A. K., Mohd, N., & Park, Y. (2022). Healthcare 5.0 Security Framework: Applications, Issues and Future Research Directions. *IEEE Access*, *10*, 129429–129442. https://doi.org/10.1109/ACCESS.2022.3228505

Wilmoth, P., & Sundaravadivel, P. (2021). An Interactive IoT-based framework for Resource Management in Assisted living during pandemic. 2021 22nd International Symposium on Quality Electronic Design (ISQED), 571–575. https://doi.org/10.1109/ISQED51717.2021.9424323

5 Blockchain for Trust, Privacy, and Security in Assisted Living

Shikha Mittal, Chetna Monga, Suvarna Sharma and Kashish Mukhija

5.1 INTRODUCTION

Traditional living spaces are becoming intelligent settings due to the increasing integration of information and communication technology (ICT) in healthcare, particularly for the senior population. This adjustment not only improves living quality but also lessens reliance on outside help. Nevertheless, implementing these cutting-edge technologies presents several difficulties, particularly in the areas of security, privacy, and trust. With its decentralized and secure architecture, blockchain technology presents a viable way to allay these worries in assisted living settings.

5.1.1 Assisted Living

Utilizing information and communication technology (ICT) can transform the homes of older adults into intelligent living spaces, reducing their reliance on external assistance and enhancing overall quality of life. Nevertheless, the adoption of novel technologies remains uncertain. This study focuses on assessing a blockchain framework specifically tailored for extensive, distributed consortia and cross-national collaborations.

5.1.2 Blockchain Technology

Blockchain technology is revolutionizing healthcare data management with its underlying concepts and growing uses. Fundamentally, blockchain is a distributed, decentralized ledger technology that guarantees data transactions' security, immutability, and transparency. It functions using a peer-to-peer network that uses cryptographic principles to ensure consensus. Each member, or node, owns a copy of the whole blockchain. The robustness and trustworthiness of blockchain are largely due to its underlying concepts, which include cryptographic hashing, proof-of-work or proof-of-stake consensus methods, and smart contracts. Blockchain's decentralized architecture and cryptographic algorithms are the foundation of its security (Kaswan et al., 2022).

 DOI: 10.1201/9781003520184-7

5.1.2.1 Blockchain Fundamentals

Blockchain is an emerging technology, often known as the Internet of Value. A sequence of "blocks" that each contain data is referred to as a "blockchain". It keeps an ever-expanding list of immutable blocks in storage using a distributed database system. There is no need for intermediates in the communication between end users and suppliers because of blockchain's open communication and transaction capabilities (Sharma et al., 2021; Sharma & Priya, 2024). Every node in the blockchain network mirrors the blockchain. Any node in the network has access to read the transactions. Blockchain basic architecture is depicted in Figure 5.1.

Every financial transaction on a blockchain is confirmed and approved before being added to the open ledger or record. Millions of nodes, or computers, are supposed to form a decentralized network called a blockchain.

5.1.2.2 Key Features of Blockchain

Blockchain technology has completely changed how information is exchanged, reserved, and protected. It stands apart from conventional databases and systems because of its special mix of features. The main qualities and elements of blockchain technology may be generally grouped into these categories, with each component adding to the overall functioning and advantages of the system. Gaining an understanding of these characteristics is essential to understanding how blockchain technology may be applied in a variety of applications to improve security, efficiency, and transparency.

5.1.2.3 Blockchain Components

The components of a blockchain, such as node, transaction, block, chain, miner, and consensus algorithms, work together to maintain the integrity and functionality of the network. These elements are used to ensure secure data storage, transaction verification, and efficient operation of a blockchain system (Sharma et al., 2023).

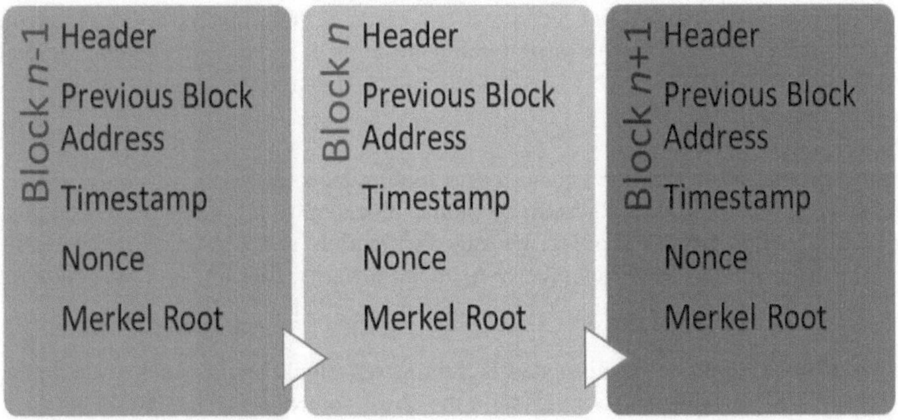

FIGURE 5.1 Blockchain basic architecture.

- **Nodes** – One of the most important components of a blockchain network is a blockchain node, which processes transactions and validates new blocks to maintain the distributed ledger.
- **Transactions** – Transactions are the fundamental exchanges that occur within a blockchain network. The core building blocks of a blockchain are transactions, which are utilized for digital asset transfers, smart contract execution, and data recording. Each transaction includes relevant information such as the sender and destination addresses, the amount, a date, and a digital signature for confirmation.
- **Block** – The blockchain is a chronological sequence of blocks made up of groups of transactions. Every block holds a collection of transactions together with a hash, which is a special identification.
- **Chain** – Evaluation of block's hash depends on the content of the current block and hash of the previous block. This creates a sequence of blocks in a specific order. This sequence is known as chain. This sequence guarantees the blockchain's immutability.
- **Consensus** (consensus protocol) – It is used to keep the blockchain in a uniform and agreed-upon state across all nodes. Proof of Work (PoW), Proof of Stake (PoS), and Delegated Proof of Stake (DPoS) are some general examples of consensus procedures.
- **Smart Contacts** – Self-executing programs on the blockchain are known as smart contracts. When certain requirements are satisfied, they automatically operate, encoding the terms and conditions of an agreement. Without the need for middlemen, smart contracts allow for the decentralized and trustless implementation of agreements. They are built in languages designed specifically for the blockchain programming framework.

5.1.2.4 Types of Blockchain

Based on their applications and thresholds, blockchains are divided into three categories: public (permissionless) chains, private (permissioned) chains, and consortium (hybrid) chains (Dinh et al., 2018; Tasca & Tessone, 2019) depicted in Figure 5.2. From totally decentralized public systems to more regulated commercial or consortium-based frameworks, each kind reflects a distinct governance and access control approach.

Public Blockchain: The blockchain that is totally decentralized is known as public blockchain. In a distributed system of public blockchain any node can participate in each action of the data reading, writing, verification, and consensus mechanisms and for their contributions they receive financial rewards. Bitcoin is an example of a public chain (Craggs & Rashid, 2019; Nembe et al., 2024).

Private Blockchain: A permissioned or centralized blockchain is the private chain. All the access permissions to the data on the chain controls by the central authority, and the permission of reading can be issued selectively to the public, usually for the

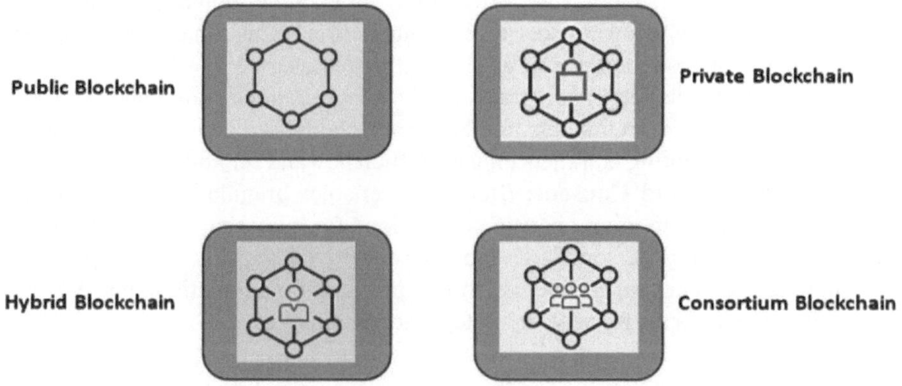

FIGURE 5.2 Different types of blockchain.

purpose of internal data management or auditing of specific organizations. Examples of private blockchain are Hyperledger Fabric, MultiChain (Dinh et al., 2018; Sankar et al., 2017).

Consortium Blockchain: The mixture of a public and private blockchain is called a consortium blockchain. Several companies get together to create a decentralized network in a consortium blockchain. Some examples of consortium blockchain are R3 corda, B3i, and Komgo (Dinh et al., 2018; Sankar et al., 2017).

Hybrid Blockchain: Hybrid blockchains are a combination of the functionalities of public and private blockchain. On the same blockchain, these networks enable private and public transactions. Some examples of hybrid blockchain are Ardor, Quorum, and Dragonchain (Lin & Liao, 2017; Zheng et al., 2017).

5.1.3 The Intersection of Blockchain and Assisted Living

Blockchain technology has the potential to significantly impact ambient assisted living (AAL) applications. AAL aims to enhance everyday environments by collecting data from various sensors, understanding people's activities and behavior, and proactively addressing identified issues. Here's how blockchain can contribute to AAL:

- **Data Security and Privacy:** Blockchain ensures secure and tamper-proof storage of data related to health monitoring, activity tracking, and other AAL aspects. It provides a decentralized and transparent system, reducing privacy concerns.
- **Interoperability and Integration:** By integrating blockchain with AAL systems, we can enhance interoperability across different care services. Legacy systems can seamlessly communicate with blockchain-based solutions, improving coordination and continuity of care.

- **Decentralization:** Blockchain's decentralized nature eliminates the need for a central authority, allowing peer-to-peer interactions. This can enhance trust and reduce reliance on intermediaries in AAL processes.
- **Smart Contracts:** Smart contracts on the blockchain can automate processes such as medication reminders, appointment scheduling, and emergency alerts. These self-executing contracts enhance efficiency and reliability.
- **Data Sharing and Consent:** Blockchain enables granular control over data sharing. Users can grant specific permissions for accessing their health information, ensuring personalized and consent-driven data disclosure paths. In summary, blockchain technology holds promise for revolutionizing AAL by addressing security, privacy, and integration challenges.

5.2 TRUST ISSUES IN ASSISTED LIVING

Active assisted living (AAL), which is defined as "all technology, devices, and wearables connected to the Internet, that enable the collection and exchange of data, and are used for health monitoring or to enhance the daily life of individuals", is one of the fields that IoT technologies and connected devices can greatly improve and support (Velmovitsky, Padses, et al., 2020).

5.2.1 Current Trust Challenges

Overcoming these problems of trust defines the use and adoption of blockchain technology across the different fields. It is often called the Internet of Value. There is no concrete view regarding its potential worth as there are some voices who put much focus on the opinion that new technologies can bring more negative changes than the Internet, with others who argue about how much significance this has (Makridakis & Christodoulou, 2019). Protecting against threats should be a top concern when handling any technology that deals with sensitive data and financial processes. Specifically, the risk of "51-percent attacks", where the mining authority in the network could exploit this control to either manipulate or completely dominate a blockchain-based system, is a worrisome issue (Kuba Nembe et al., 2024).

5.2.2 Impact of Trust Issues

The blockchain can be applied to create a record that includes all necessary and displayed certifications regarding a product which has all records of its receiving and owning up. Firms could also resist using blockchain in their operations because of doubts of blockchain's reliability, security, and impact on income taxes. This may not really be positive to the general progress and implementation of blockchain technology. In a blockchain, a new concept of truthfulness results from operational experience of a pseudonymous P2P-based network. Indeed, once a transaction has been stored in the blockchain it becomes information stored that everybody in the network knows has been made (Craggs & Rashid, 2019). We might end up in a situation where blockchain projects are not willing to interface or share data with another blockchain project creating multiple blockchains silos instead of a connected system. When the users have low confidence in the technology then it becomes challenging for them to interact and comprehend blockchain systems. This slows down the agility with which products are brought to the public and can cause a poor user experience, which discourages wider usage.

5.2.3 Blockchain as a Trust Enabler

The ongoing pursuit of increased security in the digital era has led to the emergence of blockchain technology as a game-changing force. It provides a strong resistance against the shortcomings of traditional centralized systems because of its immutability, transparency, and distributed structure. As we continue to navigate the shifting cybersecurity landscape in the digital age, blockchain technology is a beacon of security and confidence.

5.3 PRIVACY CONCERNS IN ASSISTED LIVING

As the population gets older, privacy problems in assisted living facilities are becoming more and more of a problem. These institutions must strike a balance between honoring residents' rights to privacy and autonomy and delivering the essential care.

5.3.1 Data Protection and Confidentiality

Privacy is a critical concern in the healthcare sector since medical records contain sensitive information that must be kept private. Unauthorized access to such data may have negative effects on patients, and healthcare providers may be subject to legal action. A vast amount of sensitive data is gathered in assisted living settings by several heterogeneous and networked devices. However, because most of these devices have low memory and computing capability, traditional privacy solutions cannot be deployed in them. To protect the residents' well-being, it is also crucial to understand what information should be shared with outside organizations, such medical services, and when to do so (Gupta et al., 2022). Numerous communication protocols, including ZigBee, Z-Wave, Insteon, LoRa, and KNX, have been employed in assisted living settings, as mentioned by references (Chinchero et al., 2020; Condado & Lobo, 2015).

5.3.2 Enhancing Privacy with Blockchain

It is imperative that older persons understand the nature of their permission and how to withdraw it at any moment. Enhancing patient data security and privacy is one of the many healthcare-related challenges for which blockchain technology has been suggested as a potential solution. It is feasible to create a reasonably safe assisted living environment that guards against hacker attacks and data leaks even in the face of technological limitations. In the following, we state how blockchain technology works:

- Blockchain offers a cutting-edge way to store medical data, carry out medical transactions, and establish trust for the integration and interchange of medical data in a decentralized open healthcare network.
- Blockchain technology has the potential to revolutionize patient data sharing and storage in the healthcare industry, improving operational efficiency and safety.
- Blockchain technology has the potential to strike a balance between health data access and privacy. This system functions as a peer-to-peer computer network-operated distributed ledger composed of blocks, or data structures, that are cryptographically equipped to allow confidence between parties.

5.4 SECURITY RISKS IN ASSISTED LIVING

Although they are related but distinct ideas, data security and privacy are sometimes conflated. A collection of procedures that guarantee the privacy, availability, and integrity of data is referred to as data security. Preventing data loss and unauthorized access is crucial. Therefore, access to and control over one's assisted living environment should only be granted to authorized users. A lot of issues need to be taken care of to ensure residents' privacy. Given that data security is a need for privacy, assisted living facilities must meet the following key security requirements: confidentiality, integrity, availability, authenticity, authorization, and non-repudiation.

5.4.1 Identifying Security Risks

Data collected in smart environments is susceptible to serious security and privacy abuses, so identifying these security issues is essential to taking the necessary steps to mitigate them and improve the security of the data collected within these homes. Security is a significant concern in smart home environments, particularly in situations where these environments could store and release sensitive data to third parties. Few of the frequent cyberattacks that senior home facilities currently facing are (MADISON MINER, 2023):

- Zero-Day Threats – arise when a cybercriminal exploits an unidentified security flaw in an IT network.
- Phishing attacks – use fake URLs and information requests, which are frequently delivered in emails and text messages, to get personal information from a target.
- Ransomware attacks are types of malwares, or computer-controlling software, in which a hacker demands money in exchange for unlocking a victim's device.
- Insider threats – are risks to cybersecurity posed by those who get unauthorized access to your system and utilize it for illicit activities.

- Social Engineering – A simple cyberattack is combined with interpersonal communication and the establishment of trust with a victim to create social engineering.

5.4.2 Consequences of Security Breaches

It is crucial to ensure the security of the entire ecosystem, which includes the doctors, remote assistants, receivers, and suppliers as well as the systems they use and the underlying computing and communication infrastructure that supports it. Knowing exactly how to apply appropriate cyber risk management in senior living facilities and best practices for protecting senior citizens from internet attacks is crucial as new cybersecurity threats surface. A cyberattack might have catastrophic consequences.

- For both the inhabitants and the facility operations of a senior living community due to the abundance of personally identifiable information (PII) and financial account data stored on the network.
- Healthcare records belonging to a patient might be compromised.
- Bank account hacks could result in monetary losses.
- Additionally, the facility's reputation can be harmed.

5.4.3 Blockchain for Enhanced Security

There are several important factors to consider when using blockchain to improve security in assisted living. As listed in Figure 5.3, assisted living facilities can improve security, privacy, and transparency by utilizing blockchain technology, which will ultimately result in a more dependable and secure environment for residents.

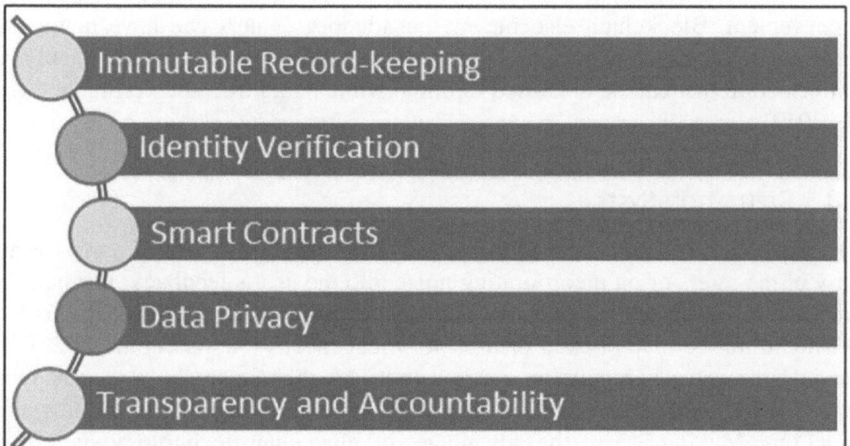

FIGURE 5.3 Security enhancement using blockchain.

The healthcare sector can gain greatly from blockchain technology in terms of data security and transparency. Its decentralized, immutable, and encrypted features make it the greatest choice for safeguarding private patient data.

5.5 BLOCKCHAIN SOLUTIONS FOR TRUST IN ASSISTED LIVING

To improve trust in assisted living settings, blockchain technology offers a robust foundation. Blockchain may successfully solve trust difficulties and encourage a more dependable and secure system for handling sensitive health data and protecting privacy by guaranteeing data immutability, transparency, and safe peer-to-peer interactions.

5.5.1 Transparent Record Tracking

Blockchain is a brilliant innovation that can bring in a tamper proof, distributed, public, safe, and accountable record. Occurrences in a supply chain network can be recorded in a way that makes them a part of transactions within the chronologically arranged blocks of a blockchain. In general, each transaction that is processed and carried out by one of the participants in the supply chain can be viewed and confirmed by other participants in the network, which guarantees the level of transparency in the entirety of the network (Aydar et al., 2019; Sunny et al., 2020).

5.5.2 Identity Verification

Blockchain transactions are permanent or more appropriately, appended, which signifies that it is nearly impossible to erase something that has been written on the blockchain once it is written. This helps in maintaining the accuracy of the identity information. Applying identity verification on the blockchain has implications on the way identities are created, protected, and accessed, which are safer, more transparent, and convenient. Blockchain also means that identity owners can have power over their own identity-based personal records, control who gets access to them, and make the information that can be disclosed minimal while being true and verifiable (Aydar et al., 2019).

5.5.3 Reputation Systems

Modern reputation systems are normally based on some trusted third party for anonymity of the raters or on incorporating noise into the user's feedback. Furthermore, the reputation values depend on the honesty of the users' feedback or input; this feedback should not be manipulated or used for other means (Arshad et al., 2022). The reviewed approaches to reputation systems on the blockchain present a promising and generally dependable model for the regulation of trust and credibility in networked transactions. Making use of the advantages of blockchain technology such as the transparency, the security, and the decentralization, such systems can generate and offer much more credible and impartial reputation scores, which are good for a lot of different fields and uses

5.6 PRIVACY ENHANCEMENTS THROUGH BLOCKCHAIN

With its decentralized approach to data management, blockchain technology has the potential to significantly improve privacy in assisted living facilities. Blockchain protects resident data from illegal access while enabling essential healthcare professionals to obtain the data they require. It does this by offering secure, permissioned access to sensitive information.

5.6.1 Data Encryption and Security

In the arena of the blockchain, symmetric encryption requires the usage of a single key for the purpose of both encryption and decryption and the commonly used algorithm underlying this is AES. While asymmetric encryption uses paired keys, one being public that is used to encrypt the text, and the other private used to decrypt the text, examples being RSA and ECC. SHA-256 and other hash functions for data validation, which takes a data input and produces a fixed number of bits for the resulting hash value. We assume that secure communication between cloud server provider and blockchain can be achieved through standard security protocols such as Secure Sockets Layer (SSL) as neither of these is a constrained node. Therefore, the aspect of the description that outlines the security mechanisms falls between the IoT sensor and the cloud server provider (Manzoor et al., 2021).

5.6.2 Decentralized Data Storage

Decentralized data storage on a blockchain is a particularly special approach to the distribution of data across the nodes of a particular network and not a single server. It is a shift from the conventional storage systems, which are much more public, insecure, and susceptible to failures. Sharding and making blocks bigger are two other options if the blockchain needs to be changed on a technical level. Huge block is actually the process that builds the block size enhancement necessary for the big block (Karaarslan & Konacaklı, 2020). Increasing the size of blocks increases the transmission limit but large blocks require very high processing power, which will also enhance an increase in the transmission cost. The verification, account, storage, maintenance, and transmission of the blockchain are based on the distributed system structure rather than establishing the judgment and trust relationship to the nodes with a centralized scheme, which constitute the decentralization feature.

5.6.3 Access Controls with Smart Contacts

Every time a subject makes an access request to him, a proper transaction on the blockchain takes place through our service. This transaction contains a reference, which checks the evaluation of the smart policy and gives the associated access decision (Bernal Bernabe et al., 2019). Smart contracts of blockchain as an open distributed ledger can introduce rules that can be used for setting permissions and regulating access to the data and other resources. Smart contracts are formal agreements where the terms of the contract are coded within the contract and this makes it possible to program the execution of the contractual terms and conditions automatically while at the same time ensuring that there is no interference with the access controls in the process.

5.7 SECURITY IMPROVEMENTS WITH BLOCKCHAIN

Healthcare institutions may now safely, confidentially, and interoperability communicate patient data, thanks to blockchain technology. Blockchain-based systems offer a tamper-proof record of patient data, facilitating safe data exchange between healthcare providers, reducing administrative costs, and improving patient care.

5.7.1 Immutable Records and Audit Trails

One of the most radical technologies of the 21st century is distributed ledgers, which allows multiple parties to have access to the same data. A distributed ledger's immutable audit trail is a record of every transaction that has taken place. A transaction cannot be changed or removed from the ledger after it has been entered. By doing this, all transactions are guaranteed to have a permanent record that can be consulted during an audit. The audit trail's immutability ensures that the data is trustworthy and dependable by making it difficult for anyone to tamper with it. Since the healthcare sector handles sensitive patient data, keeping an unchangeable audit trail is essential. All medical records can be made sure to be accurate, full, and secure with the help of immutable audit trails. This can aid in the prevention of insurance fraud, medical identity theft, and other types of healthcare fraud. Best practice for starting an audit trail, deciding what to log – identify objectives, regulatory requirements, risk assessment, data assessment, data sensitivity, user roles and privileges, critical systems and assets, consult with stakeholders. As shown in Figure 5.4, a suitable permissions checklist has been used to capture and store patient health records in the blockchain. The data owner must give their authorization when a healthcare provider or other user requests access to this recorded data.

5.7.2 Resilience Against Cyber Attacks

Senior care businesses must deal with new goods and services, interoperability issues, and a continuously changing technological landscape. For skilled care facilities and nursing homes, providing vital services, and handling sensitive data make enhancing cyber-resilience a necessity rather than just an option. The frequency of cyberattacks directed on skilled care facilities and nursing homes has increased. Because these institutions hold a lot of sensitive information, such as financial information, medical records, and personally identifying information about the residents, they are

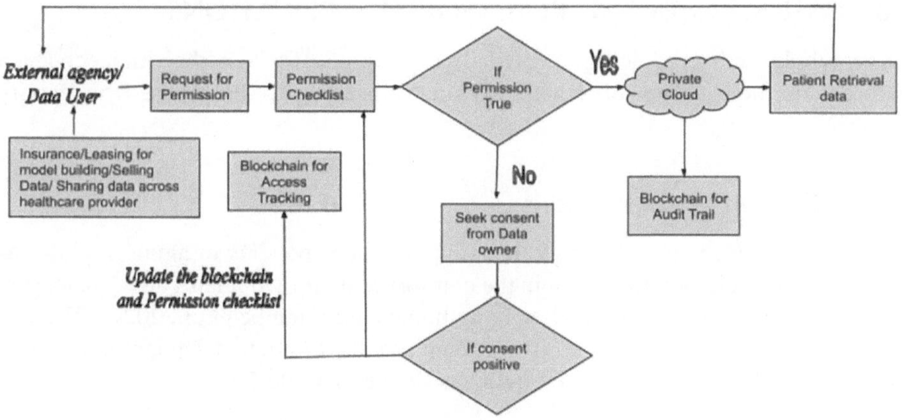

FIGURE 5.4 Patient data approval process (Jennath et al., 2020).

particularly appealing targets for cybercriminals. Cybersecurity needs to be given top organizational priority in nursing homes and skilled nursing facilities to reduce the risk of cyberattacks. This comprises the following:

- Investing in a strong cybersecurity framework.
- Enhancing staff training and awareness.
- Conducting regular security assessments.
- Establishing incident response plans.

5.7.3 Proactive Security Measures

Preventing assaults before they occur is the aim of proactive security, which lessens the burden on response procedures.

Vulnerability Assessment Scanning – Rather than wasting a lot more time and resources defending against attacks one after another, vulnerability assessment scanning is a proactive technology that enables you to foresee weaknesses and keep attackers away.

Threat Intelligence – Another example of proactive security measures is threat intelligence. Threat intelligence seeks to keep an eye out for dangerous malware, hackers, and exploits that could be sent into your networks.

Intrusion Detection System – Intelligent environment intrusion detection systems are vital tools for protecting home automation networks, or IoT networks, from many forms of intrusion. Proactive steps can be taken to reduce the likelihood of security events by identifying possible threats (Condado & Lobo, 2023).

5.8 CASE STUDIES AND REAL-WORLD APPLICATIONS

Many people with chronic age-related illnesses gradually lose their independence and become more reliant on others, eventually needing 24-hour care from family members or carers.

5.8.1 Existing Implementations

It is critical to develop technology that supports older persons in aging in place, as 89% of them would like to remain in the comfort of their own homes and considering the high expenses associated with nursing home care (Nembe et al., 2024). There is already enough work being done on blockchain for the Internet of Things applications and in the field of ambient assisted living as shown in Table 5.1.

5.8.2 Success Stories

Blockchain technology has the potential to transform the assisted living industry by enhancing transparency, security, and efficiency in managing health records, supply chains, and other essential services. Here are some success stories of assisted living facilities using blockchain:

- **Mediledger:** Blockchain is used by MediLedger as a verification system in the pharmaceutical sector. To expedite the ability to confirm the legitimacy of a prescription drug or goods in a sale, or more precisely, a return, the network organizes stakeholders into groups. It can take up to 48 hours to authenticate medications before reselling them following a return. But MediLedger uses barcode scanners and a blockchain network to drastically reduce this

TABLE 5.1
Blockchain for the Security and Privacy in Assisted Living

Blockchain Usage	References
GDPR compliant applications	(Haque et al., 2021; Ichikawa et al., 2017; Kakarlapudi & Mahmoud, 2021; Taralunga & Florea, 2021)
Informed consent management	(Aujla et al., 2020; Kakarlapudi & Mahmoud, 2021; Kumar & Tripathi, 2021; Mamdouh et al., 2021; Nasr Esfahani et al., 2021)
Data privacy and identity management	(Attarian & Hashemi, 2021; Dwivedi et al., 2022; Husnoo et al., 2021; Nasr Esfahani et al., 2021; Swathi & Venkatesan, 2021)
Security and confidentiality	(Calvillo-Arbizu et al., 2021; ElRahman & Alluhaidan, 2021; Satamraju & Malarkodi, 2021; Swathi & Venkatesan, 2021)

Source: Florea et al. (2022).

process. Serial numbers are used in this step for verification (Premkumar & Srimathi, 2020).

- **Longenesis:** Longenesis is a digital platform that connects patients, healthcare professionals, and life science businesses for post-market research and patient involvement (Longenesis, 2024). By using blockchain, Longenesis has enabled secure and transparent data sharing among healthcare providers while ensuring that residents' consent is properly recorded and managed (Somerville, 2020).
- **Solve.Care:** Whether a patient, employer, insurance, or government agency is paying for healthcare, Solve.Care enables direct communication between consumers, insurers, and service providers to enhance healthcare access, save costs, and streamline payments (Estonia: Narva, 2023). The Solve.Care platform can handle the functions of the existing processing and management systems for 3% of the total spend, which can minimize system processing and administration as well as potentially lower overall spend (Nadendla & Buckanavage, 2023).
- **Chronicled** uses blockchain to track the provenance and maintenance of medical devices used in assisted living facilities. By providing a tamper-proof record of the history and maintenance of medical devices, Chronicled has enhanced the reliability and safety of these devices (Jafri & Singh, 2022; Somerville, 2020).
- **Guardtime** leverages blockchain to secure health data against breaches and tampering in various healthcare settings, including assisted living. By ensuring the integrity and security of health data, Guardtime has helped assisted living facilities protect sensitive resident information from cyber threats (Guardtime, 2024; Rot & Blaicke, 2019).

These examples illustrate the diverse ways in which blockchain technology is being applied to improve the quality, efficiency, and security of services in assisted living facilities.

5.9 CHALLENGES AND CONSIDERATIONS

There are several problems and challenges associated with the use of blockchain technology in assisted living homes. Part of the process involves providing people with clear information about how their data is used, shared, and safeguarded (Velmovitsky et al., 2020). The legal framework dictating patient data ownership is evolving. Patients should have discretion over who can access and share their data on blockchain, according to research (Albalwy et al., 2021). Beside these there are some technical challenges also:

(1) While data encryption can increase privacy, it also complicates blockchain deployments. Ensuring that data is encrypted both in transit and at rest is vital, despite its technical difficulties.
(2) The lack of industry-standard protocols and data formats for blockchain in the healthcare sector may make it difficult to achieve smooth data transfer across several platforms.

(3) The volume of data generated by assisted living facilities, including sensor, medical, and administrative data, may overwhelm blockchain networks. The networks' efficiency and performance would suffer as a result.
(4) Blockchain activities can be resource-intensive, requiring a large amount of processing power and energy, especially when they involve proof-of-work consensus processes.
(5) Making interfaces that are easy to use and intuitive for non-techies like patients and healthcare professionals is important, but it can be challenging.
(6) Ensuring data integrity and availability while preventing redundant storage throughout the blockchain might be challenging from a technical standpoint.
(7) Blockchain networks can be energy-intensive, which raises questions regarding sustainability and operating expenses. This is especially true for networks that use proof-of-work consensus processes.

5.10 FUTURE DIRECTIONS AND OPPORTUNITIES

Facilities will use IoT devices and smart home technologies to monitor residents' health and safety in real-time, improving the quality of care and residents' peace of mind. Personalized care plans will be developed using data-driven insights, ensuring that each resident receives support tailored to their individual needs. The ease of access to medical professionals provided by telehealth services and mobile health units will reduce the need for hospital stays. Blockchain technology secures and streamlines data sharing, which will increase privacy and operational efficiency. Furthermore, housing environments that are sustainable, universally accessible, and strongly emphasize social and community involvement will create an environment that is both enriching and nurturing for residents. By taking an integrated approach, assisted living facilities can make sure that their residents' medical requirements are met while also promoting their general independence and well-being. By addressing the following areas, blockchain technology can significantly enhance the efficiency, security, and quality of care in assisted living facilities.

(1) Improving privacy by using zero-knowledge proofs to enable data verification without disclosing the real data.
(2) Utilizing sharding techniques to divide the blockchain into smaller, more manageable pieces, improving transaction throughput and data processing capabilities.
(3) Ensuring that blockchain solutions are accessible via mobile devices, making it easier for caregivers and patients to access and update information on the go.
(4) Developing advanced consent management solutions that make it simple for patients to provide, withdraw, and monitor their consent for data sharing.
(5) Implementing blockchain solutions for automated billing and claims processing to reduce errors, fraud, and administrative costs.

5.11 CONCLUSION

There are several significant benefits to using blockchain technology in assisted care homes. It greatly enhances the confidentiality and privacy of private health information while also making the processes of billing and providing care more transparent. Care plans become more comprehensive and efficient when several caregivers may collaborate more easily through the use of technology. Better consent management systems and the application of smart contracts can help individuals become more independent. Additionally, by facilitating more effective medication administration and supply chain tracking, blockchain reduces errors and enhances safety. The most exciting aspect is arguably how tokenization creates opportunities for innovative care models that have the potential to fundamentally alter how assisted living facilities treat their residents and compensate their personnel. However, other issues are also there to consider, such as implementation costs and technological difficulty, regulation observance, especially with regard to data security, guaranteeing the ease of use of services for senior citizens and staff, ethical concerns around data privacy and ownership and integration with the existing healthcare infrastructure. In summary, blockchain technology exhibits great promise in mitigating numerous contemporary issues in assisted living. However, its effective integration would necessitate meticulous arrangement, active involvement of stakeholders, and continuous assessment to guarantee that it genuinely improves the standard of care and living for occupants.

REFERENCES

Albalwy, F., Brass, A., & Davies, A. (2021). A Blockchain-based dynamic consent architecture to support clinical genomic data sharing (ConsentChain): Proof-of-concept study. *JMIR Medical Informatics*, *9*(11). https://doi.org/10.2196/27816

Arshad, J., Azad, M. A., Prince, A., Ali, J., & Papaioannou, T. G. (2022). REPUTABLE-A decentralized reputation system for blockchain-based ecosystems. *IEEE Access*, *10*. https://doi.org/10.1109/ACCESS.2022.3194038

Attarian, R., & Hashemi, S. (2021). An anonymity communication protocol for security and privacy of clients in IoT-based mobile health transactions. *Computer Networks*, *190*. https://doi.org/10.1016/j.comnet.2021.107976

Aujla, G. S., Singh, M., Bose, A., Kumar, N., Han, G., & Buyya, R. (2020). BlockSDN: Blockchain as a service for software defined networking in smart city applications. *IEEE Network*, *34*(2). https://doi.org/10.1109/MNET.001.1900151

Aydar, M., Ayvaz, S., & Cetin, S. C. (2019). Towards a Blockchain based digital identity verification, record attestation and record sharing system. *ArXiv Preprint ArXiv:1906.09791*.

Bernal Bernabe, J., Canovas, J. L., Hernandez-Ramos, J. L., Torres Moreno, R., & Skarmeta, A. (2019). Privacy-Preserving Solutions for Blockchain: Review and Challenges. *IEEE Access*, *7*. https://doi.org/10.1109/ACCESS.2019.2950872

Calvillo-Arbizu, J., Román-Martínez, I., & Reina-Tosina, J. (2021). Internet of things in health: Requirements, issues, and gaps. Computer Methods and Programs in Biomedicine, 208. https://doi.org/10.1016/j.cmpb.2021.106231

Chinchero, H. F., Alonso, J. M., & Ortiz T, H. (2020). LED lighting systems for smart buildings: A review. *IET Smart Cities*, *2*(3). https://doi.org/10.1049/iet-smc.2020.0061

Condado, P. A., & Lobo, F. G. (2015). A system for controlling assisted living environments using mobile devices. ASSETS 2015 – Proceedings of the 17th International ACM

SIGACCESS Conference on Computers and Accessibility. https://doi.org/10.1145/2700648.2809839

Condado, P. A., & Lobo, F. G. (2023). Security and privacy concerns in assisted living environments. *Journal of Smart Cities and Society*, *2*(2). https://doi.org/10.3233/scs-230015

Craggs, B., & Rashid, A. (2019). Trust beyond computation alone: Human aspects of trust in blockchain technologies. Proceedings – 2019 IEEE/ACM 41st International Conference on Software Engineering: Software Engineering in Society, ICSE-SEIS 2019. https://doi.org/10.1109/ICSE-SEIS.2019.00011

Dinh, T. T. A., Liu, R., Zhang, M., Chen, G., Ooi, B. C., & Wang, J. (2018). Untangling blockchain: A data processing view of blockchain systems. *IEEE Transactions on Knowledge and Data Engineering*, *30*(7). https://doi.org/10.1109/TKDE.2017.2781227

Dwivedi, A. D., Singh, R., Ghosh, U., Mukkamala, R. R., Tolba, A., & Said, O. (2022). Privacy preserving authentication system based on non-interactive zero knowledge proof suitable for Internet of Things. *Journal of Ambient Intelligence and Humanized Computing*, *13*(10). https://doi.org/10.1007/s12652-021-03459-4

ElRahman, S. A., & Alluhaidan, A. S. (2021). Blockchain technology and IoT-edge framework for sharing healthcare services. *Soft Computing*, *25*(21). https://doi.org/10.1007/s00500-021-06041-4

Estonia: Narva. (2023). *Global Blockchain Platform For Digital Health Networks.* https://solve.care/wp-content/uploads/2024/05/SC_Whitepaper_2024.pdf

Florea, A. I., Anghel, I., & Cioara, T. (2022). A Review of Blockchain Technology Applications in Ambient Assisted Living. *Future Internet*, *14*(5). https://doi.org/10.3390/fi14050150

Guardtime. (2024). *Research – Guardtime*. Guardtime. https://guardtime.com/research

Gupta, S., Sharma, H. K., & Kapoor, M. (2022). Integration of IoMT and Blockchain in Smart Healthcare System. In *Blockchain for Secure Healthcare Using Internet of Medical Things (IoMT)*. Springer. https://doi.org/10.1007/978-3-031-18896-1

Haque, A. B., Islam, A. K. M. N., Hyrynsalmi, S., Naqvi, B., & Smolander, K. (2021). GDPR Compliant Blockchains-a Systematic Literature Review. *IEEE Access*, *9*. https://doi.org/10.1109/ACCESS.2021.3069877

Husnoo, M. A., Anwar, A., Chakrabortty, R. K., Doss, R., & Ryan, M. J. (2021). Differential privacy for IoT-enabled critical infrastructure: A comprehensive survey. *IEEE Access*, *9*. https://doi.org/10.1109/ACCESS.2021.3124309

Ichikawa, D., Kashiyama, M., & Ueno, T. (2017). Tamper-resistant mobile health using blockchain technology. *JMIR MHealth and UHealth*, *5*(7). https://doi.org/10.2196/mhealth.7938

Jafri, R., & Singh, S. (2022). Blockchain Applications for the Healthcare Sector: Uses beyond Bitcoin. In S. Tanwar (Ed.), *Blockchain Applications for Healthcare Informatics: beyond 5G*. Academic Press. https://doi.org/10.1016/B978-0-323-90615-9.00022-0

Jennath, H. S., Anoop, V. S., & Asharaf, S. (2020). Blockchain for healthcare: Securing patient data and enabling trusted artificial intelligence. *International Journal of Interactive Multimedia and Artificial Intelligence*, *6*(3). https://doi.org/10.9781/ijimai.2020.07.002

Kakarlapudi, P. V., & Mahmoud, Q. H. (2021). A Systematic Review of Blockchain for Consent Management. *Healthcare (Switzerland)*, *9*(2). https://doi.org/10.3390/healthcare9020137

Karaarslan, E., & Konacaklı, E. (2020). Data Storage in the Decentralized World: Blockchain and Derivatives. In S. Gülseçen, S. K. Sharma, & E. Akadal (Eds.), *Who Runs the World: Data*. Istanbul University Press. https://doi.org/10.26650/b/et06.2020.011.03

Kaswan, K. S., Dhatterwal, J. S., Sood, K., & Balusamy, B. (2022). Role of Blockchain Technology in the Modern Era. In K. Sood, R. K. Dhanaraj, B. Balusamy, & S. Kadry

(Eds.), *Blockchain Technology in Corporate Governance: Transforming Business and Industries*. Wiley Online Library. https://doi.org/10.1002/9781119865247.ch1

Kumar, R., & Tripathi, R. (2021). Towards design and implementation of security and privacy framework for Internet of Medical Things (IoMT) by leveraging blockchain and IPFS technology. *Journal of Supercomputing*, *77*(8). https://doi.org/10.1007/s11227-020-03570-x

Lin, I. C., & Liao, T. C. (2017). A survey of blockchain security issues and challenges. *International Journal of Network Security*, *19*(5). https://doi.org/10.6633/IJNS.201709.19(5).01

Longenesis. (2024, July). *Unlock Patient-Centric Solutions With Longenesis*. Longenesis. https://longenesis.com/

MADISON MINER. (2023, July 18). *Safeguarding Senior Living Centers: Assessing Cyber Risks*. Systems Solution, Inc. https://insider.ssi-net.com/insights/safeguarding-senior-living-centers-assessing-cyber-risks#:~:text=Consequences%20of%20Cyberattacks%20on%20Senior%20Living%20Communities&text=A%20patient%20may%20have%20their,suffer%20damage%20to%20its%20reputation

Makridakis, S., & Christodoulou, K. (2019). Blockchain: Current Challenges and Future Prospects/Applications. *Future Internet*, *11*(12). https://doi.org/10.3390/FI11120258

Mamdouh, M., Awad, A. I., Khalaf, A. A. M., & Hamed, H. F. A. (2021). Authentication and Identity Management of IoHT Devices: Achievements, Challenges, and Future Directions. *Computers and Security*, *111*. https://doi.org/10.1016/j.cose.2021.102491

Manzoor, A., Braeken, A., Kanhere, S. S., Ylianttila, M., & Liyanage, M. (2021). Proxy re-encryption enabled secure and anonymous IoT data sharing platform based on blockchain. *Journal of Network and Computer Applications*, 176. https://doi.org/10.1016/j.jnca.2020.102917

Nadendla, R., & Buckanavage, J. (2023). *Blockchain in Healthcare: A Cure for Administrative Costs and Innovation Barriers*. George Washington University.

Nasr Esfahani, M., Shahgholi Ghahfarokhi, B., & Etemadi Borujeni, S. (2021). End-to-end privacy preserving scheme for IoT-based healthcare systems. *Wireless Networks*, *27*(6). https://doi.org/10.1007/s11276-021-02652-9

Nembe, J. K., Atadoga, J. O., Adelakun, B. O., Odeyemi, O., & Oguejiofor, B. B. (2024). Legal implications of blockchain technology for tax compliance and financial regulation. *Finance & Accounting Research Journal*, *6*(2). https://doi.org/10.51594/farj.v6i2.824

Premkumar, A., & Srimathi, C. (2020). Application of blockchain and IoT towards pharmaceutical industry. 2020 6th International Conference on Advanced Computing and Communication Systems, ICACCS 2020. https://doi.org/10.1109/ICACCS48705.2020.9074264

Rot, A., & Blaicke, B. (2019). Blockchain's future role in cybersecurity. Analysis of defensive and offensive potential leveraging Blockchain-Based platforms. Proceedings – International Conference on Advanced Computer Information Technologies, ACIT. https://doi.org/10.1109/ACITT.2019.8779855

Sankar, L. S., Sindhu, M., & Sethumadhavan, M. (2017). Survey of consensus protocols on blockchain applications. 2017 4th International Conference on Advanced Computing and Communication Systems, ICACCS 2017. https://doi.org/10.1109/ICACCS.2017.8014672

Satamraju, K. P., & Malarkodi, B. (2021). A decentralized framework for device authentication and data security in the next generation internet of medical things. *Computer Communications*, 180. https://doi.org/10.1016/j.comcom.2021.09.012

Sharma, S., & Priya, A. (2024). A Study of Blockchain Technology: Architecture, Challenges and Future Trends. Artificial Intelligence, Blockchain, Computing and Security – Proceedings of the International Conference on Artificial Intelligence, Blockchain, Computing and Security, ICABCS 2023, 2. https://doi.org/10.1201/9781032684994-23

Sharma, S., Rosmin, P., & Bhagat, A. (2021). Blockchain Technology: Limitations and Future Possibilities. In H. Patel & G. S. Thakur (Eds.), *Blockchain Applications in IoT Security*, 1st ed. (pp. 140–151). IGI Global. https://doi.org/10.4018/978-1-7998-2414-5.ch009

Sharma, S., Sharma, O., & Arora, J. (2023). Consensus Mechanisms Analysis: A Remedy for the Byzantine Generals Problem. Proceedings – International Conference on Technological Advancements in Computational Sciences, ICTACS 2023. https://doi.org/10.1109/ICTACS59847.2023.10390006

Sunny, J., Undralla, N., & Madhusudanan Pillai, V. (2020). Supply chain transparency through blockchain-based traceability: An overview with demonstration. *Computers and Industrial Engineering*, 150. https://doi.org/10.1016/j.cie.2020.106895

Susanne Somerville. (2020, August 27). MediLedger Network: How Blockchain-Enabled Solutions Will Change How Companies Do Business, Together. Chronicled. www.chronicled.com/content-resources/mediledger-network-how-blockchain-enabled-solutions-will-change-how-companies-do-business-together

Swathi, P., & Venkatesan, M. (2021). Scalability improvement and analysis of permissioned-blockchain. *ICT Express*, *7*(3). https://doi.org/10.1016/j.icte.2021.08.015

Taralunga, D. D., & Florea, B. C. (2021). A blockchain-enabled framework for mhealth systems. *Sensors*, *21*(8). https://doi.org/10.3390/s21082828

Tasca, P., & Tessone, C. J. (2019). A Taxonomy of Blockchain Technologies: Principles of Identification and Classification. *Ledger*, *4*. https://doi.org/10.5195/LEDGER.2019.140

Velmovitsky, P. E., Padses, M., Vaillancourt, H., Donovska, T., Teague, J., & Morita, P. P. (2020). Blockchain and IoT: a conceptual framework for a blockchain consent platform in active assisted living. *Journal of Medical Internet Research*, *22*, e20832.

Velmovitsky, P. E., Souza Miranda, P. A. D. S. E., Vaillancourt, H., Donovska, T., Teague, J., & Morita, P. P. (2020). A blockchain-based consent platform for active assisted living: Modeling study and conceptual framework. *Journal of Medical Internet Research*, *22*(12). https://doi.org/10.2196/20832

Zheng, Z., Xie, S., Dai, H., Chen, X., & Wang, H. (2017). An Overview of Blockchain Technology: Architecture, Consensus, and Future Trends. Proceedings – 2017 IEEE 6th International Congress on Big Data, BigData Congress 2017. https://doi.org/10.1109/BigDataCongress.2017.85

Section III

Artificial Intelligence (AI) for Data Analysis for Assisted Living in Healthcare 5.0

6 Human Fall Detection Using One-Class Support Vector Machine Classifier and Feature Ranking

Rashmi Gupta and Jeetendra Kumar

6.1 INTRODUCTION

Ambient assisted living technology is enabling older adults to carry out their everyday tasks on their own. A subset of ambient assisted living technology is human fall detection. Human fall detection techniques use machine-learning algorithms and sensor data to automatically identify unintended human falls. Because the fall detection system alerts the caregiver to fall occurrences so they may take the appropriate action as soon as possible, human fall detection is essential to lessen the severity of falls. Elderly persons who live alone may experience major health issues as a result of inadvertent falls. This research relates to fog computing's detection of human falls. Although there are several causes of falls, aging and domestic difficulties are among the most frequent ones. People's bodies change significantly as they age, leaving them more susceptible to injury and increased risk of falling. For more than ten years, fall-detection (FD) and fall-prevention (FP) systems have been the focus of the most research. There are several obstacles involved in creating and executing a successful FD or FP system. Interference, occlusion, many individuals (cameras), aging (changing filming qualities over time), privacy, technological challenges, expenses, noise, and threshold description (threshold-based systems) are a few of the issues they deal with. Wearable or external sensors are used in the design of fall detection and prevention systems. People are surrounded by external sensors that are installed, and they also wear wearable sensors.

Fall-detection methods can be categorized into three categories. (1) Vision based; (2) ambient sensor based; (3) fusion sensor based. In vision-based fall-detection methods, camera sensors are utilized for fall detection. Camera images or live camera streaming data are utilized to detect falls. In ambient sensor-based fall detection, wearable sensors like accelerometers, magnetometers, gyroscopes, etc., are utilized

DOI: 10.1201/9781003520184-9

for fall detection. In fusion-based sensors, fusion of various sensors like accelerometer, pressure sensor, radar sensor, etc., are utilized for fall detection.

Several characteristics have been computed from raw data during fall detection in order to use machine-learning methods. It is crucial to assign a ranking to each of these criteria. A crucial step in the categorization process is feature ranking. The ranking will be helpful and the characteristics may be simply deleted from the feature set depending on their significance whenever a big number of features determine the efficacy of prediction models. Numerous benefits result from ranking the features to determine, which is best: fewer features mean less messy features, a predictive model with a shorter training period, less overfitting, and less resources needed for model training.

The ranking of variables based on how they affect the prediction model is known as feature ranking or variable ranking in machine learning. It is necessary to understand how features affect the model as each variable has a unique effect on models. Feature ranking assigns a value to each feature based on how significant it is to the model, as features might occasionally be redundant or unimportant. The ordering of features based on their ratings is another definition of feature ranking. The relevance of features is gauged using scores. The primary goal of this chapter is to order the computed characteristics based on relevance. This chapter presents a feature ranking approach that evaluates the impact of five computed characteristics on fall detection.

Numerous algorithms for feature rating and selection are now in use. In order to rank the feature, the existing feature-ranking algorithms often employ the linear regression methodology, random forest technique, and several other techniques. Occasionally, the feature-ranking techniques that are now accessible fail to accurately rank the features in accordance with the actual categorization model. A feature-ranking method has been suggested for this purpose, taking into account the model being used for classification and rating the features based on how well they perform in the classification. The existing fall-detection models rank features using a feature-selection approach that is independent of the classifier that will be used for training, using a set of all predictors and classes. A few features will be utilized for training. After the model has been trained, the impact of features on the fall-detection model has been examined in this suggested technique. While there are a number of feature-rating techniques available, the outcomes vary. The suggested technique leverages the post-classification performance of the features on the fall-detection model and ranks the features. F1 score has been utilized as a performance metric for feature ranking since accuracy is not a reliable indicator of performance for imbalanced classes and can occasionally lead to biased findings.

6.2 RELATED WORK

A lot of research works have been done on fall detection. But there are very less works that have explored feature ranking in fall detection. Wu & Wang (2016) proposed online feature selection for fall detection. They have a used accelerometer sensor placed in the chest, waist, and legs. Their model was able to learn with partial data. They found that their proposed method of online feature calculation has fewer mistakes for activity prediction. Howcroft et al. (2017) proposed fall detection in older people with feature selection. For feature selection they used Relief-F, correlation-based feature selection, and fast correlation-based filter algorithms. For classification purpose, they used NB, MLP, and SVM classifiers. They found that using feature-selection performance of the model was improved. Fu et al. (2017) proposed somatotype-based feature selection for the identification of fall activity. They grouped the users based on their somatotype features and for each group the best features were calculated. They found that their selected features performed better than another unified classification model.

Xiong et al. (2018) proposed standard binary particle swarm optimization based feature-selection methods for fall detection. With their SBPSO-based feature selection and SVM-based classification, they have achieved 99% accuracy. Li et al. (2018) compared the performance of various feature-selection methods for human activity recognition. After experimenting on two publically available datasets, they found the highest accuracy with the hybrid feature-selection method. In 2019, Putra & Vesilo (2019) proposed a genetic algorithm-based feature-selection method that selects the best features having the low computational cost and having better prediction in terms of F1 score. They have achieved 97.7% F1 score and the method performs better than RFE and SelectKBest techniques.

In 2020, Liu et al. (2020) proposed daily activity feature selection in smart homes. Their feature-selection method was based on Pearson correlation coefficient. They removed redundant feature by relation degree between daily activity features. Using the proposed method, F score was improved with 1.56%. In 2020, Ahmed et al. (2020) proposed to identify human activities using fusion of feature-selection models. They used sequential floating forward search to extract features. For classification purpose, they used a multiclass SVM. Using the proposed method, they achieved 98.13% accuracy. In 2021, Le et al. (2021) proposed a feature-selection method for fall detection with various classifiers. They proposed a novel feature-selection approach to reduce the number of effective features. They performed feature selection using two optimization strategies: (1) particle swarm optimization and (2) gray wolf optimization. Six different classifiers were used by them for the classification of fall activities. Using the proposed method, they achieved highest 99.4% accuracy. In 2023, Zhang et al. (2023) proposed human activity recognition using feature selection. They performed feature selection using oppositional and chaos particle swarm optimization method. For classification, they used a 1D-CNN network and deep decision fusion. They found that deep decision fusion method achieved 97.81% accuracy.

6.3 METHODOLOGY

Machine learning is a collection of algorithms that uses features to discriminate the data into two classes or multiple classes. The feature is meaningful measurable data that can be used by learning algorithms. Using simple raw data for classification tasks is not an appropriate classification method. There are always some meaningful features that can be calculated from that raw data. Calculation of features reduces the volume of data as well as signifies the actual features, which can be used for the classification task. There is no limit on the number of features. In some research task, there is fewer features and in some research tasks, there are many features. Every feature has some impact on the accuracy of the classification model. Some features are less important and some features are more important. In the proposed method, three datasets have been used. The proposed fall-detection model has been trained on ADL (activity of daily living) data and tested on ADL data as well as fall data of dataset 2 and dataset 3.

6.3.1 Datasets Used

For building and testing the fall-detection model, three datasets have been used. Dataset 1 contains data of both fall and ADL activities, and dataset 2 contains data of only fall activities and dataset 3 contains data of only ADL activities. Table 6.1 shows brief details of the dataset used.

6.3.2 Data Preprocessing

It is a major step in classification. The accelerometer has acceleration in x, y, and z direction. Suppose A_x, A_y, and A_z are accelerations values in x, y, and z direction then

$$\text{Resultant acceleration} = \sqrt{A_x^2 + A_y^2 + A_z^2} \tag{1}$$

TABLE 6.1
Brief Details of Datasets

Dataset	Dataset 1 (Medrano et al., 2014)	Dataset 2 (Klenk et al., 2016)	Dataset 3 (Shrivastava & Pandey, 2021)
Number of volunteers	10	22	27
Male	07	10	17
Female	03	12	10
Weight of volunteer (Kg)	54–98	75.59 (mean)	39–77
Height of volunteer (cm)	161–181	167 (mean)	150–180
Age of volunteer (year)	20–42	69.5 (mean)	19–26
Device specification	Samsung Galaxy Smartphone with Android Operating System 2.2	AcitvePal3, mini mode and hybrid	Any smartphone
Sensor used	Accelerometer	Accelerometer, gyroscope, and magnetometer	Accelerometer
Position of device	Left or right pocket	Lower back and thighs	Left or right pocket
Sampling rate	45±12 Hz Average 50 Hz	20 Hz 100 Hz	50 Hz
Total instances of activities	7816 (ADL activities) 503 (fall activities)	22 (fall activities)	2821 (ADL activities)

In the proposed method, a total 301 values, i.e., 150 values before and 150 values after peak acceleration value have been saved. Thus total of 6-second (301 values) accelerometer data is considered as one instance in the dataset. Before calculating features, the fast Fourier transformation was applied to all three datasets.

6.3.3 Feature Calculation

Feature calculation is extracting important information from a large volume of data. So there is a need to calculate five features for every instance of data. Then five features are calculated as follows.

Post Impact (PI): Most of the time individuals in a fall remain motionless on the ground for a while following their fall activity, the accelerometer readings are largely consistent after the fall, making post impact the most discriminative characteristic between fall and activities of daily living (ADL).

$$\text{Post impact} = \frac{\sum_{i=201}^{301} (\mu i - A)^2}{N} \tag{2}$$

A: mean of μi from 201th value to 301th value.
N: No. of data points

Mean Frequency (MF) – It is sum of the product of accelerometer value in given range divided by sum of accelerometer values.

$$\text{Mean frequency} = \frac{\sum_{i=126}^{176} \text{inten}_i \, . \, \text{freq}_i}{\sum_{i=126}^{176} \text{inten}_i} \tag{3}$$

where freq_i = frequency of signal at ith bin, inten_i = intensity of signal at ith bin.

Median Frequency (M_dF): The frequency at which the signal spectrum splits into two equal segments with the same amplitude is known as the median frequency.

Peak-to-Peak Distance (P2P): It is the difference between the highest and lowest values of signals.

Peak to RMS (P2R): It is the proportion between the data's RMS value and greatest absolute value.

6.3.4 Classification

For the classification of fall activities from ADL activities, support vector machine classifier has been used. SVM divides given data into distinct classes based on feature vectors. One of the SVM classifier's variations is the one class SVM. The target data point in feature space F is classified using a one-class SVM apart from an anomaly data point. In areas with training data, the one class classification yields +1, while in other areas, it yields 0 values. Schölkopf et al. (2000) proposed a one-class SVM to classify one class data.

Let $x_1, x_2, x_3, x_4, \ldots\ldots\ldots\ldots x_n \in X$ is training with n observations. Let function Θ is a mapping function that transforms the input data into a higher-dimensional space, allowing for the possibility of non-linear decision boundaries. Kernel ker(x,y) is calculated as follows:

$$\ker(x,y) = (\Theta(x).\ \Theta(y)) \tag{4}$$

For given training data $x_i \in R^n$, $i = 1,\ldots,1$ without any class label, the primal problem of one-class SVM is

$$\min \frac{1}{2}\|w\|^2 - \rho + \frac{1}{vl}\sum_{i=1}^{l}\xi i \tag{5}$$

$$w \epsilon F,\ \xi \epsilon R^l,\ \rho \epsilon R$$

$$\text{subject to} \left(W.\Theta(xi)\right) \geq \rho - \xi i \tag{6}$$

$$\xi i \geq 0,\ i = 1 \ldots\ldots\ l$$

$$f(x) = sgn\left(\sum_{i=1}^{l} \alpha i K(xi, x) - \rho\right) \tag{7}$$

Using w and p, this approach builds a hyper-plane in feature space F with a maximum distance from the origin. The approach suggested by Shrivastava & Pandey (2021) has been used to build the kernel matrix for this one class SVM.

6.3.5 Algorithm for Feature Importance Ranking

After following the aforementioned procedures, the following algorithm has been used to determine each feature's significance inside the fall-detection model.

STEP 1: Calculate five features. Let feature set $F = \{f_{t1}, f_{t2}, f_{t3}, f_{t4} \ldots\ldots f_m\}$
STEP 2: Generate all possible subsets of feature set F of length at least 3.
STEP 3: Train the model using each subset and calculate F1 score for every model.
STEP 4: Arrange the feature set in decreasing order of their F1 score.
STEP 5: Rescale the F1 scores of all models in –5 to +5 range. This will be considered as weight.
STEP 6: Prepare the matrix of features and set of features. In matrix elements put 1 where feature occurs in feature set for specific model otherwise 0.

Feature

Subset of Feature Set *F*	f_{t1}	f_{t2}	f_{t3}	f_{t4}	.	.	f_{tn}
$\{f_{t1}, f_{t2}, f_{t3}\}$	1	1	1	0	.	.	0
$\{f_{t1}, f_{t2}, f_{t4})$	1	1	0	1	.	.	0
$\{f_{t2}, f_{t3}, f_{t4}\}$	0	1	1	1	.	.	0
*N*th Subset	–	–	–	–	–	–	–

STEP 7: Multiply the corresponding element of the matrix with the pre-calculated W_1, $W_{2,}$ W_3…… .W_n) of each subset.

Feature

Subset of Feature	$f_{t1} \times W_1$	$f_{t2} \times W_2$	$f_{t3} \times W_3$	$f_{t4} \times W_4$	.	$f_{tn} \times W_n$
$\{f_{t1}, f_{t2}, f_{t3}\}$	$1 \times W_1$	$1 \times W_2$	$1 \times W_3$	$0 \times W_4$	.	$0 \times W_n$
$\{f_{t1}, f_{t2}, f_{t4})$	$1 \times W_1$	$1 \times W_2$	$0 \times W_3$	$1 \times W_4$	.	$0 \times W_n$
$\{f_{t2}, f_{t3}, f_{t4}\}$	$0 \times W_1$	$1 \times W_2$	$1 \times W_3$	$1 \times W_4$	.	$0 \times W_n$
	–	–	–	–	–	–

STEP 8: Calculate S_1 = sum of weights of top half rows for every feature and S_2 = sum weights of bottom half rows for every feature. Score = $S_1 - S_2$ for each feature. High-score features are more important than low-score feature.

Features

Subset of Feature	f_{t1}	f_{t2}	f_{t3}	.	$f_{tn} \times$ **weight**$_n$
$\{f_{t1}, f_{t2}, f_{t3}\}$	$1 \times W_1$	$1 \times W_2$	$1 \times W_3$	.	$0 \times W_n$
$\{f_{t1}, f_{t2}, f_{t4})$	$1 \times W_1$	$1 \times W_2$	$0 \times W_3$	.	$0 \times W_n$
$\{f_{t2}, f_{t3}, f_{t4}\}$	$0 \times W_1$	$1 \times W_2$	$1 \times W_3$	.	$0 \times W_n$
	.	.	.	.	..
	.	.	.	.	..
S_1	$\sum_1^{n/2} f_{t1}$	$\sum_1^{n/2} f_{t2}$	$\sum_1^{n/2} f_{t3}$		$\sum_1^{n/2} f_{tn}$
S_2	$\sum_{n/2}^{n} f_{t1}$	$\sum_{n/2}^{n} f_{t2}$	$\sum_{n/2}^{n} f_{t3}$		$\sum_{n/2}^{n} f_{tn}$
Score	$S_2 - S_1$	$S_2 - S_1$	$S_2 - S_1$		$S_2 - S_1$

After above calculation, features having higher scores are more important than features having lower scores.

6.4 RESULTS

During the application of the above algorithm on different combinations of feature sets some calculations have been performed as shown in Tables 6.2 and Table 6.3 shows the ranking of features based on their scores.

TABLE 6.2
Calculation While Applying Feature Ranking Algorithm on the Feature Set

Feature			PI		MF		M_dF		P2P		P2R	
Set #	F1 Score	Weight (w)	M_1	$M_1 \times$	M_2	$M_2 \times w$	M_3	$M_3 \times w$	M_4	$M_4 \times w$	M_5	$M_5 \times w$
[1 2 3 4 5]	93.821	5	1	5	1	5	1	5	1	5	1	5
[1 2 3 4]	93.821	5	1	5	1	5	1	5	1	5	0	0
[1 2 4 5]	93.821	5	1	5	1	5	0	0	1	5	1	5
[1 3 4 5]	93.821	5	1	5	0	0	1	5	1	5	1	5
[1 3 4]	93.821	5	1	5	0	0	1	5	1	5	0	0
[1 2 4]	93.790	4.9931	1	4.994	1	4.993	0	0	1	4.993	1	4.993
[1 4 5]	93.790	4.9931	1	4.994	0	0	0	0	1	4.993	1	4.993
[1 2 3 5]	93.730	4.9809	1	4.981	1	4.980	1	4.980	0	0	1	4.980
[1 2 3]	93.730	4.9809	1	4.981	1	4.980	1	4.980	0	0	0	0
[1 2 5]	93.730	4.9809	1	4.981	1	4.980	0	0	0	0	1	4.981
[1 3 5]	93.730	4.9809	1	4.981	0	0	1	4.980	0	0	1	4.981
[2 4 5]	91.211	4.4495	0	0	1	4.449	0	0	1	4.449	1	4.449
[3 4 5]	91.178	4.4411	0	0	0	0	1	4.441	1	4.441	1	4.442
[2 3 4 5]	91.170	4.4399	0	0	1	4.439	1	4.439	1	4.439	1	4.440
[2 3 4]	91.011	4.4117	0	0	1	4.411	1	4.411	1	4.411	0	0
[2 3 5]	41.503	–5.0000	0	0	1	–5	1	–5	0	0	1	–5
Sum of top $n/2$ rows (S_1)				**39.97**		**24.97**		**24.98**		**34.99**		**29.97**
Sum of bottom $n/2$ rows (S_2)				**14.94**		**18.27**		**18.21**		**17.75**		**18.29**
Score (S_1–S_2)				**25.03**		**1.71**		**1.72**		**17.24**		**11.18**

Note: M_1, M_2, M_3, M_4, and M_5 are matrix elements. Feature 1 – PI, 2 – MF, 3 – M_dF, 4 – P2P, 5 – P2R.

TABLE 6.3
Ranking of Features Based on Their Scores

Feature	Rank	Score
Post impact (PI)	1	25.03
Peak-to-peak distance (P2P)	2	17.24
Peak-to-RMS distance (P2R)	3	11.18
Median frequency (M_dF)	4	1.72
Mean frequency (MF)	5	1.71

It can be seen from Table 6.3 that the post impact feature is highly important for this fall-detection model with the highest score 25.03. The next important scores are peak-to-peak distance with 17.24 score, peak-to-RMS distance with 11.18 score. Mean frequency with 1.72 score and the least important feature is the mean frequency with 1.71 score. The features, which are having high scores, are highly important and without that feature the performance of the fall-detection model will be degraded a lot.

6.5 CONCLUSION

Fall-detection techniques can detect human falls using sensor-generated data. The fall-detection method mostly relies on machine-learning techniques and thresholding techniques. Machine-learning techniques mostly require the calculation of some meaningful features from raw data as a data preprocessing step. Every feature has a different impact on the fall-detection model. Some features are important, some are less important and even some features are not required in the fall-detection model. The importance of previously calculated features in the fall-detection model has been calculated using a proposed method. This method calculates the importance of features for post-model training. The feature importance was found in the order of post-impact, peak-to-peak distance, peak-to-RMS, median frequency, mean frequency with scores 25.03, 17.24, 11.18, 1.72, and 1.71, respectively.

REFERENCES

Ahmed, N., Rafiq, J. I., & Islam, M. R. (2020). Enhanced Human Activity Recognition Based on Smartphone Sensor Data Using Hybrid Feature Selection Model. *Sensors*, *20*(1), 317. https://doi.org/10.3390/S20010317

Fu, X., Tan, Z., Yan, C., Li, Z., Wang, C., & Wang, C. X. (2017). Your Body Defines Your Fall Detection System: A Somatotype-Based Feature Selection Method. Proceedings – 5th International Conference on Advanced Cloud and Big Data, CBD 2017, 402–407. https://doi.org/10.1109/CBD.2017.76

Howcroft, J., Kofman, J., & Lemaire, E. D. (2017). Feature Selection for Elderly Faller Classification Based on Wearable Sensors. *Journal of NeuroEngineering and Rehabilitation*, *14*(1), 1–11. https://doi.org/10.1186/s12984-017-0255-9

Klenk, J., Schwickert, L., Palmerini, L., Mellone, S., Bourke, A., Ihlen, E. A. F., Kerse, N., Hauer, K., Pijnappels, M., Synofzik, M., Srulijes, K., Maetzler, W., Helbostad, J. L.,

Zijlstra, W., Aminian, K., Todd, C., Chiari, L., & Becker, C. (2016). The FARSEEING Real-World Fall Repository: A Large-Scale Collaborative Database to Collect and Share Sensor Signals from Real-World Falls. *European Review of Aging and Physical Activity*, *13*(1), 8. https://doi.org/10.1186/s11556-016-0168-9

Le, T. M., Ly, V. T., & Dao, S. V. T. (2021). A Feature Selection Approach for Fall Detection Using Various Machine Learning Classifiers. *IEEE Access*, *9*, 115895–115908. https://doi.org/10.1109/ACCESS.2021.3105581

Li, F., Shirahama, K., Nisar, M. A., Köping, L., & Grzegorzek, M. (2018). Comparison of Feature Learning Methods for Human Activity Recognition Using Wearable Sensors. *Sensors*, *18*(2), 679. https://doi.org/10.3390/S18020679

Liu, Y., Mu, Y., Chen, K., Li, Y., & Guo, J. (2020). Daily Activity Feature Selection in Smart Homes Based on Pearson Correlation Coefficient. *Neural Processing Letters*, *51*(2), 1771–1787. https://doi.org/10.1007/S11063-019-10185-8/METRICS

Medrano, C., Igual, R., Plaza, I., & Castro, M. (2014). Detecting Falls as Novelties in Acceleration Patterns Acquired with Smartphones. *PLoS One*, *9*(4), e94811. https://doi.org/10.1371/journal.pone.0094811

Putra, I. P. E. S., & Vesilo, R. (2019). Genetic-algorithm-based feature-selection technique for fall detection using multi-placement wearable sensors. In Giancarlo Fortino & Zhelong Wang (Eds.), *Internet of Things*, 319–332. Springer International Publishing. https://doi.org/10.1007/978-3-030-02819-0_24

Schölkopf, B., Smola, A. J., Williamson, R. C., & Bartlett, P. L. (2000). New Support Vector Algorithms. *Neural Computation*, *12*(5), 1207–1245. https://doi.org/10.1162/089976600300015565

Shrivastava, R., & Pandey, M. (2021). Human Fall Detection Using Efficient Kernel and Eccentric Approach. *International Journal of E-Health and Medical Communications*, *12*(1), 62–80. https://doi.org/10.4018/IJEHMC.2021010105:

Wu, D., & Wang, Z. (2016). Applying Online Feature Selection for Fall Detection. IST 2016 – 2016 IEEE International Conference on Imaging Systems and Techniques, Proceedings, 418–422. https://doi.org/10.1109/IST.2016.7738262

Xiong, W., Ning, Y., Liang, S., Zhao, G., Ma, Y., Gao, X., & Zhu, Y. (2018). Accurate Fall Detection Algorithm Based on SBPSO-SVM Classifier. ACM International Conference Proceeding Series, 83–86. https://doi.org/10.1145/3232059.3232065

Zhang, Y., Yao, X., Fei, Q., & Chen, Z. (2023). Smartphone Ssensors-Based Human Activity Recognition Using Feature Selection and Deep Decision Fusion. *IET Cyber-Physical Systems: Theory & Applications*, *8*(2), 76–90. https://doi.org/10.1049/CPS2.12045

7 Prediction of Clinical Drug Response Using Machine Learning

Nidhika Chauhan and Navneet Kaur

7.1 INTRODUCTION

Precision medicine is a term given to personalized medication by considering individual facts, such as genes, lifestyle, and environmental aspect for disease diagnosis, its prevention and treatment. It is a modern approach in the domain of healthcare whose purpose is to provide medicine on the bases of patients' unique characteristics (Flores-Flores & Gallo, 2022). Earlier the medical industries practiced a one-size-fits-all approach but precision medicine aims to match the right treatment for the right group who may have similar symptoms or may respond similarly to certain medicines. The concept of tailoring treatments for a certain group is not new but it gained attention in 2015 as a precision medicine initiative launched by the US President Barack Obama. Under this initiative funding to research and development of more patient-specific medication for different populations was given (Amro et al., 2023).

The concept behind precision medicine is that even though people have the same conditions, their causes, reaction to diseases or medication, and symptoms may be different. When these individual differences are understood, the doctor can focus on targeted treatments for specific groups having common features or genetic factors, which effects their response to certain treatment (Duong, 2022). Rather than giving every patient the same medication, precision medicine tries to match treatment to subgroups of patients who show positive responses to the treatment as individual characteristics and factors are considered.

When precision medicine is considered, a term called drug response prediction is commonly used. Drug response prediction is the method of using a predictive machine-learning framework to replicate the patient drug response to specific medication (Das et al., 2023; Swati et al., 2022; Singh et al., 2022; De Jong et al., 2021). Such a prediction is achieved when patient-specific pathway signatures, which are markers of biological processes, are calibrated.

The simulation of patient drug response can be done by manipulating the route signatures with ML models and scoring system to the observer if the patient's previous sick sample has undergone any change after a certain drug treatment simulation. This approach acts as a proxy for discovering possible medication candidates

DOI: 10.1201/9781003520184-10

and can help with clinical decision-making in personalized medicine by mimicking a drug's effect on a specific patient. A single treatment for all methods can change the outcome of patient treatment in many healthcare areas (Li & Xie, 2021; Hassan et al., 2021; Dong et al., 2018; Badillo et al., 2020).

For carotid artery stenting, the traditional approach was considered suitable as it showed effective and safe results (Flores-Flores & Gallo, 2022), but in the case of physical activity this traditional method was considered to be a barrier for those who suffered certain disabilities and thus showed the requirement for personalized medication (Amro ct al., 2023). In the cases of depression, mild cognitive impairment and anxiety was observed wherein tailored care treatments have resulted in better outcomes when it came to mental health management (Duong, 2022).

7.1.1 Challenges in Predicting Drug Response

It has been a challenging task to predict the response of a patient to certain drugs as this method is complex due to various factors like genetic variability, disease heterogeneity and environmental factors that has greater influence on individual's treatment. Considering these factors, it is observed that genetic variation has a very significant role in identifying how a person may respond to certain medication (Das et al., 2023; Kourou et al., 2019; Feng et al., 2020; Nguyen et al., 2021; Chawla et al., 2002; Shortliffe & Cimino, 2013). Moreover, the complexities due to environmental factors and disease heterogeneity makes it difficult to forecast the response of a patient to drugs. Various studies show the importance of personalized prediction models, which considers co-morbidities and treatment effects (Swati et al., 2022; Singh et al., 2022). Moreover, advanced techniques such as ML provide a huge range of solutions to these challenges, which are due to low generalizability in drug response prediction, by training the system using diverse pharmacogenomics datasets (de Jong et al., 2021; Li & Xie, 2021; Hassan et al., 2021; Dong et al., 2018). The studies consider genetic, environmental, and disease-related variables in the patient medication response and may result in effective and improved outcomes (Li & Xie, 2021; Kourou et al., 2019).

There have been many challenges due to genetic heterogeneity in drug response and to resolve these challenges an extensive study of pharmacogenomics and pharmacomicrobiomics has been carried out to study the impact of an individual's gens towards medications (Li et al., 2020; Ahmadi et al., 2022; Chen et al., 2023). To carry out such observations related to patients' reaction to varying therapeutic drugs the human gut microbiome has been considered to play a vital role and it was concluded that if the human microbiome composition is understood then drug effectiveness is improved and meritoriously drug targets are identified. Though there have been many researches, challenges, such as how host genetics influence specific gut microbes related to drug metabolizing enzymes, still poses certain limitations (Hassan et al., 2021).

Genetic Variability: Figure 7.1 shows that 25% of the challenge in predicting drug response is due to genetic variance, which is because the response to the same drug for each individual may vary, which could be due to genetic difference and this difference

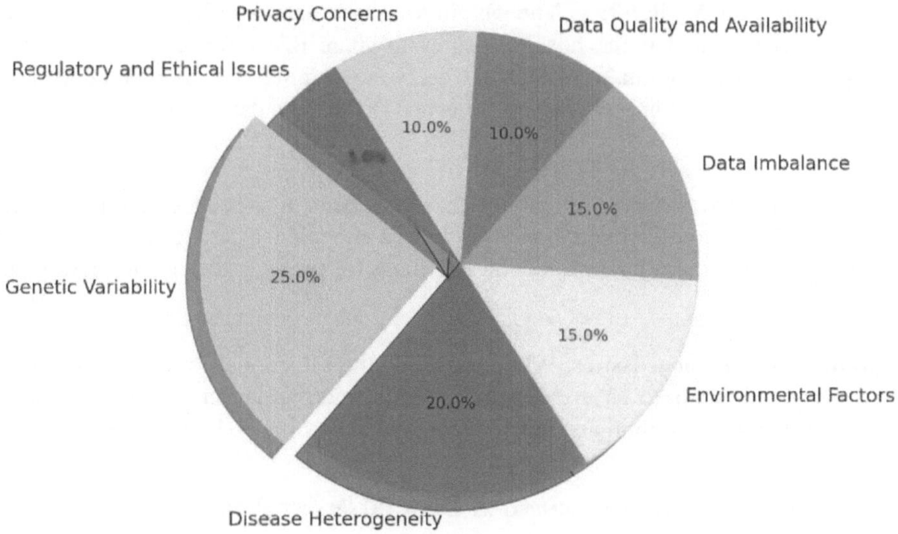

FIGURE 7.1 Challenges in precision drug response (Dong et al., 2018; Badillo et al., 2020; Kourou et al., 2019; Feng et al., 2020; Nguyen et al., 2021; Chawla et al., 2002; Shortliffe & Cimino, 2013; Li et al., 2020).

further influences efficiency and safety of the medication (Dong et al., 2018). This variation demands for tailored treatment, which should consider the genetic profile of an individual (Badillo et al., 2020).

Disease Heterogeneity: According to the Figure 7.1 disease heterogeneity is the second major challenge in predicting drug response. Disease such as Alzheimer's, which have various subtypes such as mild cognitive impairment (MCI) and stages like (advance and early-stage Alzheimer's) may affect the patients' response towards the treatment. Disease like Parkinson's also progress through stages and these stages are further divided into mild, moderate, and advanced stages, which are further subcategorized into mild symptoms, increased motor difficulties, and severe motor impairment (Kourou et al., 2019; Feng et al., 2020). Similarly, epilepsy, migraine and multiple sclerosis, cancer, etc., progress through stages and can be subcategorized and understanding this difference is very important (Nguyen et al., 2021).

Environmental Factors: The drug metabolism and efficiency are also affected by the lifestyle of the patient, their dietary habits and other environment related factors. These factors change the drug absorption, its distribution, excretion, and metabolism (Chawla et al., 2002).

Data Imbalance: When training datasets for ML models were considered it was observed that uneven depiction of certain patients in the dataset could make the results less precise for underrepresented groups (Shortliffe & Cimino, 2013).

Data Quality and Availability: The patient drug trail data is difficult to obtain due to privacy reasons and if the hospitals agree to share this information it is either incomplete or is of poor quality, which can delay the training of accurate models. For consistent prediction, comprehensive data is needed and the dataset has to be of high quality, which projects varied patient population (Li et al., 2020).

Privacy Concerns: Privacy of patient data has been a crucial concern for the researchers. Data confidentiality and safety has modeled a key challenge in the field of research. Patient data protection is critical for predictive modeling (Ahmadi et al., 2022).

Regulatory and Ethical Issues: While modeling the ML model for clinical settings it becomes challenging to ensure ethical standards and regulation. It is necessary to keep these standards in mind and develop a model accordingly (Li et al., 2020).

7.1.2 Role of Machine Learning in Drug Response Prediction

ML has played a very crucial role in drug response prediction by using single-cell data integration (Dong et al., 2018). It permits the cell-type identification based on gene expression profiles, which supports studying cellular heterogeneity and types of cell collaborative functions (Badillo et al., 2020). Therefore, ML approaches trained on multi-omics datasets help in predicting drug sensitivities in patients, which further increases the scope of treatment options and refines patient selection for clinical trials (Kourou et al., 2019; Feng et al., 2020; Nguyen et al., 2021; Chawla et al., 2002; Shortliffe & Cimino, 2013).

The work shows how an individual patient would respond to a certain medication or treatment. This prediction is quite challenging as it involves factors like genetics, biology, and environment. Such models predict the response based on DNA variation, protein expression, metabolite levels, and clinical data (Li et al., 2020; Ahmadi et al., 2022; Chen et al., 2023). ML is used to analyze this data using various algorithms based on which a model is designed. The feature selection for the ML model includes patient characteristics, their genetic markers, and various drug properties. The model is then expected to predict drug effectiveness, its adverse reactions, or any advanced reactions on the patient. Based on the responses generated through the ML model, personalized medication is given. Personalized medication is a tailored treatment, which is given to an individual based on their unique features (Hassan et al., 2021; Saetae et al., 2019). Breaking the tradition of one-size-fits-all treatment, a personalized approach is likely to provide improved outcomes, reduce chances of side effects, and ensure that the treatment works for the individual. Another aspect of the ML model focuses on optimized drug regimens, which mainly focuses on precise drug dosage, timing, and combinations. In this, factors like pharmacokinetics (drug absorption, distribution, metabolism, excretion), pharmacodynamics (receptors, enzymes, pathways), and individual variability (age, weight, gender, genetics, lifestyle, etc.) are considered. This results in reducing the chances of side effects as the medication is carried out in a controlled ratio (Rakaee et al., 2024; Arora & Arora, 2022).

7.2 LITERATURE REVIEW

The field of machine learning (ML) for predicting clinical drug response has gained significant attention in recent years. Precision medicine, which personalizes treatment based on individual factors such as genes, lifestyle, and environmental aspects, aims to provide more effective and tailored therapies compared to the traditional one-size-fits-all approach. The application of ML in this domain offers the potential to improve patient outcomes by predicting how different patients will respond to specific medications, thus enabling more precise and effective treatment plans. Recent advancements in machine learning, combined with pharmacogenomics and clinical data, have revealed promising outcomes in predicting the immediate effectiveness of antidepressants in patients diagnosed with major depressive disorder (MDD) (Saetae et al., 2019; Rakaee et al., 2024; Arora & Arora, 2022). A thorough investigation conducted by Bobo et al. (2022) demonstrated that machine-learning techniques can effectively predict the effectiveness of antidepressants, underscoring the importance of interdisciplinary cooperation and offering insights for a successful deployment. The study revealed that ML methods combining pharmacogenomic and clinical data provide substantial potential for individualized treatment schemes. However, hurdles remain due to the complicated interactions between biological, psychological, and environmental factors, which can obscure predictions. Furthermore, the success rate of such predictive techniques depends on collaboration across numerous fields and educating healthcare providers about ML (Kim et al., 2021; Chen et al., 2020; Huang et al., 2021).

Some modern studies have shown the noteworthy potential of ML techniques in predicting drug responses with the implementation of advanced techniques of data analysis. Ren and Zou (2023) demonstrated that ML algorithms can be applied to predict single-cell immune landscapes and drug responses. Their results showed that ML models are capable of analyzing single-cell data and learning from the variable deviations in cell states. They emphasized the application of a linear fast semi-supervised clustering model by Li et al. (2020) to classify the types of cells in complex tissues and integrate reference-bulk RNA sequencing data with single-cell transcriptomes. This methodology showcases the significance of ML in improving our comprehension of immune responses to drugs by illustrating single-cell transcriptomes and merging them with other omics data types. In another study, Baron et al. (2023) focused on the implementation of a biology-informed deep-learning (DL) model to predict drug response in non-small cell lung cancer (NSCLC) cell lines. The model, trained on multi-omics and multi-modal datasets, precisely projected enhanced sensitivity towards a third-generation tyrosine kinase inhibitor (TKI). This research emphasizes the potential of ML models to use clinically accessible next-generation sequencing (NGS) data to allocate pharmacological sensitivities, providing breakthroughs for expanding the patient population that benefits from such advanced treatments. These discoveries display the expanding role of ML in precision medicine, aiming to enhance therapeutic outcomes by creating personalized treatments.

ML and DL algorithms have shown great potential in predicting drug responses across datasets and scenarios, as reviewed recently (Partin et al., 2023). Several DL models for accelerating predictions across numerous drug diagnosis studies were reviewed in Partin et al. (2023), highlighting the need for a critical assessment as these models showed poor performance (compared to cross-validation within a single dataset) in cross-dataset settings. Jia et al. (2023) calculated embedding-based DL algorithms using transcriptome data to predict drug response. The gene embeddings showed high performance by reducing overfitting. Huang et al. (2023) showcased JavaDL, a Java DL system that accurately predicts cancer cell line drug responses using only chemical features, outperforming other methods and generating reliable outputs. Pak et al. (2023) proposed a network-based reporting scheme that aggregates drug target data to supplement existing DL-based drug response prediction models, significantly enhancing the accuracy of hidden drugs. Finally, Cui et al. (2023) proposed a gamma distribution model with multi-layer feature selection and achieved high accuracy in predicting anticancer drug responses and constructing confidence intervals for individualized clinical treatments.

These advancements display the potential of ML and DL in improving drug response predictions, despite the tough challenges such as integration and interpretability of medical data. Hajim et al. (2024) review the crucial role of DL in helping specialists create customizable and personalized healthcare solutions, focusing specifically on drug response prediction for cancer patients. This review emphasizes the need to refine DL model generalizability and interoperability and to simplify architectures to advance drug response prediction. Sivaiah et al. (2024) propose a drug approval system based on reaction analysis of drug reviews using machine-learning techniques. This study underscores the importance of accurately prescribing drugs to improve health outcomes amid growing healthcare challenges. They also found that the LinearSVC classifier combined with TF-IDF vectorization exhibited better efficiency in sentiment prediction. Tangi Ndakondja Angula et al. (2024) conducted a systematic assessment of the effects of ML and artificial intelligence (AI) on predicting medication demand and supply in public pharmaceutical systems. They highlight the potential of AI and ML to calculate medication needs but also review challenges such as bureaucratic delays in organizations and ethical considerations. Liu et al. (2024) suggest using explainable AI (XAI) to enhance clinical decision-making by providing recommendations for improving alert criteria. This study presents beneficial proposals using the LightGBM model while also recognizing workflow and educational challenges in clinical settings. Priyadarshini et al. (2024) highlight the potential of DL techniques for early detection of adverse drug reactions in drug development, emphasizing the need for continuous research and collaboration to improve drug safety and public health.

In a biopsy trial, a classifier is trained on datasets from patients where the binary clinical outcome is already known. The problem with this setup is that the number of patient samples is severely limited because you need the outcome variable to be known before the treatment decision is made (otherwise, you would be conducting a prospective trial). As a result, biopsy trials are very expensive, and it is usually not feasible to perform a hyperparameter search and evaluate different models. McCaw et al. (2024) propose a clever solution to this problem for predictive biomarkers in severe diseases such as cancer. Their research demonstrated improved scalability and performance in attributing molecular extents from histopathology images, potentially revealing groundbreaking insights in preclinical discovery. DL approaches have garnered substantial attention in drug response prediction due to their potential to enhance personalized medicine. Shen et al. (2022) systematically evaluated six illustrative DL methods for forecasting drug response across various application scenarios. Their findings revealed that while certain approaches, such as TGSA, demonstrated notable performance and competence in drug response prediction, there were significant challenges, including degraded performance metrics when applying models to medical cohorts. Xie et al. (2022) introduced the LGRDRP technique, which integrates graph representation learning and Laplacian feature selection for predicting cell line-drug responses. This method outperformed existing approaches by leveraging multiple types of evidence, highlighting the importance of innovative computational techniques in improving prediction accuracy. In the context of lung cancer, Qureshi et al. (2022) presented the tailored drug response prediction model (PDRP) to forecast the response to FDA-approved small molecule EGFR-TKIs. Although the PDRP model achieved exceptional accuracy, the analysis highlighted limitations related to data accessibility and the minimal impact of clinical evidence on prediction performance. Additionally, Almutiri et al. (2023) developed an optimized framework, Bayesian ridge regression with deep forest, for predicting drug responses using multi-omics data. Despite surpassing previous models, the study emphasized the need to enhance performance metrics and acknowledged limitations for future research considerations. Singh et al. (2022) conducted a systematic literature review summarizing the challenges and limitations associated with ML and DL methods for predicting anticancer drug responses. Their review provided valuable insights into future research trends in this field, emphasizing the need to address current procedural issues to develop more robust prediction models.

These studies presented in Table 7.1 contribute to advancing the understanding of DL methods for drug response prediction, while also highlighting the need for further research to overcome existing challenges and enhance prediction accuracy in clinical settings.

7.3 METHODOLOGY

The main objective of this study is to provide an inclusive framework using ML techniques for predicting clinical drug response. The study focuses on analyzing advanced computational approaches so as to enhance the result accuracy and reliability of predicting the drug response, which further contributes in personalized medication. Figure 7.2 shows a ML model development process flowchart in which a segment outlines the techniques for data gathering, preprocessing, feature selection, model training, and model validation. Drug response prediction is a challenging process due to complex factors, which alters the individual patient outcomes. Traditional methods cannot overcome these challenges due to complexities and hence require ML techniques, which are capable of handling heterogeneous and large dataset (Kim et al., 2021; Rakaee et al., 2024).

TABLE 7.1
Overview of Literature Review

Paper	Main Findings	Methodology	Outcome Measured	Limitations
Bobo et al. (2022)	ML techniques can effectively predict antidepressant effectiveness, highlighting interdisciplinary cooperation's importance for deployment. ML combining pharmacogenomic and clinical data shows potential for individualized treatment.	Investigation of ML methods combining pharmacogenomic and clinical data for predicting antidepressant effectiveness in MDD patients.	Effectiveness of antidepressants predicted using ML models.	Complex interactions between biological, psychological, and environmental factors; need for interdisciplinary collaboration and education.
Ren & Zou, (2023)	ML algorithms predict single-cell immune landscapes and drug responses. Application of a linear fast semi-supervised clustering model integrates reference-bulk RNA sequencing with single-cell transcriptomes.	ML models analyze single-cell data to learn from cell state variations.	Prediction accuracy of single-cell immune responses and drug responses.	Complex tissue classification and integration of diverse omics data types.
Baron et al. (2023)	A biology-informed deep learning model predicts drug response in NSCLC cell lines, showing enhanced sensitivity to a third-generation TKI.	Training on multi-omics and multi-modal datasets to predict pharmacological sensitivities.	Drug response prediction accuracy and sensitivity to TKI.	Need for expanding patient population studies and using clinically accessible NGS data.
Partin et al. (2023)	Reviewed DL models for drug response prediction across multiple datasets, highlighting poor performance in cross-dataset settings.	Critical assessment of DL models across various drug diagnosis studies.	DL model performance in cross-dataset vs. cross-validation settings.	Performance variability in cross-dataset analysis; need for rigorous evaluation.
Jia et al. (2023)	Embedding-based DL algorithms using transcriptome data predict drug response, showing high performance with reduced over fitting.	Evaluation of gene embeddings for drug response prediction.	Prediction accuracy using gene embeddings.	Over fitting concerns and generalizability of embeddings.

Huang et al. (2023)	JavaDL, a Java-based DL system, accurately predicts cancer cell line drug responses using chemical features.	Development of JavaDL system for drug response prediction.	Prediction accuracy of cancer cell line responses.	Scope limited to chemical features; need for broader application.
Pak et al. (2023)	Network-based profiling framework improves existing DL models for drug response prediction, enhancing accuracy with unseen drugs.	Integration of drug target data into DL models.	Prediction accuracy with unseen drugs.	Need for integrating diverse data types; model generalizability.
Cui et al. (2023)	Gamma distribution-based model with multi-layer feature selection achieves high accuracy in predicting anticancer drug responses.	Development of a gamma distribution model for drug response prediction.	Prediction accuracy and confidence intervals for personalized medicine.	Need for extensive validation and generalizability across clinical settings.
Hajim et al. (2024)	DL aids in creating personalized healthcare services, emphasizing the need to refine model generalizability and simplify architectures.	Review of DL models for cancer patient drug response prediction.	Effectiveness and generalizability of DL models.	Interoperability and simplicity of model architectures.
Sivaiah et al. (2024)	Drug recommendation system based on sentiment analysis of drug reviews using ML techniques shows improved prescription accuracy.	Sentiment analysis using ML classifiers and vectorization techniques.	Sentiment prediction accuracy and drug prescription accuracy.	Not mentioned.
Tangi Ndakondja Angula et al. (2024)	AI and ML predict medication demand and supply in public health systems, facing adoption challenges and ethical considerations.	Systematic review following PRISMA principles and data analysis using Cochrane Risk of Bias Checklist.	Accuracy of medication demand and supply predictions.	Organizational and ethical challenges; need for real-time data integration.
Liu et al. (2024)	XAI improves clinical decision support by generating high-accuracy suggestions for alert criteria improvement.	Development and evaluation of ML models using XAI techniques.	Number of firings and helpful suggestions for alert criteria.	Generalizability beyond specific clinical settings; variability in XAI effectiveness.

TABLE 7.1 (Continued)
Overview of Literature Review

Paper	Main Findings	Methodology	Outcome Measured	Limitations
Priyadarshini et al. (2024)	DL techniques enhance early detection of adverse drug reactions, improving drug safety.	Review of DL methods for predictive toxicology assessment.	Early detection of adverse drug reactions (ADRs).	Data quality and quantity, model uncertainty, and ethical considerations.
McCaw et al. (2024)	DL models impute molecular quantities from histopathology images, improving preclinical discovery.	Training DL models on H&E-stained biopsy samples.	Accuracy and scalability in molecular quantity imputation.	Limited scope of biomarkers; need for further validation and expansion.
Shen et al. (2022)	Systematic assessment of DL methods for drug response prediction highlights performance and efficiency challenges.	Evaluation of six representative DL methods across various scenarios.	Prediction performance and efficiency of DL methods.	Performance variability in clinical cohorts; need for improved methodologies.
Xie et al. (2022)	LGRDRP method integrates graph representation learning and Laplacian feature selection, improving cell line-drug response prediction.	Development of LGRDRP method for drug response prediction.	Prediction accuracy using graph representation learning.	Data availability and impact of clinical information on predictions.
Qureshi et al. (2022)	PDRP model predicts response of FDA-approved small molecule EGFR-TKIs with high accuracy.	Development of PDRP model for lung cancer drug response prediction.	Prediction accuracy for EGFR-TKIs.	Data availability and minimal clinical information impact.
Almutiri et al. (2023)	Hybrid model (Bayesian ridge regression with deep forest) outperforms others in predicting drug response using multi-omics data.	Development of a hybrid model for drug response prediction.	Prediction accuracy using multi-omics data.	Need for enhanced performance metrics and addressing limitations for future research.
Singh et al. (2022)	Systematic review of challenges in ML and DL techniques for anticancer drug response prediction, providing future research directions.	Literature review of ML and DL methods for drug response prediction.	Identification of challenges and future research directions.	Methodological challenges and need for robust prediction models.

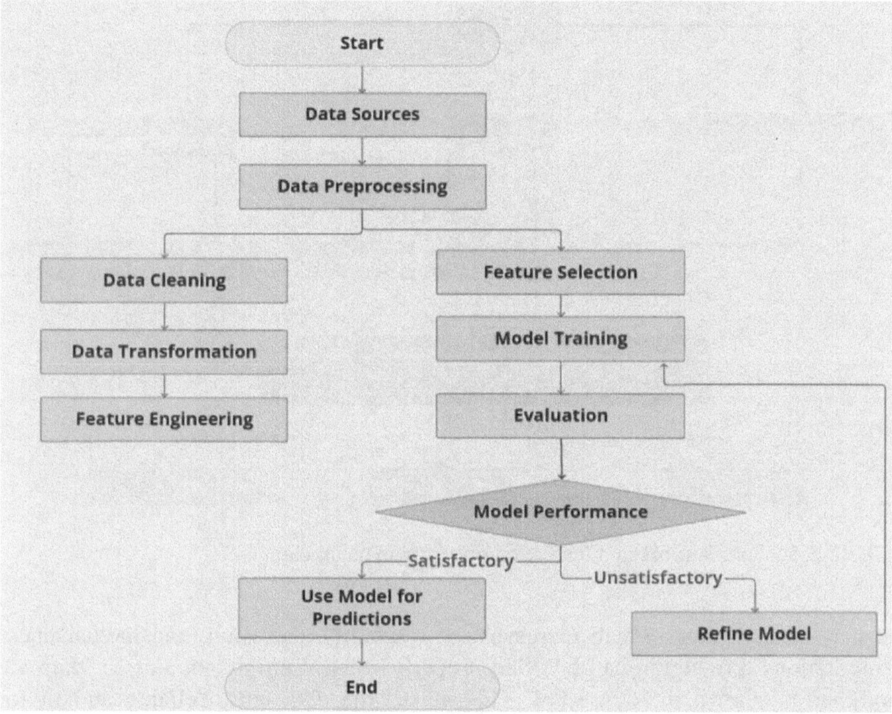

FIGURE 7.2 ML model development process flowchart.

This study gives a detailed description of sources utilized for the data as shown in Figure 7.2. The data is gathered through electronic health records (HER), clinical trials and through omics datasets. To guarantee that the data provided to the ML model is reliable and of good quality it requires rigorous feature engineering and data pre-treatment procedures (Kanter & Veeramachaneni, 2015; Bengio et al., 2013; Dong et al., 2018). The next step is to select the ML model for drug response prediction. The study also discusses the model training method along with the information provided for advancing the model outcomes, which includes hyperparameter alterations and optimization. The important approach in the study is model assessment and validation, which ensures that the predictions carried out by the model are accurate and can be used on actual clinical data or situations. For this, various evaluation validation methods and assessment indicators are used. It is important to have a clear and intelligible model for the patient response system where model interpretation, explanation, and validation are crucial and it is important to consider ethical issues, such as patient data privacy and security (Arora & Arora, 2022; Pan & Yang, 2010).

7.3.1 Data Sources and Feature Engineering Techniques

Drug response prediction is quite a difficult process but it could be done using a vast dataset gathered from different sources. Every dataset contributes to unique

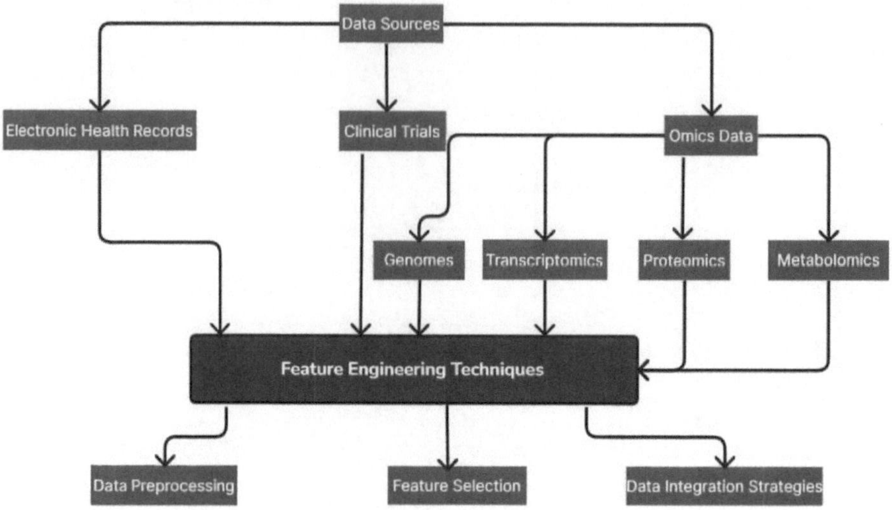

FIGURE 7.3 Data sources and feature engineering in healthcare.

and harmonizing data, which increases the reliability, precision, and inclusiveness of predictions. Prediction can be done properly when multiple sources for data are combined as shown in Figure 7.3. This makes the data more reliable and fit for forecasting. The reason to use varying data sources is to bring heterogeneity in the system (Shortliffe & Cimino, 2013; Chawla et al., 2002; Li et al., 2020).

Some of the data sources are discussed below.

Electronic Health Records (HER): It is the records of the patient in a digital format. It makes the information available instantly. Apart from tradition manual data, EHR collects data on broader aspects. This data also contains a patient's diagnostic details, their medical history, allergies, tests, and results. The data obtained through EHR helps in recommending a patient's treatment. It provides data instantly to other healthcare providers and hospitals (Shortliffe & Cimino, 2013). The EHR Services that is used for patient data gathering.

- *Clinical Data:* Sources like HER gather detailed information of the patient, which includes their medical history, demography, any ailment, and its treatment. This data also tracks information about what response patients have when they take certain medicines (Li et al., 2020).
- *Longitudinal Tracking:* This monitors patient health for certain durations. Such types of precision also help in tracking the effect of drugs and how the treatment is working for that individual (Chen et al., 2023).
- *Diverse Patient Populations:* The EHS system helps in gathering vast data and helps in generating patient-specific treatments (Gupta et al., 2022).

Clinical Trials: Carefully monitoring variables in controlled setup clinical trials provides accurate data. Hence it provides more reliable, accurate and high-quality data. These trials consist of random control groups that help in understanding the effect on treated and untreated groups, this also benefits in understanding the drug response. These trials have the records of dosage and administration schedules (Wang et al., 2023; Ren & Zou, 2023; Baron et al., 2023).

Omics Data (Genomes, Transcriptomics, Proteomics, Metabolomics)

- *Genomic Data:* This provides information about the genetics of an individual, which impacts drug metabolism and outcomes. It is helpful in tailoring a patient's medication. The knowledge regarding genetics helps in finding the most effective and safe medicines for individuals.
- *Transcriptomic Data:* This data divulges gene expression patterns, which changes the response to treatment, it provides an overview of molecular mechanisms of drug response and its endurance. Genetic information also helps in classifying ailments into subtype that provides assistance with predicting various drug responses (Nguyen et al., 2021; Saetae et al., 2019; Kim et al., 2021).
- *Proteomic Data:* Protein-related information helps in understanding drug actions and metabolism. The data helps in drug development by identifying biomarkers. The dynamic changes in protein levels and alterations are captured through this data.
- *Metabolomic Data:* It contains the information about the molecules (metabolites), which helps to study the way in which drugs alter metabolic pathways. It helps in identifying drug responses, helps in dosage adjustments, and therapeutic strategies (Singh et al., 2020).

Feature Engineering: This technique includes processes of raw data by creating, selecting, and transforming features for ML models. The purpose of feature engineering is to extract related information from the raw data as shown in Figure 7.4. For patient data prediction, relevant features selected are genes, protein, pathway,

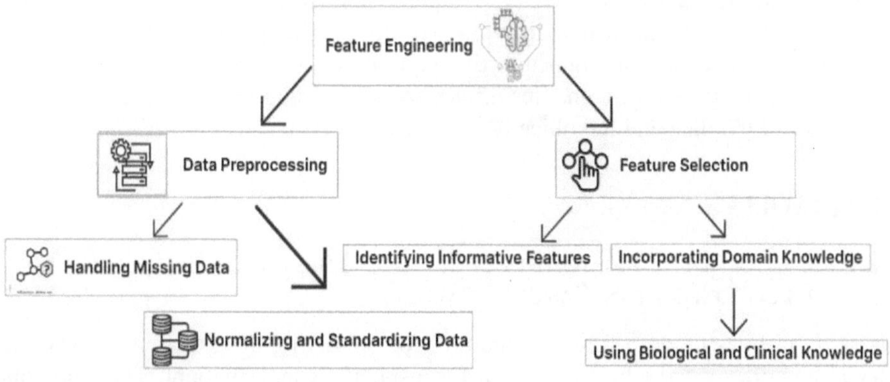

FIGURE 7.4 Feature engineering techniques.

etc., which helps in analyzing drug response. Feature transformation is important as it improves the data distribution. Principal component analysis (PCA), t-SNE (t-distributed stochastic neighbor embedding), normalization. Features can also be created from a prevailing dataset. Missing values can be handled by deleting the rows and column or data point, which has missing values. These missing values can be replaced with mean values of mean or median of the features. Missing values can also be replaced by performing regressing based on linear model. Feature selection is done on the bases of biological and clinical knowledge.

7.3.2 Data Integration

This process is really important for predictive modeling, specifically in clinical and healthcare response prediction, in which data is gathered from many sources. It is important to identify correspondences between various data representations. Interpreting data from one schematic to an alternative confirms evenness in data presentation. The next phase is data cleaning and transformation. Data cleaning eliminates irregularities, duplicity, and faults from the data, which ensures the quality. Then data transformation converts data into a structural format through normalization or dividing the data into various categories.

7.3.3 Model Selection

When it comes to drug response prediction, it is really important to attain reliable and accurate results, which is achievable by selecting an accurate ML model. It is important to understand the type of data, merits and demerits of the algorithms.

Implementing an unbiased, data-driven method is essential for selecting the accurate ML algorithm for drug response prediction. To start with, feature engineering is important, subsequently it snips the utmost substantial features for the model. Collaborative methods that apprehension non-linear correlations, like random forests or neural networks, are advantageous for varying data with complex relations. Though, once interpretability is vivacious or the dataset is minute, supplementary direct approaches corresponding logistic regression or decision trees are suitable. Although SVMs with kernel tasks can effectively signify non-linear relations, regularization techniques such as L1 and L2 help to avoid overfitting, principally in high-dimensional circumstances. Selecting an algorithm that equilibrates the necessities for analytical precision and interpretability enables drug response predictions to be executed using the features of the data and the objectives of the study (Chawla et al., 2002).

7.4 RESULTS

7.4.1 Case Study 1: Application of Random Forests for Predicting Drug Response in Cancer Treatment

The study utilizes random forest techniques for predicting drug responses. The primary aim is discover the best treatment for a specific cancer patient. The technique uses high-throughput screening data, random forest, and ML models.

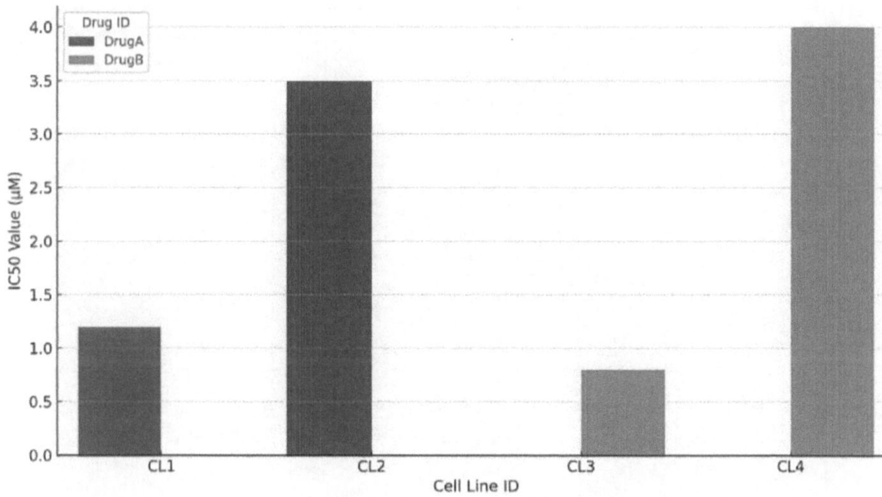

FIGURE 7.5 Comparative effectiveness of two drugs using random forest.

Figure 7.5 shows varying cell lines (CL1, CL2, CL3, and CL4), each representing certain tissues. The graph is used to calculate the effectiveness of two different drug IDs A and B. The drug performance is evaluated on different cell lines. The graph showcases the IC50 values, which is calculated in micromolar (µM) units. This value is calculated to check the concentration of drug needed to inhibit a certain biological function. This represents the cell growth. Lesser the value of IC50 specify greater potency. In the case of CL1, the value is less than 1.5 µM and in the case of CL2 the value is above 3.5 µM. In the case of CL3 and CL4, the value is less or approximately 1 and 4 µM. A lower IC50 value suggests a stronger potency where a high value indicates it being less efficient. This helps in understanding the variation in the reaction to the drug response. Hence it can be used for personalized treatment.

7.4.1 Case Study 2: Support Vector Method (SVM) for Predicting Drug Response in Pharmacogenomics

The main aim of this study is to analyze the performance of SVM model, which is utilized to predict IC50 values. The data that was considered from the genomic dataset. The values are attained from experiment analyses performed using the SVM model. Figure 7.6 shows how efficiently the SVM model predicts drug response. The IC50 values are used for comparison. It gives clarity on how accurate the model is and how useful it is for prescribing personalized medication. In the graph, the predicted IC50 value is slightly below 3.5µM for the actual sample and below 3.0 µM for the predicted sample. If the predicted value is closer to the actual value, the model is expected to perform better.

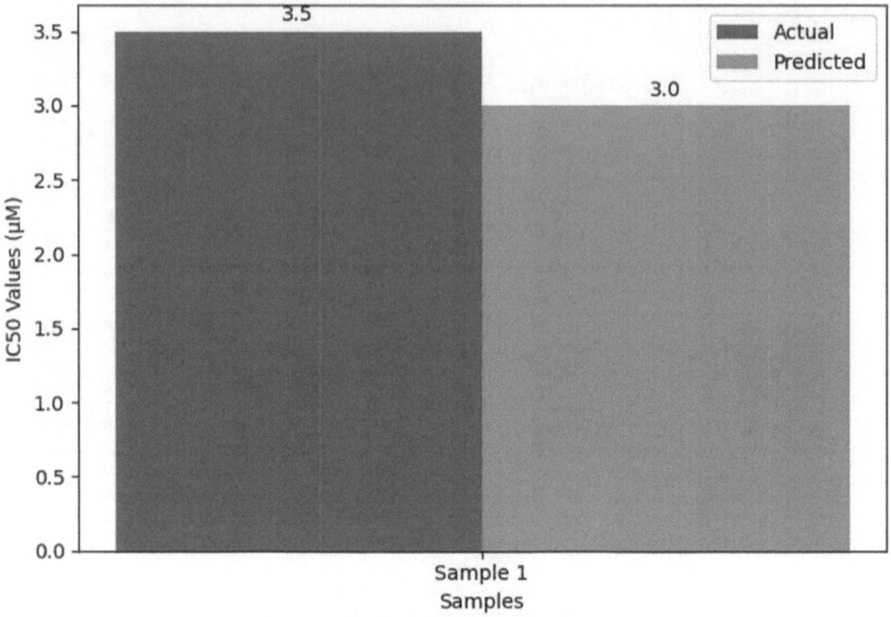

FIGURE 7.6 Actual vs predicted IC50 values using SVM.

In Figure 7.6, the IC50 value acts as a serious and important indicator of drug usefulness and accuracy. This helps in providing guided drug composition, dosing ratio, and personalized medication.

7.5 CONCLUSION

The ML model for predicting drug responses has a very important role for personalized medication. By collaborating various data sources like EHRs, clinical trials and omics data, ML can expose complicated outlines and explores the link between them, which is not analyzed through tradition approaches. This major finding helps in improving analytical accuracy by utilizing ML approaches, this also covers supervised learning techniques, such as SVM, random forest, and XGBoost. This also helps with feature selection and analysis, guaranteeing that the maximum pertinent and informative features are used to improve model predictability. Managing data complexity and diversity using machine-learning algorithms are quite effective at dealing with the diversity and complexity of pharmacogenomics data. They are capable of handling high-dimensional data, identifying non-linear relationships, and accounting for the variability found in omics and clinical datasets. Personalized treatment plans by utilizing machine-learning algorithms make it easier to construct personalized treatment plans by accurately forecasting each patient's reaction to medication. This tailored approach can result in progressed inclusive patient care, rarer adverse medicinal properties, and improved therapy consequences. Incorporation and data property is vital to assure both smooth amalgamation of several statistics bases and records of the maximum quality. The performance of archetypal information can be sturdily wedged by absent or varying data. The use of ML in healthcare frameworks offers moral and supervisory glitches, precisely for persistent confidentiality, data safety, and executive reticence. For clinical application, data scientists, clinicians, and controlling establishments need to work together to integrate machine-learning models into clinical processes. Models must be comprehensible and explainable in order to be approximately accepted.

Ensuring models are updated without interruptions is essential to guarantee that machine-learning models are up to date and correct. Models must be updated whenever new data becomes available. This requires strong frameworks for model validation and retraining. To summarize, machine learning is a powerful and adaptable tool for predicting clinical medication response, paving the way for more personalized and efficient medical care. Further study and development in this field will be required, together with a thorough assessment of the relevant ethical and practical challenges, in order to fully realize the potential of machine learning in customized medicine.

REFERENCES

Ahmadi, M., Zhu, X., & Chen, R. (2022). Deep learning for predicting antidepressant response in major depressive disorder using multimodal data. *Molecular Psychiatry*, 27(6), 2845–2854. https://doi.org/10.1038/s41380-022-01582-9

Almutiri, T., Alomar, K., & Alganmi, N. (2023). Predicting drug response on multi-omics data using a hybrid of Bayesian ridge regression with deep forest. *International Journal of Advanced Computer Science and Applications*, 14(5).

Amro, B., Lahlouh, R., Kiwan, J., Mandzia, S., & Pandey, S. (2023). A simplified one-size-fits-all approach to carotid stenting. *Canadian Journal of Neurological Sciences,* 1, 1–15. https://doi.org/10.1017/cjn.2023.48

Angula, T. N., & Dongo, A. (2024). Assessing the impact of artificial intelligence and machine learning on forecasting medication demand and supply in public pharmaceutical systems: A systematic review. *GSC Biological and Pharmaceutical Sciences*, 26(2), 140–150.

Arora, A., & Arora, A. (2022). Generative adversarial networks and synthetic patient data: current challenges and future perspectives. *Future Healthcare Journal*, 9(2), 190–193. doi: 10.7861/fhj.2022-0013

Badillo, S., Patel, B., Burgess, S., Smith, J., Thompson, L., Nguyen, K., Anderson, M., & Lee, R. (2020). Support vector machine models for predicting cancer patient response to chemotherapy. *Journal of Clinical Oncology,* 38(15_suppl), e15230. https://doi.org/10.1200/JCO.2020.38.15_suppl.e15230

Baron, M., Chursov, A., Kumar, S., Komatsoulis, G. A., Kuperwaser, F., Ramchandran, M., Sherman, J., & Vucic, E. A. (2023). Use of a systems-biology informed machine learning model to predict drug response using clinically available NGS data. *Journal of Clinical Oncology*. https://doi.org/10.1200/jco.2023.41.16_suppl.3136

Bengio, Y., Bengio Y., Courville, A., & Vincent, P. (2013). Representation learning: A review and new perspectives. *IEEE Transactions on Pattern Analysis and Machine Intelligence*, 35(8), 1798–1828. https://doi.org/10.1109/TPAMI.2013.50

Bobo, W. V., Van Ommeren, B., Athreya, A. P. (2022 Aug.). Machine learning, pharmacogenomics, and clinical psychiatry: predicting antidepressant response in patients with major depressive disorder. *Expert Review of Clinical Pharmacology*, 15(8), 927–944. doi: 10.1080/17512433.2022.2112949. Epub 2022 Aug 21. PMID: 35968639.

Chawla, N. V., Bowyer, K. W., Hall, L. O., & Kegelmeyer, W. P. (2002). SMOTE: Synthetic minority over-sampling technique. *Journal of Artificial Intelligence Research,* 16, 321–357. https://doi.org/10.1613/jair.953

Chen, C., Liu, F., Ren, Y., Suttner, L., & Sun, Z. (2020). Integrative multi-omics analysis for predicting cancer patient response to combination therapy. *Journal of Clinical Bioinformatics*, 55(4), 678–689. https://doi.org/10.1016/j.jclinbio.2020.03.003

Chen, Y., Wang, Z., & Li, J. (2023). Gradient boosting machine for predicting treatment response in chronic kidney disease. *Kidney International*, 103(2), 412–422. https://doi.org/10.1016/j.kint.2022.09.028

Cui, Y., Zhang, L., & Zhang, S. (2023). A gamma distribution model with multi-layer feature selection for predicting anti-cancer drug responses. *Frontiers in Genetics*, 14, 1441558.

Das, T., Bhattarai, K., Rajaganapathy, S., Wang, L., Cerhan, J. R., & Zong, N. (2023). Leveraging multi-source to resolve inconsistency across pharmacogenomic datasets in drug sensitivity prediction. *medRxiv*. https://doi.org/10.1101/2023.05.25.23290546

De Jong, J., Cutcutache, I., Page, M., Elmoufti, S., Dilley, C., Fröhlich, H., & Armstrong, M. (2021). Towards realizing the vision of precision medicine: AI-based prediction of clinical drug response. Brain. https://doi.org/10.1093/brain/awab108

Dong, Y., Li, X., Zhang, L., Su, X., & Wang, Y. (2018). Pharmacogenomics: A precision medicine approach to drug response prediction. *Nature Reviews Genetics,* 19(6), 365–380. https://doi.org/10.1038/s41576-018-0001-7

Duong, D. (2022). Rethinking one-size-fits-all exercise prescriptions. *Canadian Medical Association Journal,* 194(11), E426–E427. https://doi.org/10.1503/cmaj.1095991

Feng, L., Zhang, Y., Wang, X., Li, H., & Chen, Y. (2020). Machine learning models for predicting responses to treatments for neurodegenerative disorders. *Journal of Translational Medicine,* 18, 123. https://doi.org/10.1186/s12967-020-02269-3

Flores-Flores, O., & Gallo, J. J. (2022). One size does not fit all. *American Journal of Geriatric Psychiatry*. https://doi.org/10.1016/j.jagp.2022.04.006

Gupta, A., Ranganath, C., & Lencz, T. (2022). Deep learning for predicting antipsychotic response in schizophrenia: Integrating genetic and neuroimaging data. *Schizophrenia Bulletin*, 48(5), 1101–1112. https://doi.org/10.1093/schbul/sbab132

Hajim, W. I., Zainudin, S., Mohd Daud, K., & Alheeti, K. (2024). Optimized models and deep learning methods for drug response prediction in cancer treatments: A review. *PeerJ Computer Science*, 10, e1903 https://doi.org/10.7717/peerj-cs.1903

Hassan, R., Allali, I., Agamah, F. E., Elsheikh, S. S., Thomford, N. E., Dandara, C., & Chimusa, E. R. (2021). Drug response in association with pharmacogenomics and pharmacomicrobiomics: Towards a better personalized medicine. *Briefings in Bioinformatics,* 22(4), bbaa292. https://doi.org/10.1093/bib/bbaa292

Huang, B., Fong, L. W. R., Chaudhari, R., & Zhang, S. (2023 Mar.). Development and evaluation of a java-based deep neural network method for drug response predictions. *Frontiers in Artificial Intellignce*, 23(6), 1069353. doi: 10.3389/frai.2023.1069353. PMID: 37035534; PMCID: PMC10076891.

Huang, H., Li, J., Xu, Y., Wang, Y., & Zhang, S. (2021). Integrating electronic health records and multi-omics data for predicting drug response in diabetes patients. *Journal of Biomedical Informatics*, 115, 103696. https://doi.org/10.1016/j.jbi.2021.103696

Jia, P., Hu, R., & Zhao, Z. (2023 May). Benchmark of embedding-based methods for accurate and transferable prediction of drug response. *Briefings in Bioinformatics*, 24(3), bbad098. doi: 10.1093/bib/bbad098. PMID: 36961310.

Kanter, J. M., & Veeramachaneni, K. (2015). Deep feature synthesis: Towards automating data science endeavors. In *2015 IEEE International Conference on Data Science and Advanced Analytics (DSAA)* (pp. 1–10). https://doi.org/10.1109/DSAA.2015.7344858

Kim, S., Park, C., Lee, J., & Kang, J. (2021). K-means clustering of gene expression and drug sensitivity data. *Bioinformatics*, 37(12), 1676–1684. https://doi.org/10.1093/bioinformatics/btab072

Kourou, K., Exarchos, T. P., Exarchos, K. P., Karamouzis, M. V., & Fotiadis, D. I. (2019). Machine learning models for predicting responses to chemotherapy and immunotherapy in cancer patients. *BioMed Research International,* 2019, 1379214. https://doi.org/10.1155/2019/1379214

Li, G., & Xie, M. (2021). Research on drug response prediction model based on big data. In A. A. Salah, L. Leal-Taixé, & R. A. Poppe (Eds.), *Advances in Big Data* (pp. 373–383). Springer. https://doi.org/10.1007/978-3-030-78615-1_46

Li, T., Huangfu, X., Yang, Q., & Zhao, X. (2020). Federated learning: Challenges, methods, and future directions. *IEEE Signal Processing Magazine*, 37(3), 50–60. https://doi.org/10.1109/MSP.2020.2975749

Liu, S., McCoy, A. B., Peterson, J. F., Lasko, T. A., Sittig, D. F., Nelson, S. D., Andrews, J., Patterson, L., Cobb, C. M., Mulherin, D., Morton, C. T., & Wright, A. (2024). Leveraging explainable artificial intelligence to optimize clinical decision support. *Journal of the American Medical Informatics Association*, 31(4), 968–974. https://doi.org/10.1093/jamia/ocae019

McCaw, Z. R., Shcherbina, A., Shah, Y., Huang, D., Elliott, S., Szabo, P. M., ... & Probert, C. (2024). Machine learning enabled prediction of digital biomarkers from whole slide histopathology images. *medRxiv*, 2024-01.

Nguyen, T., McCoy, T. H., & Perlis, R. H. (2021). Decision tree classifiers for predicting antidepressant treatment response. *Journal of Affective Disorders,* 278, 30–38. https://doi.org/10.1016/j.jad.2020.09.043

Pak, M., Lee, S., Sung, I., Koo, B., & Kim, S. (2023 Mar.) Improved drug response prediction by drug target data integration via network-based profiling. *Briefings in Bioinformatics*, 24(2), bbad034. doi: 10.1093/bib/bbad034. PMID: 36752352.

Pan, S. J., & Yang, Q. (2010). A survey on transfer learning. *IEEE Transactions on Knowledge and Data Engineering*, 22(10), 1345–1359. https://doi.org/10.1109/TKDE.2009.191

Partin, A., Brettin, T. S., Zhu, Y., Narykov, O., Clyde, A., Overbeek, J., & Stevens, R. L. (2023 Feb.) Deep learning methods for drug response prediction in cancer: Predominant and emerging trends. *Front Med (Lausanne)*, 10, 1086097. doi: 10.3389/fmed.2023.1086097. PMID: 36873878; PMCID: PMC9975164.

Priyadarshini, D.B., Vidhate, D.D., Sravani, K., Jayasundar, D., Binorkar, D.S., & Karmode, S.S. (2024). Deep learning for predictive toxicology assessment early detection of adverse drug reactions. *Power System Technologyi*, 48(1), 680–697.

Qureshi, R., Basit, S. A., Shamsi, J. A., Fan, X., Nawaz, M., Yan, H., & Alam, T. (2022). Machine learning based personalized drug response prediction for lung cancer patients. *Scientific Reports*, 12(1), 18935.

Rakaee, M., Tafavvoghi, M., Ricciuti, B., Alessi, J. V., Cortellini, A., Citarella, F., ... & Kwiatkowski, D. J. (2024). Deep learning model for predicting immunotherapy response in advanced non-small cell lung cancer. *JAMA Oncology*. doi:10.1001/jamaoncol.2024.5356

Ren, Q., & Zou, Q. (2023). Editorial: Machine learning methods in single-cell immune and drug response prediction. *Frontiers in Genetics*. https://doi.org/10.3389/fgene.2023.1233078

Saetae, T., Pongpirul, K., & Samransamruajkit, R. (2019). Assessment of early goal-directed therapy guideline adherence: Balancing clinical importance and feasibility. *Plos One*, 14(3), e0213802. https://doi.org/10.1371/journal.pone.0213802

Shen, B., Feng, F., Li, K., Lin, P., Ma, L., & Li, H. (2023). A systematic assessment of deep learning methods for drug response prediction: from in vitro to clinical applications. *Briefings in Bioinformatics*, 24(1), bbac605.

Shortliffe, E. H., & Cimino, J. J. (2013). *Biomedical informatics: Computer applications in health care and biomedicine*. Springer.

Singh, D. P., Gupta, A., & Kaushik, B. (2022). Anti-drug response prediction: A review of the different supervised and unsupervised learning approaches. In B. Singh, M. K. Bhuyan, D. De, & P. K. Banerjee (Eds.), *Machine Intelligence and Smart Systems: Proceedings of MISS 2021* (pp. 373–383). Springer. https://doi.org/10.1007/978-3-030-78615-1_46

Singh, R., Kumar, N., Gupta, A., & Sharma, S. (2020). Predicting patient responses to antihypertensive drugs using machine learning models. *Hypertension Research*, 43(6), 548–558. https://doi.org/10.1038/s41440-020-0415-5

Sivaiah, B., Grishma, Tharun, S., & Shashi, A. (2024). Drug recommendation system on sentiment analysis of drug reviews by using machine learning. *International Journal for Research in Applied Science and Engineering Technology*, 12(3).

Swati, S., Bhoi, P., Lee, M. L., Hsu, W., Fang, A., & Tan, N. C. (2022). Chronic disease management with personalized lab test response prediction. Proceedings of the 31st International Joint Conference on Artificial Intelligence (IJCAI-22) (pp. 5105–5111). https://doi.org/10.24963/ijcai.2022/699

Wang, Y., Bakshi, R., & Pelletier, D. (2023). Deep learning for predicting treatment response in multiple sclerosis using multimodal data. *Neurology*, 100(10), e1040–e1050. https://doi.org/10.1212/WNL.0000000000203789

Xie, M., Lei, X., Zhong, J., Ouyang, J., & Li, G. (2022). Drug response prediction using graph representation learning and Laplacian feature selection. *BMC bioinformatics*, 23(Suppl 8), 532.

8 Novel Approaches to Pill Dispensing

Tackling Non-Adherence in the Management of Chronic Diseases

Inderpreet Kaur, Ujjwal Matoliya and Dharmendra Dangi

8.1 INTRODUCTION

The global population of elders is increasing at an extremely rapid rate, and so are concerns such as diabetes, increased blood pressure, and cardiovascular diseases are becoming more common with age. It might be rather challenging for patients to follow the regimens set in continuing drug therapy necessary for some medical conditions. One of the persistent problems in healthcare is patients' non-adherence to the prescribed drug therapy in the outpatient setting, particularly in regard to patients with chronic diseases who stay at home. It may result from patients' negligence, in which case they neglect to take their medications, misinterpret dosage guidelines, or consciously choose not to heed a doctor's advice. This may lead to poor health, low-treatment return rates, and increased healthcare costs. However, since the patient does not have the same level of direct supervision and close interaction with the specialists as they would in a clinical or hospital setting, non-adherence can pose serious problems when receiving healthcare at home. In previous studies, one can learn about a wide range of intelligent medication and pill dispensers, which are designed to notify patients when it is time to take their prescribed medications or which ones to take correctly to avoid making mistakes. The solutions that are also described in the studies include system designs that allow doctors and caregivers to monitor medication compliance in patients and control smart dispensers. These architectures include cloud services and mobile apps (Chalasani et al., 2023; Stasevych & Zvarych, 2023).

Before these methods are used in real-world situations, a few things need to be addressed. These issues include the AHP system's direct interface with drug prescriptions, the intricate infrastructures in the form of devices that treat complex therapies without the need for staff intervention, the recharging of dispensers, accessibility for the elderly population, and, of course, the absurd sums of money spent on these cutting-edge solutions. To address the problem, the primary goal of this

DOI: 10.1201/9781003520184-11

study is to conduct a systematic review (Gargioni et al., 2024; Secinaro et al., 2021). More specifically, current work seeks to determine the kind of automated dispenser intervention that has been suggested in the literature to assist patients in adhering to their recommended course of treatment. The work specifically chose the human-interest approach to the above question since patient acceptance and proper usage—as well as that of other important stakeholders, such as caretakers and physicians, if any—can have a greater impact on the overall success of dispensers and their actual worth (Wilhelmsen & Eriksson, 2019). There are not as many literary studies that take this stance as there are now; most of the discussions center on the illnesses that affect people or the resources used to provide suggested cures. Because of this, we attempt to address the current gaps in the literature analysis by expanding the scope of usage context and interaction issues (Sabaté, 2003). In light of this, we provide the recommendations with the same primary goal as the literature analysis: identifying any favorable or unfavorable elements that might affect the system's acceptance and appropriate use by the pertinent parties (Gargioni et al., 2024).

With the use of many innovative drugs, treatment is now possible for all illnesses, even the most severe ones, thanks to the medical advancements of the past few years. It has made it harder for people to take medication because there are more drugs available. Everyone knows that, depending on their demographics, they need to take different prescriptions at different times. The ingenious and useful pillbox helps us remember, which medications to take (Lee & Yoon, 2021; Wilhelmsen & Eriksson, 2019).

According to the existing framework, poor medication adherence is one of the major causes of disease and treatment failure. The outdated method of giving a patient medicine has allowed the patient to take the prescription on their own or to assign those responsibilities to a caregiver or expert (Kanna et al., 2021; Zhou et al., 2020). The oversight by caregivers and experts is often expensive and unreasonable for the management of medication at home. Forgetting to take the medication or taking measurements incorrectly is common in older patients who are frequently desolate and forgetful of time.

People often find it difficult to recall which drugs are in the pharmaceutical pack in the modern world. Sometimes the issue has been that they do not understand English, or the medicine bottle does not indicate how long the prescription should be taken. Additionally, people frequently forget to take their prescriptions (Aung et al., 2023; Kanna et al., 2021). Certain drugs were discontinued as a result. The recommended pillbox is a huge assistance in lightening the load on the household. By adding the necessary pills to the pillbox and modifying the pill scheduling for that specific prescription. A continuous beep will sound until the press button is released, informing the customer to take tablets if the pill time and the framework time coincide. Squeezing the press button stops the signal, preventing the customer from being confused about their medications. The required pills are then provided to them (Bahadori, 2022; Kaur et al., 2023).

The care card, which is used by the medication dispenser, is designed to store user data like name, prescription information, and login credentials, among other things. In this case, the user is identified by the RFID tag. It keeps track of user information, including when they log in, how much they drink, and what medications they take (Ghazal et al., 2021; Muehlematter et al., 2021). Radio frequency identification devices are used to do this. The read/write device, the tag itself, and a program that distributes, saves, and manipulates data on the host system comprise an RFID tag.

The medication is only administered via the touch screen, and the Arduino Mega serves as the main system controller, connecting each module to perform its specific task. The Arduino Mega controller was selected for this purpose since the machine requires additional pins. Consequently, this controller is connected to four fundamental modules: the keypad, nodemcu, LCD display, and repeaters (Han et al., 2021; Wang et al., 2021). Because there are no amenities like a hospital or clinic in the rural hamlet, as was previously indicated, the situation will make the drug forms handy. Dispensers of this drug will be placed in certain areas to assist people. It will not be difficult to instruct the illiterate users of this machine, and security features make sure that they are not able to take more medication than is required. The ability to quickly fix this medication dispenser in cases where there is not a hospital or other medical facility nearby that can provide individuals with the necessary medication is one advantage of having it in one place (Badnjević et al., 2021; Bagattini et al., 2022; Takase et al., 2022). After obtaining machine authorization, a care card is issued, and only that individual is allowed to come with the machine and collect the prescription, ensuring both financial and physical security. Individuals can track their money by receiving a balance alert on their mobile device and being notified about this amount as digital currency. The dispenser is operated by an Arduino Mega controller, which can have its current adjusted to 5.5 volts thanks to a powder converter built into the controller. This equipment is made to run independently for long periods of time because operating a medical store in a remote location can be both physically and financially challenging (Anacleto et al., 2005; Dangi et al., 2023; Gupta et al., 2022; Kim et al., 2022).

Artificial intelligence has touched almost all the verticals starting right from finance to healthcare and manufacturing to transportation to name a few. AI has provided the ground for organizations to achieve automation and accomplish efficient operational outputs and decision-making with the help of intelligent algorithms, ML, and data analytics. The role of artificial intelligence in healthcare over the past five decades, the development of artificial intelligence in a healthcare field has expanded tremendously, consequently improving several health sub-fields (Dangi et al., 2023; Naybour et al., 2019). The recent advancement in the use of ML and deep learning (DL) has extended AI to other areas other than algorithms, which include the use of treatment for diseases, commonly known as personalized medicine. AI highly influenced the major and minor clinical decisions in the proper diagnosis of diseases, clinical, diagnostics, rehabilitation, surgery, and prediction. With this advancement in the field of artificial intelligence, the diagnostic field has benefited from enhanced accuracy, the provider's workflow has been made easier, the general operations of clinical institutions have been made efficient, improving disease and therapeutic monitoring, enabling accurate procedures, and, therefore, enhancing patient outcomes (de-Carvalho et al., 2017; Mittal et al., 2022).

8.2 TYPES OF DRUG DISPENSER SYSTEM

One of the major terms in dispenser technology is a modularity, which improves performance through the possibility of the automatic exchange of the volume, the geometric configuration of the tips or heads of dispensers.

8.2.1 Automated Dispensing Cabinet System

Based on the Joint Commission on Accreditation of Healthcare Organizations or JCAHO the safe practice of administering medication is the recommended means by which patient safety can be enhanced. However, there are still 400,000 drug-related adverse events in the United States yearly and the annual costs is estimated to be US $3.5 billion. The Ministry of Health and Welfare of Taiwan has estimated more than 20,000 adverse drug events (ADEs) annually from the year 2014 to 2019. To minimize these errors the follow innovations has been implemented, including computerized physician order entry (CPOE), electronic medication administration record (eMAR), automated dispensing cabinets (ADCs), and barcode medication administration (BCMA). More than 98% of hospitals in the United States used ADC and BCMA as of 2015 and these facilitate the nurses in getting the medicines correctly and minimizes the possibility of errands when medicines are placed in ADC.

Robotic drug conveyance systems that are utilized in growth facilities to stock and dispense drug have made it feasible for the change and screen of the drugs. The administration of drugs to and from the pharmacy and waiting for them thereby makes the inpatient drug administration process efficient, less prone to errors, and full of time, hence the need to enhance the use of ADC systems. While the concept of 'ADC systems' can be familiar to American organizations, they are scarce in Taiwan thanks to the investments required and the organizational alterations associated with this system (Ali & Alrobaian, 2024).

A study was conducted at the National Taiwan University Hospital (NTUH), a medical facility in Taipei, Taiwan. Pharmacy employees in the facilities who dose the medications required for a single day use an eMAR in conjunction with a daily unit dose-dispensing device. It indicates that every package is set up with drugs inside, categorized according to the physicians' prescriptions. With the use of order set templates or single orders, doctors enter prescription orders in an electronic format. Through a two-way link, the pharmacist receives these orders and reviews them. Since 2018, the idea of an extended analytical term of two years has been used to assess improvements in clinical outcomes and patient safety. The University Hospital, with its East, West, and Children's Hospital sections, was the one that was identified. The present investigation included one ward each from the East, West, and Specialty ICU districts in the East. The ADC maintained a compliance rate of between 80% and 88% with regard to prescription medication compliance.

The nursing department's nursing information team created a questionnaire that was used to collect data from clinical observations and nurse surveys, which were conducted using a cross-sectional research design. The NTUH Research Ethics Committee gave its approval for this study to be carried out, and no informed consent form from the patient was needed. All nurses who took part in the study were initially sent an email with information on the study's goal and the fact that participation was voluntary. The study notes that although there was no signed consent form, the individuals' completion of the surveys was taken as their agreement.

8.2.2 Smart Pump

Aspects of the ADC integration with nurses' medication preparation operations were timed and monitored during data collection activities. The percentage of patients compared to nurses involved in medicine preparation made up a sample of medication preparation time. Delineation of drug preparation duration subsequent to ADC deployment: The time that the nurse finished preparing the medication for a specific patient, including the time that the nurse spent looking for the medication from different locations, was also calculated, as was the time that the consultant of the ADC computer indicated the nurse was ready to pull the medication for a particular patient.

In today's healthcare companies, mistakes are a big worry. The IOM has suggested that a more forgiving attitude should be taken when treating these errors. Medication errors can happen at any stage of the medication usage process, including ordering the medication, writing the prescription, compounding or dispensing the medication, and even giving it out. Electronic methods, such as robotic medicine dispensers and CPOE, have been put in place to target dispensing inconsistencies and minimize prescription discrepancies. Thus, the fact that monitoring medication delivery is particularly difficult, especially in the patient populations listed, and the necessity of vital medications are among the additional problems noted.

In order to improve safety when giving cardiovascular medication, infusion pump technology was initially used in the healthcare field 45 years ago to monitor the rate and volume of IV medications. Research conducted in 2018 revealed that just 5% of US hospitals use smart pump technology, with institutions with 600 beds or more reporting 100% usage. Intelligent pumps are equipped with DERS, important software that is suggested to remove infusion setting fluctuations and notify the end user by maintaining the drug library. The following are thus included in a general library of drugs: drug parameters, dosing limits (minimum and maximum doses), duration rate, and concentration rates. Adverse medication reactions, home healthcare, and the avoidance of infusion errors are outcomes of employing smart pump technology. A two-year research study reported a 70% reduction in reporting errors linked to basic drug infusions, while another study showed an 80% reduction in drug errors connected to infusions.

Implementing smart infusion pump technologies to hospitals may overwhelm healthcare organizations because smart IV pumps must be smart, and users must be taught new ways continuously while ensuring its drug library's accuracy. Partially, the effectiveness of smart pump technology in preventing IV drug-related errors is proved by the results of several studies, nevertheless, smart pump systems turn out to have varying effectiveness rates. Since the subjects engaging with the drug library are less likely to adhere to the rule, the alerts are triggered more often.

The current status of smart pump technology is assessed, whether there are more advantages than disadvantages is determined, strategies to boost the smart pump's benefits and lower its incidence rate are identified, and lastly the workarounds related to the technology are discussed. Search criteria were established to retrieve studies published between January 2000 and November 2019 from the databases of Scopus, PUBMED, Web of Science, and Science Direct.

Home healthcare, undesirable drug effects, and a decrease in infusion errors are consequences associated with smart pump technology. In one study, the rate of drug errors linked to infusions was reduced by 80%, and in another, over the course of two years, there were 70% fewer reported errors pertaining to common drug infusions. Smart pump infusion technology can, however, not completely eliminate medication errors during infusions and may even introduce new kinds of problems. The most often reported types of IV administration errors were drug (17%), dose (14%), pump rate (almost 20%), incorrect medication (not administered; 23% caused by open tubing failures), and medication delivery. More than half of the basic smart pump infusions employed small IV infusion profiles. Nevertheless, by not paying attention to the medication's name, the physicians might override the medication maximums. Partly, one of the risk factors for alerts during infusion is nurse shift. Alerts cannot be produced by continuous infusions when the medication limits are exceeded. The main purpose of second medicine administration is to enable the continuation of primary infusions in the event that the secondary infusion is completed.

8.2.3 Robotic Dispensing Systems

A single hospital-based care module is being replaced by a community-based regional collaborative care system in healthcare systems. From inpatient to outpatient treatment, pharmacists are essential to optimizing patient safety and medication effectiveness. A notification entitled "The conception of medication dispensing" was sent to pharmacists by the Japanese Ministry of Health, Labor, and Welfare in April 2019 to make sure they had enough time for patient care. One task that pharmacists can assign to pharmacy support personnel is preparing medications. Japan has already used automated dispensing robots, which have significantly decreased dispensing errors and increased the effectiveness of dispensing procedures. Pharmacists' clinical roles are enhanced by the ability of robots to dispense medication quickly and accurately, freeing up more time for clinical patient care. In Japan, the effectiveness and safety of these devices have not yet been thoroughly assessed (Mitchell et al., 2009).

According to a study conducted at Kobe City Medical Center General Hospital, a 768-bed acute phase hospital in Japan, the hospital pharmacy handles 500 prescriptions a day on average, with each prescription involving one or more pharmaceutical orders. The study looked at how much shorter the dispensing times and errors were before and after the robotic dispensing system, which used a collaborative working approach with pharmacists and pharmacy support staff, was implemented. Three components of the robotic dispensing system were incorporated in the study: a bar-coded pharmaceutical dispensing support system with personal digital assistance (PDA), an automated dispensing robot for powdered medicine, and an automated dispensing robot operated by pharmacy support staff. Pharmacy assistants using the robotic dispensing system's automated dispensing robot to prepare prescription drugs. Since there is not a separate association for pharmacy technicians in Japan, pharmacy support employees have received training on working alongside pharmacists to dispense medications.

According to the study, robots can assist pharmacists and pharmacy support staff in appropriately preparing drugs. The Pharmacy and Therapeutic Committee (P&T Committee) accepted 749 oral or topical medications for the hospital formulary;

623 (83.2%) of these medications are kept in the automated dispensing robot. The robot was unable to store the remaining 126 medications because of stringent legal regulations, low-temperature storage specifications, or bulky packaging. Additionally, a PDA-based bar-coded pharmaceutical dispensing support system was put into place, which uses PDA to collate and bar-code medications in order to control prescriptions and medicine packages. Dispensing errors were significantly minimized by this system.

8.3 TECHNOLOGIES USED IN THE DRUG DISPENSING SYSTEM

This section has been organized and clarified by being divided into four distinct categories: hardware, communication, software, and electronics, with the goal of better understanding their design. The components within each category have been organized based on their appropriate roles. Five main classes of electronic components were distinguished and include microcontrollers, and communication-related components, sensors, the real-time clock, and the storage. Figure 8.1 depicts the components used in drug dispensing system.

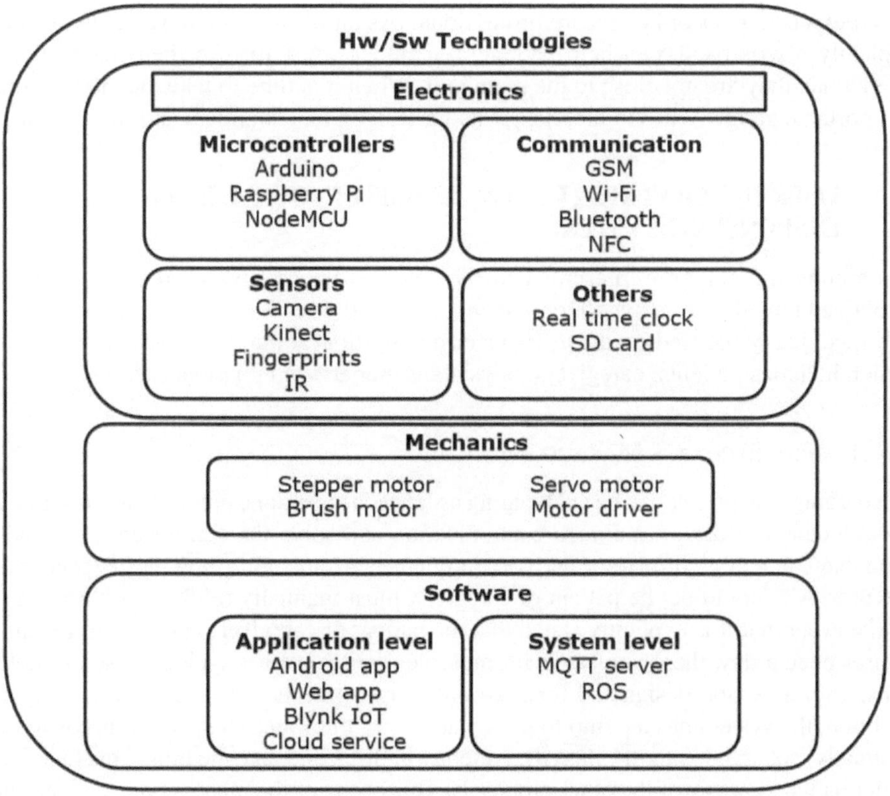

FIGURE 8.1 Components used in the drug dispensing system.

8.3.1 Interaction Through Separate Devices

The other device can be a smart phone, a personal computer, a robot, any wearable device. Communications are in-app and occur when it is time for pills or when the dispenser requires maintenance or the patient has not taken the pills and the dispenser is run by a caregiver/health professional. Communications are made to the user's smart phone through the simple service messages (SMS) and no mobile application is required. On a computer, a specific software program is installed, controlling the device. It is likely that all medication compliance records are stored here, and emails with instructions to caregivers are sent. It is worth noting that the identical software package might be utilized for scheduling times and dosages of medications. Specifically, Mobile Robot is aimed to address the deficiency of human–robot interaction in the context of COVID-19 by designing a robot that could create an indoor map and administer medication to patients. As demonstrated in the aforementioned publications, all three methods make use of a mobile robot in tandem with a smartphone application that controls the robot's operation and allows for the setting of drug timings. Wearable technology takes the shape of metabolizers, which record and monitor daily routines, physical activity, and health. The capacity to monitor medication data and notify users when it is time to take their medicines should be flexible. Additionally, in the event that treatment is received at home, the gathered data may be given to a caregiver or healthcare professional. As an illustration, a wearable device, typically a wristband, can help patients remember when to take their medications even when they are not close to the main unit. When it is time to take the medication, the portable gadget will vibrate, flicker its LED light, and sound an auditory alarm.

8.4 USER INVOLVEMENT IS ENVISAGED IN THE DRUG DISPENSING SYSTEM

Examining the solutions presented in the selected papers, we tried to see if they explained how the medicine therapy is managed and how the dispenser is recharged. We specifically focused on the user-performed portion of the previously listed tasks, which includes patients, caregivers, physicians, nurses, and pharmacists.

8.4.1 Pill Recharge Management

Recharging a dispenser can be challenging as it needs to be done precisely as prescribed by a doctor in order to minimize contamination and solve the component that holds the tablets in a straightforward and secure manner. Almost all of the papers state that the user, who could be the patient or caregiver, must manually refill the refilling unit. In the event that it is explicitly stated that the patient or caregiver must pre-fill the dispenser once a day, there is a box with multiple sections that is typically used to hold pills, with a section designated for each pill to be taken at a specific time of day. In addition, the system has a pump to pour water from the water tank, which needs to be manually recharged, into the glass the patient will drink and take the pills. This function is not included in any of the other proposals. This is one of the most antiquated ideas in one of the proposals, which requires a caregiver to place pills in system canisters: sets of three should go to the canisters. Medicine is stored in plastic containers, and a patient may take up to three containers each day—one in the morning, one in the middle of the day, and one in the evening. After that, the pillboxes must be inserted into the appropriate device, which has three vertical slots for morning, noon, and night. To put it simply, the user merely needs to press a button on the device to release the pillbox when it is time to take the medication; the pillbox then returns to its original position within the dispenser.

Pill recharge methodology

- Manually by patient/caregiver
- Manually, supported by software application
- Manually by healthcare professionals
- Prepackaged medication bags

Manually filling three containers—one for each time of day—using an online application as a guide. One area where the prototype needs improvement is the requirement for qualified pharmacists to refill the dispenser boxes based on doctor-defined prescriptions and timings. This can be achieved by creating a suitable software program that simplifies the refilling process and reduces complexity.

8.4.2 Therapy Management

With the aid of the dispensers, which are covered in this chapter, a variety of patients take part in the therapeutic setting, with the study of their medicine intake patterns and the assessment of their level of meal adherence. As a result, many kinds of tactics were developed and employed by the consumers to start therapy or data.

Physician order entry entails a pill dispenser entering the prescription details while another pill dispenser sets the other device parameters, including the time, phone number, and Wi-Fi network, into the web-based program that runs on the smart device's microcontroller. The medical staff uses an online application to prescribe the patient's medication, including the frequency and dosage. The application also has the capability to verify the patient's medication compliance and other physiological parameters. The developed web application resides in the cloud, and both patients and physicians can access its database to manage pill consumption. Physicians can enter medication dosages into the cloud database linked to the dispenser's controller, ensuring the latter operates properly.

One healthcare professional can communicate with multiple patients with corresponding pill timings and receive alerts regarding medication intake thanks to an Android mobile application that has been developed. The application opens a Firebase resource through which the patient can interact with the dispenser, which in turn modifies Firebase's status and updates the application itself. The patient can also control the dispenser and manage all of their personal information and schedule. This one shows up when the user logs into the app. Here, the user configures the therapy, which consists of the number of pills to take each day, the dosage and time of the pills, any associated alarms, and—most importantly—where the pills should be placed in the connected dispenser. Because the information provided by the app indicates the quantity of pills remaining, the user may also control the replenishment of the dispenser using it. The user must align their smartphone with the app near the pill dispenser in order for it to be Bluetooth-compatible. Then, the smartphone sends signals to the dispenser indicating when the container needs to be opened. With this system, caregivers play a passive role; they enter their phone numbers on the app and get notified via SMS each time a patient forgets to take their medication. It uses Wi-Fi to connect to the dispenser, and patients can use it to check the medication present in the dispenser, schedule medication and receive related alerts. If the patient forgets to take a pill, the caregiver receives an email alert.

A mobile cross-platform application offering two distinct user profiles. It consists of two sections: one that must be completed by the caregiver and the elderly patient together. In certain situations, the patient is allowed to change the timing and recharge the dispenser by using the app. The patient can also control the times at which the tablets are desired and receive instructions when the tablets need to be ingested. Taking care of the appropriate user profile, the app lets you schedule your pill intake, pause one or more pills, and get alerts when you need to use the cutter or are not in compliance.

The user must physically interact with the dispenser via the touch screen, touchpad, or other unique buttons in some cases, and less commonly within the chosen papers, in order to initiate the therapy. The medication dispenser shown in this study has a touch screen and graphical user interface so that patients can control when their medications are taken and receive important information. A method based on interruptions is executed; the user can specify one to five interrupts, which control the time and give alerts when pills are taken, with the aid of the GUI. Instead, the medication timings are set using an LCD display and a keypad in the dispenser that is being offered. A keyboard and LCD combination that lets the user enter the prescription schedule and choose a few items from a pre-made list. The timings can be programmed to run for up to four periods a day for a week.

The majority of the features on a separate PC connected to the dispenser are software programs intended to manage patients and provide them pre-recorded orders. In order to create control signals for the hardware components of the dispensers and send email messages to the caregiver, a medical adherence controller, for example, retrieves the medication therapy from a database and data from the storage unit's sensors. It also updates the database with clients' medication adherence information. Because of this, the app also assists caretakers with monitoring patients' schedules and administering medications.

8.5 OPEN ISSUES AND CHALLENGES

As previously demonstrated, pill and drug dispensers continue to be a challenging topic due to the fact that they are potentially life-saving devices and have multiple uses. The following significant features stand out among the numerous approaches that have been highlighted in the literature, as the writers have pointed out.

8.5.1 Integration

The two proposed prototypes have several packages and subsystems, such as sensors, medicine tracking software, and the dispensing mechanism. These components are often designed independently and are not always coordinated in an efficient manner. There may be limitations on compatibility and integration as well as obstacles to working capacity as a result of this absence and separation. The effective application of these technologies is vital, and developers and manufacturers must devote their efforts to making sure that the components operate together and interact in a harmonious manner. Achieving integration will enable them to provide consumers with a more positive experience, which will improve patient care and medication management in addition. It also alludes to a better, more open market for these kinds of products (Um et al., 2024).

8.5.2 Authentication and Security

These factors are not as crucial when creating the application's prototype, but they become crucial in any actual use case for the technology, particularly in large-scale applications. On the one hand, only those who are permitted to be in this area must be able to walk up and speak with the dispenser. This is vitally necessary in situations like the case study entities, but it is particularly significant in cases like those in hospitals. However, this is also applicable in domestic environments, particularly those with children present. Even while this need is arguably self-evident, it becomes somewhat problematic because elderly individuals may find it difficult to use traditional modes of verification. However, issues with insecurity become apparent if the dispensers are once more linked to the network. Therefore, proper preventive and control measures are necessary for any attack that could potentially impair the dispensers' ability to work and directly affect life. It is consequently necessary to establish and implement appropriate business strategies that are inclusive of all segments of society.

8.5.3 Dependability and Safety

For certain patients, medication dispensers are often essential medical devices. Consequently, as technology advances, corresponding analyses of dependability and fault tolerance issues will also become more sophisticated. Consolidating the engineering methods may lead to the dispenser design being considered again. The dispenser needs to be able to perform certain tasks, such as working within; it should also take into account the absence of other parts or services (like in the case of no networks) and the ease with which it may be switched (like the Wi-Fi connection settings). This is especially important if the dispenser stays on the property for an extended period of time while goods given to the customer must be moved from one place to another (for example, if the patient needs to relocate for a job, vacation, or hospital stay—there was not one for him or his family). For the consumer, the term "safe" refers to a product that has been branded, and as such, it is defined by the features listed below. The flow and pattern of interactions must be designed with usage considerations in mind. The concept of providing end consumers with adequate utility is then contested by the operation's main objective, which is to avoid taking any risky positions.

8.5.4 Scalability

Since small-scale and individual use are more typical of these analytical levels, they serve as a foundation for all uses and a testing ground for solutions that are still in the early stages of development. However, it is imperative that the scalability question—which is important in many applications—be approached thoughtfully. It is possible that in the coming years, medium-sized and larger organizations, such as hospitals and homes, may implement it. In the event that a portion of the procedure is not completed by each individual, for example, the majority of dispensers are trained specifically for pharmacies. Client suggestions for possible enhancements to the current business model also include refrigeration and dispensing equipment for numerous separate dispensers. Scalability analysis ought to be used for every facet of a solution's design (Yuan et al., 2023). In particular, we see that a longer spatial dispersion throughout the dispenser's preparation and filling phase will likewise result in a longer final spatial dispersion. Because of this, if they involve manual labor, they may become a significant obstacle to this area of operational expansion.

8.5.5 User Experience and Personalization

Learning disabilities or other medical issues can impair a child's physical and/or cognitive performance. This occurs between old patients and equipment on the assumption that other parties are underestimated. Pill dispensers using graphical user interfaces commonly seen in desktops, mobiles, or web apps often do not meet the demands of patients or are not sensitive to their needs. As the proliferation of new and progressive techniques for engagement rises with the use of speech and gestures, proper methods of engaging with dispensers may be investigated. This raises the interesting question of how many different types of interactions may be designed for the same device so that users can adjust to the one that is more desired and feels most relevant to their capabilities. This may necessitate the implementation of functions that allow caretakers, or professional personnel, to quickly customize.

8.6 REAL-TIME WORKING DRUG DISPENSER SYSTEMS

Pyxis MedStation is one of the BD group's automated solutions for decentralized drug delivery. Its features include pharmaceutical storage and tracking, user rights, automated medication stock management, connectivity with EHRs, and barcode scanning for medication identification with increased safety and better operations. Omnicell Automated Dispensing Cabinets are Point of Care Cabinets that offer secure medicine storage and convenient administration at the patient's bedside. They include drug safety, inventory management, replenishment notifications, connectivity with EHRs, and reliable transactions that improve patient safety and workflow.

TABLE 8.1
Summary of Real Time working Drug Dispenser Systems

S. No.	Real-Time Working Drug Dispenser Systems	Provide Facilities
1	Pyxis MedStation	Medication stock, tracking, user, storage, scanning, safety, pyxis
2	Omnicell Automated Dispensing Cabinets	Care cabinets, Omnicell, safety, medication, cabinets, transactions, storage, secure, replenishment, pt, point
3	ScriptPro SP 200 Robotic Prescription Dispensing System	Developed robot, client management, community pharmacies, recognition, client management information system
4	AccuDose-Rx Automated Dispensing Cabinets	Top access, instant availability, pharmacological systems, compatibility, safety
5	MedSelect Flex	EHR, password access, Medselect, ARxLUM
6	TCGRx Beacon	LTC facilities, Modifiable settings, AMM, pharmacy system

The ScriptPro SP 200 Robotic Prescription Dispensing System is a specially designed robot that has the potential to improve prescription dispensing and labeling operations in community pharmacies. It provides automatic prescription dispensing, faultless barcode identification, stock control, connectivity with client management information systems, and reduced error rates.

Baxter International Inc.'s AccuDose-Rx Automated Dispensing Cabinets for hospitals and healthcare organizations provide the organization with top access, quick availability of count, compatibility with all forms, and interoperability with clinical and pharmaceutical systems. These cabinets increase medicine safety while reducing waste and managing these drugs.

MedSelect Flex is a flexible automated dispensing system developed by ARxIUM that caters to the different healthcare settings' needs. What makes it attractive is that it is highly customizable, it has a biometric and password access, tracks real-time inventory, and is compatible with EHR and pharmacy systems. Instead, TCGRx Beacon is an AMM designed specifically for healthcare institutions like hospitals and long-term care homes. It enables storage and inventory tracking, interoperability with clinical and pharmacy systems, customizable settings, and contributes to pharmaceutical protection, inventory optimization, and legislative compliance. A summary of some real-time working drug dispenser systems are given in Table 8.1.

8.7 CONCLUSIONS

This chapter provided a systematic study on pill and prescription dispensers from a human-cantered viewpoint. To this end, works indexed in Scopus, Springer, and PubMed were reviewed. This chapter was evaluated based on the proposed solution's stage of development, the developed software and hardware technology, the type of user interaction provided by the solution, and the extent of engagement of various users in the utilization and administration of the identified solution. The study identifies many shortcomings in the development of comprehensive healthcare solutions that include pill and prescription dispensers. This analysis has identified several open issues and challenges, with future research focusing on the scalability of solutions, integration with other systems, authentication and security, dependability and safety, user experience, and personalization. Finally, two additional directions for future work have been provided as two general indications expressed at the end of the review: design approaches for ST solutions, which may include medication adherence in a broader sense and would imply the development of more holistic solutions for patients' health enhancement.

REFERENCES

Ali, A. M. A., & Alrobaian, M. M. (2024). Strengths and weaknesses of current and future prospects of artificial intelligence-mounted technologies applied in the development of pharmaceutical products and services. *Saudi Pharmaceutical Journal*, 32(5), 102043.

Anacleto, T. A., Perini, E., Rosa, M. B., & César, C. C. (2005). Medication errors and drug-dispensing systems in a hospital pharmacy. *Clinics*, *60*, 325–332.

Aung, M. M., Maneetham, D., & Chawaphan, P. (2023). Automatic pill dispenser for pharmacy. *International Journal of Engineering Trends and Technology*, *71*(12), 61–68,

Badnjević, A., Avdihodžić, H., & Gurbeta Pokvić, L. (2021). Artificial intelligence in medical devices: Past, present and future. *Psychiatria Danubina*, *33*(suppl 3), 101–106.

Bagattini, Â. M., Borges, J. L. A., Riera, R., & de Carvalho, D. C. M. F. (2022). Automation of a tertiary hospital pharmacy drug dispensing system in a lower-middle-income country: A case study and preliminary results. *Exploratory Research in Clinical and Social Pharmacy*, *6*, 100151.

Bahadori, M. K. (2022). The role of" dose-unit" drug distribution system in the professionalism of pharmacists and job satisfaction of nurses: A case study. *Journal of Health Administration*, *25*(1), 92–101.

Chalasani, S. H., Syed, J., Ramesh, M., Patil, V., & Kumar, T. M. P. (2023). Artificial intelligence in the field of pharmacy practice: A literature review. *Exploratory Research in Clinical and Social Pharmacy*, *12*, 100346.

Dangi, D., Sharma, S., & Dixit, D. K. (2023). An Effective Deep Learning Prediction Model for the COVID-19 Pandemic in India. 2023 2nd International Conference on Ambient Intelligence in Health Care (ICAIHC), 1–4.

de-Carvalho, D., Alvim-Borges, J. L., & Toscano, C. M. (2017). Impact assessment of an automated drug-dispensing system in a tertiary hospital. *Clinics*, *72*(10), 629–636.

Gargioni, L., Fogli, D., & Baroni, P. (2024). A systematic review on pill and medication dispensers from a human-centered perspective. *Journal of Healthcare Informatics Research*, *8*(2), 244–285.

Ghazal, T. M., Hasan, M. K., Alshurideh, M. T., Alzoubi, H. M., Ahmad, M., Akbar, S. S., Al Kurdi, B., & Akour, I. A. (2021). IoT for smart cities: Machine learning approaches in smart healthcare—A review. *Future Internet*, *13*(8), 218.

Gupta, V., Verma, V., Kaur, S., & Kaur, I. (2022). Amalgamation of Cloud computing with big data. 2022 Seventh International Conference on Parallel, Distributed and Grid Computing (PDGC), 67–70.

Han, Y., Chung, S.-L., Xiao, Q., Wang, J.-S., & Su, S.-F. (2021). Pharmaceutical blister package identification based on induced deep learning. *IEEE Access*, *9*, 101344–101356.

Kanna, R. K., Vasuki, R., & Kripa, N. (2021). Modern smart medicine dispenser kit based on emergency alert system. *Journal of Xi'an Shiyou University*, *64*(6), 123–137.

Kaur, G., Bindal, R., Kaur, V., Kaur, I., & Gupta, S. (2023). Bitcoin and cryptocurrency technologies: A review. *AIP Conference Proceedings*, *2782*(1).

Kim, J., Kwon, H., Kim, J., Park, J., Choi, S.-U., & Kim, S. (2022). PillGood: Automated and interactive pill dispenser using facial recognition for safe and personalized medication. IJCAI, 5920–5923.

Lee, D., & Yoon, S. N. (2021). Application of artificial intelligence-based technologies in the healthcare industry: Opportunities and challenges. *International Journal of Environmental Research and Public Health*, *18*(1), 271.

Mitchell, S. H., Veltri, M. A., & Kim, G. R. (2009). Dispensing: Pharmacy information systems. In Christoph U. Lehmann, George R. Kim, & Kevin B. Johnson (Eds.), *Pediatric Informatics: Computer Applications in Child Health* (pp. 345–355). Springer.

Mittal, S., Monga, C., Upreti, K., Kumar, N., Raut, R. D., & Alam, M. S. (2022). Light weight cryptography for cloud-based e-health records. 2022 7th International Conference on Communication and Electronics Systems (ICCES), 690–696.

Muehlematter, U. J., Daniore, P., & Vokinger, K. N. (2021). Approval of artificial intelligence and machine learning-based medical devices in the USA and Europe (2015--20): A comparative analysis. *The Lancet Digital Health*, *3*(3), e195–e203.

Naybour, M., Remenyte-Prescott, R., & Boyd, M. J. (2019). Reliability and efficiency evaluation of a community pharmacy dispensing process using a coloured Petri-net approach. *Reliability Engineering \& System Safety*, *182*, 258–268.

Sabaté, E. (2003). *Adherence to Long-Term Therapies: Evidence for Action*. World Health Organization.

Secinaro, S., Calandra, D., Secinaro, A., Muthurangu, V., & Biancone, P. (2021). The role of artificial intelligence in healthcare: A structured literature review. *BMC Medical Informatics and Decision Making*, *21*, 1–23.

Stasevych, M., & Zvarych, V. (2023). Innovative robotic technologies and artificial intelligence in pharmacy and medicine: Paving the way for the future of health care—a review. *Big Data and Cognitive Computing*, *7*(3), 147.

Takase, T., Masumoto, N., Shibatani, N., Matsuoka, Y., Tanaka, F., Hirabatake, M., Kashiwagi, H., Nishioka, I., Ikesue, H., Hashida, T., & Koide, N. (2022). Evaluating the safety and efficiency of robotic dispensing systems. *Journal of Pharmaceutical Health Care and Sciences*, *8*(1), 24.

Um, I. S., Clough, A., & Tan, E. C. K. (2024). Dispensing error rates in pharmacy: A systematic review and meta-analysis. *Research in Social and Administrative Pharmacy*, *20*(1), 1–9.

Wang, Y.-C., Tsan, C.-Y., Chen, M.-C., & others. (2021). Implementation of an automated dispensing cabinet system and its impact on drug administration: Longitudinal study. *JMIR Formative Research*, *5*(9), e24542.

Wilhelmsen, N. C., & Eriksson, T. (2019). Medication adherence interventions and outcomes: An overview of systematic reviews. *European Journal of Hospital Pharmacy*, *26*(4), 187–192.

Yuan, M., Zhao, N., Wu, K., & Chen, Z. (2023). The storage location assignment problem of automated drug dispensing machines. *Computers \& Industrial Engineering*, *184*, 109578.

Zhou, Y., Wang, F., Tang, J., Nussinov, R., & Cheng, F. (2020). Artificial intelligence in COVID-19 drug repurposing. *The Lancet Digital Health*, *2*(12), e667–e676.

9 Cognitive Impairment Assessment

Role of Artificial Intelligence in Transforming Early Detection and Care

Richa Singh and Anurag Upadhyay

9.1 INTRODUCTION

Global population aging and technological advancements are the two realities of the current era. Although population aging can be considered as a human success story and the credit can be attributed to the advancements in public health, medical technology, economic and social development (United Nations, 2019). By 2050, the global population of elderly people is projected to reach 1.5 billion (United Nations, 2019), i.e., across the world out of every 6 people 1 will be above the age of 65. One of the major challenges associated with aging is the decline in cognitive functions, which leads to psychological and behavioral problems for the elderly. With age, some cognitive decline may occur, which is natural. But if this decline is more than the normative decline and gradually progresses, it may result into dementia and other neurocognitive disorders.

Since, there is not any definite treatment available for patients with cognitive impairments, dementia and other neurocognitive disorders and pharmacological interventions provide only symptomatic relief, early diagnosis is extremely important to provide care and support to such patients. Neuropsychological assessment is crucial for early diagnosis of cognitive impairment, which is more than what comes naturally with age. Traditional human-based neuropsychological assessment requires trained professionals, is time consuming, and leads to delay in assessment. Application of artificial intelligence (AI) has extremely increased in the area of cognitive neuroscience and evidences reports that AI can assist in early diagnosis, supporting rational clinical decision-making and improve patient care. AI-based neurocognitive screening tests are being developed, which will not only assist the clinical decision making but will also increase the accessibility and availability of these tests. The present chapter will focus on the applications of different models of AI like machine learning (ML), deep learning (DL), natural language processing (NLP), and virtual reality (VR) in cognitive impairment assessment along with its merits and limitations.

DOI: 10.1201/9781003520184-12

9.2 COGNITIVE IMPAIRMENT AND DEMENTIA

Impairments in brain functions like attention, learning, memory, thinking, problem solving, decision making, etc., is termed as cognitive impairment. Cognitive impairments can range from mild to severe and can deteriorate as the age progresses and can affect an individual's daily life functioning (Sarraf et al., 2019). Some decline in cognitive functions is the normal part of the biological aging process but when this decline is more than the normative decline it may result in mild cognitive impairment (MCI) (Khatun et al., 2019), which is an initial stage of dementia and may progress to neurocognitive disorders like Alzheimer's disease (AD) in aged people. Early signs of MCI may include deficits in attention, short-term memory, inability to concentrate, reduced processing speed, decreased decision-making ability, language problems, losing sense of direction, etc. (Javed et al., 2023). Figure 9.1 shows the symptoms of MCI. Problems in these cognitive functions affects an individual's daily life functioning. So, early detection of MCI is crucial for minimizing the risk of developing AD.

Dementia is a progressive disease marked by impairments in memory and other cognitive functions such as deficits in abstract thinking, language, and judgements which considerably affects an individual's ability to perform activities of daily living. AD is a gradually progressive degenerative disorder and is the most frequent form of dementia, contributing to 60–70% of total cases of dementia. According to World Health Organization (World Health Organization, 2017) it is projected that the number of older people suffering from dementia will rise from 47 million in 2015

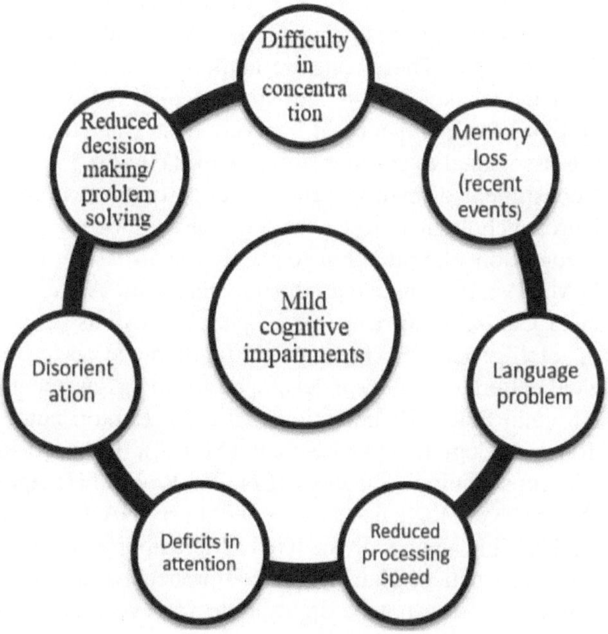

FIGURE 9.1 Symptoms of mild cognitive impairment.

to 75 million in 2030 and 132 million by 2050. Since, dementia is one of the main reasons of disability and dependency of elderly people across the globe, an increase in the number of people with dementia will lead to an increase in the cost of disease management.

Since, MCI is the early stage of dementia and AD in aged people, accurate and early diagnosis in its initial stage is essential to delay its progress and manage the disease. Despite the fact that the most commonly accepted approach to control AD at present is the MCI screening and early intervention (Javed et al., 2023), dementia remains undiagnosed worldwide and diagnosis is typically made at a relatively later stage of the disease. However, early diagnosis and interventions can lead to better management of dementia and related problems. Among the different methods like brain imaging, biomarker tracking, etc., available to assess cognitive impairment, neurocognitive tests are the most common, easy, and low-cost method to assess cognitive decline.

9.3 NEUROPSYCHOLOGICAL ASSESSMENT

Neuropsychological assessment also known as neurocognitive tests, are the non-invasive methods to assess the cognitive, emotional, and behavioral deficits. Traditionally neuropsychological assessment is carried out to assess the extent of impairment to a particular skill after brain injury or neurological illness. It assesses the important aspects of cognitive functioning that includes orientation, learning, memory, intelligence, and language, perceptual motor, and executive functions. These tests are used to assess both healthy brain functions and brain functions affected by dementia and other degenerative disorders. These assessment tools play an important role in identifying the changes in behavior and cognitive functions as disease progresses over time. These tests are administered to determine diagnosis, identify the strength and weakness of an individual's cognitive system after the diagnosis and develop plans for treatment and interventions. Thus, these tests assess the cognitive functions associated to specific structure of the brain.

The essential constituent of neuropsychological assessment is the neuropsychological tests. Neuropsychological tests can be used to assess problems in specific domains of cognition like attention (e.g., digit span test), memory (Wechsler Memory Scale, WMS-IV), language (e.g., Boston Diagnostic Aphasia test), executive function (Wilconsin Card Sorting test), visuospatial functions (e.g., Benton facial recognition test), intelligence (Wechsler Adult Intelligence scale, WAIS-IV), etc. Neuropsychological batteries have been developed for the assessment of global cognition like Mini Mental Status Examination (MMSE), Benton neuropsychological investigation, Montreal Cognitive Assessment (MoCA), Halstead-Reitan Battery, Luria Nebraska Neuropsychological battery (LNNB), Revised Hasegawa's dementia scale (HDS-R), Neuropsychological Assessment battery (NAB), etc. These batteries can be in a fixed and flexible manner. In the fixed battery approach the same set of tests is administered on every patient that gives a comprehensive assessment. However, it is time consuming and may not be appropriate for every patient. Examples of neuropsychological tests and batteries are shown in Figure 9.2. Traditionally, neuropsychological tests are manually administered by trained and specialized personnel

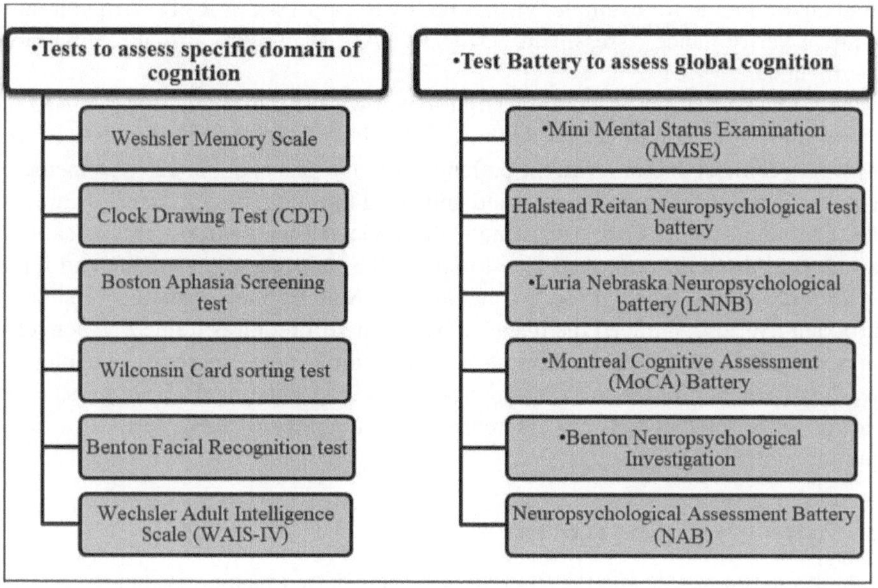

FIGURE 9.2 Examples of neuropsychological tests and batteries to assess specific domains of cognition and global cognition.

in a controlled clinical setting. The paper and pencil-based neurocognitive tests rely heavily on the administrator and are time consuming.

9.3.1 Computer-Assisted Neuropsychological Assessment

Advancements in computer programming have led to the development of computerized versions of many of the neuropsychological tests. Application of technology in neuropsychological assessment has the advantage of administering the tests in a highly structured manner thereby enhancing its reliability and efficiency. Advancements in technology had permitted many neuropsychological test batteries to be administered without clinicians being directly involved. With computerized neurocognitive tests, long-term monitoring of cognitive functions will be possible for better management of dementia.

Computers, tablets, or any digital interface can be used as an alternative to human administrator in the administration of computer-assisted neuropsychological test. Scoring and interpretation of the test results is also done using a computer program, thus minimizing the role of human examiners. Chan et al. (2018) reported that both computerized and paper-and-pencil memory tests were having comparable diagnostic performance in the detection of MCI and dementia. Examples of computerized assessment tools include Cambridge Neuropsychological Test Automated Battery (CANTAB), Cambridge Cognition Examination (CAMCOG) etc. Advancement in virtual reality has integrated computerized versions of neuropsychological tests into a virtual environment, for example, Virtual-reality Stroop Task (VRST), Virtual Reality Cognitive Performance Assessment Test (VRCPAT), leading to virtual-reality-based assessment.

Due to the COVID-19 pandemic, strict lockdown was enforced, which raised the demand for remote cognitive test. In those difficult times, telemedicine emerged as a platform to connect doctors with the patients virtually (Rai et al., 2022). Telemedicine led to overcome the distance barrier and enhanced the accessibility to healthcare services. Carotenuto et al. (2021) systematically reviewed the neuropsychological tests administered through traditional face-to-face (FTF) and via telemedicine and found no difference in the score in the two modalities. Although telemedicine versions of neurocognitive tests reduced the distance barrier it still requires trained personnel to administer. To overcome these limitations, application of AI in neuropsychological assessment can minimize the dependence on trained personnel to administer and interpret the results. It will also increase the availability of these tests to a larger population in remote areas.

9.4 ARTIFICIAL INTELLIGENCE

Artificial intelligence is an area of computer science that enables computer systems to work and react like humans. These systems can perform activities like speech recognition, problem-solving, decision-making, perception, learning, and planning. AI focuses on developing software, which empowers machines to learn from the data and accomplish tasks that involve human intelligence. AI-powered systems not only learn from the dataset, they also constantly update their learning on the availability of new data (Nevin et al., 2018). AI can work on large datasets and can yield results, which are more accurate than humans in complex situations. Application of AI in healthcare had brought a paradigm shift due to the growing availability of healthcare data and speedy progress of analytics techniques.

The main subfields of AI techniques, which is applied to healthcare data include ML, DL, NLP, virtual reality and so on. ML provides the system with the ability to improve their performance without being explicitly programmed, works on structured data and makes inferences regarding the probability of disease outcomes thereby improving prediction performance. Deep learning is a subdivision of machine learning, which enables machines to learn to think and make decisions using the complex structure of algorithms modeled on human brain. NLP enables computers to derive meaning from spoken or written texts in natural language input and works on unstructured data (Jiang et al., 2017).

Different techniques of AI like ML, DL, and NLP are gradually becoming more significant for early detection and management of diseases. Since neuropsychological batteries are time consuming, researchers are implementing AI technology in neurocognitive tests and converting the traditional paper-based test into AI-assisted neurocognitive tests (Sirilertmekasakul et al., 2023). An AI-based framework can help to differentiate normal aging from mild cognitive impairment in a personalized manner providing a cost-effective alternative to face-to-face interviews (Tang et al., 2020).

As the prevalence of dementia and other neurocognitive disorders are increasing due to population aging, the cost of its management and care has increased tremendously. Different techniques of AI can play an important role in early detection of cognitive impairments, progression, and facilitating early intervention for better outcome. AI technology can assist neuropsychologists in the diagnosis of dementia, AD and other neurodegenerative disorders by identifying the significant patterns, which is difficult to detect through the conventional methods. Therefore, integrating AI techniques into clinical practice can transform the management of neurocognitive or neurodegenerative disorders for the better (Veneziani et al., 2024). A summary of the studies using AI techniques discussed in this chapter is given in Table 9.1. In the

TABLE 9.1
Summary of Studies Using AI Technology for Neuropsychological Assessment

AI Feature Used	Type of Test	Conclusion	Author and Year
ML	LM, ADAS-Cog, Rey AVLT and (FAQ)	ML can be used to optimize tests for automatic classification of patients to diagnose clinical disorders.	Battista et al., 2017
ML and DL	Clock Drawing test (CDT)	CAD is a reliable method for the CDT assessment process.	Jiménez-Mesa et al., 2023
ML	MMSE, MoCA	The ML approach is a valuable tool for the screening of cognitive dysfunction.	Yim et al., 2020
ML	MemTrax	The ML predictive model can be used for early detection and screening of MCI and AD.	Bergeron et al., 2020
DL	CDT	DNN-based CDT can automatically detect cognitive decline.	Sato et al., 2022
ML and DL	Seoul Neuropsychological Screening Battery	ML algorithm and DL can predict cognitive impairment.	Kang et al., 2019
ML and DL models	CANTAB, EEG/MEG, Blood samples	AI mind tool can be used to identify MCI patients at the risk of dementia.	Haraldsen et al., 2024
NLP	MMSE, MoCA, GPCog, CDT, and verbal fluency	Preclinical stages of dementia can be identified using the NLP technique.	Beltrami et al., 2018
ASR (NLP)	Semantic verbal fluency (SVF)	Fine-grained analyses of SVF data can be fully automated for the screening of cognitive decline.	König et al. 2018
VR	Virtual Reality Cognitive Performance Assessment Test (VRCPAT)	VRCPAT provides a reliable and efficient method to study neurocognitive function.	Pearson et al., 2008

following section, we will discuss different studies that have integrated AI techniques with neuropsychological tests and reported promising results.

9.4.1 Neuropsychological Assessment and Machine Learning

Neuropsychological assessment helps in discriminating different degrees of cognitive impairments. The conventional method of administration and interpretation of these tests are prone to subjectivity effect along with other limitations. ML has emerged as a reliable technique to quantitatively support the diagnostic procedure. ML is being applied for automatic classification of individuals into normal and pathological category and applies the learning models for the prediction of a new subject. ML has been extensively applied in neuroimaging studies on dementia, as it can handle large and complex data (Salvatore et al., 2015). Now researchers are focusing on the implementation of ML techniques with neuropsychological test, findings of such studies are reporting a positive effect of ML both on improved accuracy and reducing testing time.

Battista et al. (2017) assessed the potential of ML in automatic classification of subjects with AD in the initial stage of disease. Measures of cognitive domains and subdomains were used as classification features. The role of 12 neuropsychological tests was evaluated in the automatic classification of subjects with AD. They reported that ML can provide an effective technology to categorize patients quantitatively and helps in diagnosis of clinical disorders using neuropsychological tests. They also concluded that ML can assist clinicians in optimizing the best measures and reduce the subjectivity in the diagnosis process. Out of 12 tests, the best dependable predictors for automatic classification of subjects with AD was found to be logical memory (LM), Alzheimer's Disease Assessment Scale-Cognitive Behavior (ADAS-Cog), measure of delayed and immediate memory, Rey Auditory Verbal Learning Test (AVLT), and functional assessment questionnaire (FAQ).

Clock drawing test (CDT) is a commonly used paper-pencil test to measure cognitive impairment. It relies heavily on subjective evaluation by trained personnel. For the automatic diagnosis of cognitive impairment Jiménez-Mesa et al. (2023) designed an AI-based computer aided diagnosis (CAD) to analyze the CDT data. To assess the patient's cognitive status, they used a preprocessing pipeline and convolutional neural network (CNN) to identify the informative patterns. They concluded that the CAD system was a reliable and appropriate method for the analysis of CDT data.

Studies are focusing on the application of ML models to neuropsychological tests for screening of individuals with cognitive impairments. Yim et al. (2020) developed a ML algorithm to identify cognitive dysfunctions based on the neuropsychological screening test results. They used MMSE and MoCA tests to evaluate their subjects. The data was analyzed using different ML algorithms and they reported screening accuracy of 93.5% for MCI, 95.5% for cognitive dysfunction and 99.9% for dementia. Thus, for the screening of individuals with cognitive dysfunction, ML-based methods can offer a valuable solution.

For the early detection of dementia and AD, memory testing is crucial. MemTrax is an online screening test for episodic memory. Bergeron et al. (2020) developed a predictive model based on ML using MemTrax performance for early detection and screening of MCI and AD. The findings revealed that MemTrax performance can be efficiently utilized in a ML classification predictive model screening application for diagnostic support for individuals experiencing cognitive impairments.

Recently, Haraldsen et al. (2024) developed an AI mind tool that involved the ML and DL models. Using the data obtained from (EEG/MEG), blood samples and CANTAB they developed AI mind connector and predictor to identify MCI patients who are at the early risk of dementia.

9.4.2 Neuropsychological Assessment and Deep Learning

DL is a subdivision of ML, which enables a machine to learn to think by using the complex structures of algorithms modeled on human brain. DL uses neural network with three or more layers to mimic human brain functioning so that it can learn from a huge amount of data. Using artificial neural network models, the decision-making process is more precise as compared to humans. Several studies have DL algorithms with a larger dataset to check the potential of neuropsychological tests for screening of cognitive impairments.

Sato et al. (2022) developed a CDT based on the deep neural network (DNN) model to automatically detect impairments in cognition of elderly people. They also explore the possibility of CDT as a screening test at mass level. The AI-assisted CDT using DNN was applied on a data of 40,000 elderly people. They reported that the accuracy of DNN-based CDT for identification of patients with decline in executive function was approximately 90% and 77% for people with probable dementia. They concluded that DNN-based CDT has the potential as a mass screening test for screening executive dysfunction or with probable dementia.

Researches have been done to assess the precision of machine-learning algorithms to predict cognitive impairment. Kang et al. (2019) used TensorFlow to train a machine-learning model with artificial neural network. Using multi-center neuropsychological test data of the Seoul Neuropsychological Screening Battery they suggested that the machine-learning algorithm has the potential to predict cognitive impairment using deep learning trained with multi-center neuropsychological test data.

9.4.3 Neuropsychological Assessment and Natural Language Processing

The field of AI that permits computer systems to comprehend human language, both written and verbal is designated as NLP. Automatic speech recognition (ASR) or speech-to-text (STT) is the most frequently used NLP technique. STT allows human speech to be recognized and comprehended by a computer system when we directly speak to the computer interface (Jiang et al., 2022). In NLP, after transforming speech to text, ML is applied for the assessment of cognitive impairments. Speech alterations are one of the early signs of cognitive impairments that can be noticed before the dysfunctions of other cognitive functions. Conventional neuropsychological tests for language dysfunction offer vague results. To detect the initial signs of speech alteration indicative of cognitive decline in elderly people Beltrami et al. (2018) used NLP technique in their study. For the screening of participants with single and multiple domains MCI and early dementia and healthy controls they used the neuropsychological tests, which included MMSE, General Practitioner Assessment of Cognition (GPCog), CDT, and test of verbal fluency (phonemic and semantic). The natural language of the participants during tasks such as describing a usual working day, describing a complex picture, and recalling the last remembered dream, were recorded, transcribed, and interpreted at various linguistic levels. The NLP technique was used to analyze the transcribed linguistic features of spontaneous speech during neuropsychological tests. They reported that healthy control subjects differ significantly from the participants of pathological conditions, i.e., MCI and early dementia. Thus, it was concluded that for the identification of preclinical phases of dementia, NLP is a promising technique.

In ASR technology, participants directly speak to smartphones or computer interfaces and AI convert speech into text, which helps to solve the problem of technology-induced anxiety among the older people and thus resolves the difficulties due to user-interface unfriendliness and technology strangeness (Sirilertmekasakul, et al., 2023). Considering the advantages of NLP, many researchers are now using NLP to automate the tests used for the screening of cognitive impairments. Semantic verbal fluency (SVF) task is one such test used for the screening of mild cognitive impairments in which within a certain time limit participants have to name as many items as possible. Traditionally task performance is measured manually adding the correct words and errors, which is time consuming. König et al. (2018) examined whether the automatic speech-based analysis of SVF task is as accurate as the manual version of the test for the screening of cognitive decline. The data on SVF task was collected from elderly healthy controls, with MCI and Alzheimer's or related dementias. The SVF data was analyzed and interpreted both manually and automatically with clusters and switches. High correlation was obtained between manually established values and automatically extracted clusters and switches and healthy controls can be distinguished from individuals with MCI and Alzheimer's or related dementias. They concluded that fine-grained analyses of SVF data can be fully automated for the assessment of cognitive decline.

9.4.4 Neuropsychological Assessment and Virtual Reality

VR provides a completely digital and computer-generated environment providing a three-dimensional (3D) view to its users. It facilitates users to step inside and interact with the 3D world that can either simulate or completely differ from the real world. It requires users to wear gears like VR Goggles, VR Headset, etc., and then enter in the virtual world. VR is another technological advancement of AI that has the potential to be used for the assessment and rehabilitation of individuals with cognitive dysfunctions.

The traditional neuropsychological tests are conducted in an artificial environment of clinical setting, which is different from the environment a person lives in. This limitation of traditional neuropsychological assessment can be reduced through the use of virtual reality. Dynamic and three-dimensional stimulus environments can be created using virtual reality in which we can record all the behavioral response. Initially VR technology was used to evaluate the different domains of cognition like attention, spatial abilities, memory and executive functions. VR technology-assisted neuropsychological tests have also created new avenues for cognitive rehabilitation because of its ability to record all the behavioral responses, reproducibility of daily life, and high level of ecological validity as compared to traditional neuropsychological tests (Veneziani et al., 2024). Virtual Reality Cognitive Performance Assessment Test (VRCPAT) is used to assess cognitive functions, which focus on enhanced ecological validity using virtual environment scenario. Pearson et al. (2008) reported significant correlation between 15 minute VRCPAT battery and traditional neuropsychological tests, which took approximately 1.5 hours to administer by a trained personnel. They concluded that VRCPAT provides a reliable and efficient method to assess cognitive function within an ecologically valid environment.

9.5 MERITS AND LIMITATIONS OF AI-ASSISTED COGNITIVE ASSESSMENT

As technological advancements influence human cognition neuropsychologists are also integrating advancements in computer programming into the assessment process to enhance the quality of assessment process. The AI-based (ML and DL) next generation of cognitive assessment is capable of classifying meaningful patterns from large data leading to efficient prediction of cognitive impairments. AI-assisted neuropsychological assessment will help in reducing the workload of clinicians, reducing subjectivity and biasness in scoring and interpretation. A digitalized version will increase the accessibility of these tests to individuals living in areas where healthcare facilities are unreachable, allowing the early detection of cognitive impairments of people living in those areas. Further the application of ASR technology can reduce the technology-induced anxiety among older people thus solving the problems of technology unfamiliarity and user interface unfriendliness

However, there are certain limitations too. Educational level, availability, and cost of internet, technology familiarity and acceptance by the elderly could limit the use of AI-assisted neuropsychological assessment. Since there are a variety of neuropsychological test batteries and screening tests available, some of the digitalized versions of these tests have been automated, however, there are many tests that need trained personnel to supervise the administration. Confidentiality and privacy of patient information security is another issue that needs special attention.

9.6 CONCLUSION

Aging of the global population has led to the increase in the incidence and prevalence of cognitive impairments and neurodegenerative disorders like dementia and related problems. The projected cost of care and management of dementia is projected to increase many times in the coming decade. With increasing age, some amount of cognitive decline is normal, but if it is more than the normative decline it may result into MCI, which is the initial stage of dementia. Since, pharmacological treatments are only symptomatic, early detection can help in the management and care of elderly people affected with neurodegenerative diseases. So early detection of changes in cognitive functions will not only help to alert the patients, caregivers, and clinicians but it will also lead to cost-effective treatment and patient care.

Neuropsychological assessment tools are used to detect the changes in cognitive functions. Traditionally, paper-and-pencil versions of these tests require trained personnel to administer, score, and interpret the results. With the advancements in computer technology, computerized versions of neuropsychological assessment measures have evolved that improved the efficiency, reliability, and cost effectiveness and permitted several neuropsychological tests that can be administered without the direct involvement of clinicians. Further advancements in AI, with its subfields including ML, DP, and NLP, can yield results that are more accurate than humans in complex situations due to its ability to work on large datasets. A growing number of studies are confirming that AI-assisted neuropsychological assessment can provide an economical substitute to face-to-face interviews to screen normal aging from MCI in a personalized manner. AI-assisted assessment will not only reduce the workload of the clinicians, it will also reduce subjectivity and biases in interpretation. However, uncontrolled test administration protocols, patient information security, and low technology familiarity of the elderly, etc., could limit its applicability for a larger population. Therefore, further studies should try to work on the limitations and enhance the applicability of neuropsychological assessment tools

REFERENCES

Battista, P., Salvatore, C., & Castiglioni, I. (2017). Optimizing Neuropsychological Assessments for Cognitive, Behavioral, and Functional Impairment Classification: A Machine Learning Study. *Behavioural Neurology*, *2017*, 1–19. https://doi.org/10.1155/2017/1850909

Beltrami, D., Gagliardi, G., Rossini Favretti, R., Ghidoni, E., Tamburini, F., &Calzà, L. (2018). Speech Analysis by Natural Language Processing Techniques: A Possible Tool for Very Early Detection of Cognitive Decline? *Frontiers in Aging Neuroscience*, *10*, 369. https://doi.org/10.3389/fnagi.2018.00369

Bergeron, M. F., Landset, S., Zhou, X., Ding, T., Khoshgoftaar, T. M., Zhao, F., Du, B., Chen, X., Wang, X., Zhong, L., Liu, X., & Ashford, J. W. (2020). Utility of MemTrax and Machine Learning Modeling in Classification of Mild Cognitive Impairment. *Journal of Alzheimer's Disease: JAD*, *77*(4), 1545–1558. https://doi.org/10.3233/JAD-191340

Carotenuto, A., Traini, E., Fasanaro, A. M., Battineni, G., & Amenta, F. (2021). Tele-Neuropsychological Assessment of Alzheimer's Disease. *Journal of Personalized Medicine*, *11*(8), 688. https://doi.org/10.3390/jpm11080688

Chan, J. Y. C., Kwong, J. S. W., Wong, A., Kwok, T. C. Y., & Tsoi, K. K. F. (2018). Comparison of Computerized and Paper-and-Pencil Memory Tests in Detection of Mild Cognitive Impairment and Dementia: A Systematic Review and Meta-analysis of Diagnostic Studies. *Journal of the American Medical Directors Association*, *19*(9), 748–756.e5. https://doi.org/10.1016/j.jamda.2018.05.010

Haraldsen, I. H., Hatlestad-Hall, C., Marra, C., Renvall, H., Maestú, F., Acosta-Hernández, J., Alfonsin, S., Andersson, V., Anand, A., Ayllón, V., Babic, A., Belhadi, A., Birck, C., Bruña, R., Caraglia, N., Carrarini, C., Christensen, E., Cicchetti, A., Daugbjerg, S., Di Bidino, R., … Rossini, P. M. (2024). Intelligent Digital Tools for Screening of Brain Connectivity and Dementia Risk Estimation in People Affected by Mild Cognitive Impairment: The AI-Mind Clinical Study Protocol. *Frontiers in Neurorobotics*, *17*, 1289406. https://doi.org/10.3389/fnbot.2023.1289406

Javed, A. R., Saadia, A., Mughal, H., Gadekallu, T. R., Rizwan, M., Maddikunta, P. K. R., Mahmud, M Liyanage, M., & Hussain, A. (2023). Artificial Intelligence for Cognitive Health Assessment: State-of-the-Art, Open Challenges and Future Directions. *Cognitive Computation*, *15*, 1767–1812 https://doi.org/10.1007/s12559-023-10153-4

Jiang, F., Jiang, Y., Zhi, H., Dong, Y., Li, H., Ma, S., Wang, Y., Dong, Q., Shen, H., & Wang, Y. (2017). Artificial Intelligence in Healthcare: Past, Present and Future. *Stroke and Vascular Neurology*, *2*(4), 230–243. https://doi.org/10.1136/svn-2017-000101

Jiang, Z., Seyedi, S., Haque, R. U., Pongos, A. L., Vickers, K. L., Manzanares, C. M., Lah, J. J., Levey, A. I., & Clifford, G. D. (2022). Automated Analysis of Facial Emotions in Subjects with Cognitive Impairment. *PloS One*, *17*(1), e0262527. https://doi.org/10.1371/journal.pone.0262527

Jiménez-Mesa, C., Arco, J. E., Valentí-Soler, M., Frades-Payo, B., Zea-Sevilla, M. A., Ortiz, A., Ávila-Villanueva, M., Castillo-Barnes, D., Ramírez, J., Del Ser-Quijano, T., Carnero-Pardo, C., &Górriz, J. M. (2023). Using Explainable Artificial Intelligence in the Clock Drawing Test to Reveal the Cognitive Impairment Pattern. *International Journal of Neural Systems*, *33*(4), 2350015. https://doi.org/10.1142/S0129065723500156

Kang, M. J., Kim, S. Y., Na, D. L., Kim, B. C., Yang, D. W., Kim, E. J., Na, H. R., Han, H. J., Lee, J. H., Kim, J. H., Park, K. H., Park, K. W., Han, S. H., Kim, S. Y., Yoon, S. J., Yoon, B., Seo, S. W., Moon, S. Y., Yang, Y., Shim, Y. S., ... Youn, Y. C. (2019). Prediction of Cognitive Impairment via Deep Learning Trained with Multi-Center Neuropsychological Test Data. *BMC Medical Informatics and Decision Making*, *19*(1), 231. https://doi.org/10.1186/s12911-019-0974-x

Khatun, S., Morshed, B. I., & Bidelman, G. M. (2019). A Single-Channel EEG-Based Approach to Detect Mild Cognitive Impairment via Speech-Evoked Brain Responses. *IEEE Transactions on Neural Systems and Rehabilitation Engineering: A Publication of the IEEE Engineering in Medicine and Biology Society*, *27*(5), 1063–1070. https://doi.org/10.1109/TNSRE.2019.2911970

König, A., Linz, N., Tröger, J., Wolters, M., Alexandersson, J., & Robert, P. (2018). Fully Automatic Speech-Based Analysis of the Semantic Verbal Fluency Task. *Dementia and Geriatric Cognitive Disorders*, *45*(3–4), 198–209. https://doi.org/10.1159/000487852

Nevin, L., & PLOS Medicine Editors (2018). Advancing the Beneficial Use of Machine Learning in Health Care and Medicine: Toward a Community Understanding. *PLoS Medicine*, *15*(11), e1002708. https://doi.org/10.1371/journal.pmed.1002708

Parsons, T. D., Silva, T. M., Pair, J., & Rizzo, A. A. (2008). Virtual Environment for Assessment of Neurocognitive Functioning: Virtual Reality Cognitive performance assessment test. *Studies in Health Technology and Informatics*, *132*, 351–356.

Rai, U., Upadhyay, A, & Singh, R. (2022). Telemedicine: A Future of Healthcare Sector in India. In T. Choudhury, A. Katal, J. Um, A. Rana& M. Al-Akaidi (Eds.). *Telemedicine: The Computer Transformation of Healthcare*. Springer Nature Singapore Pvt Ltd. https://doi.org/10.1007/978-3-030-99457-0

Salvatore, C., Cerasa, A., Battista, P., Gilardi, M. C., Quattrone, A., Castiglioni, I., & Alzheimer's Disease Neuroimaging Initiative (2015). Magnetic Resonance Imaging Biomarkers for the Early Diagnosis of Alzheimer's Disease: A Machine Learning Approach. *Frontiers in Neuroscience*, *9*, 307. https://doi.org/10.3389/fnins.2015.00307

Sarraf, S., Desouza, D. D., Anderson, J., Saverino, C., & Alzheimer's Disease Neuroimaging Initiative (2019). MCADNNet: Recognizing Stages of Cognitive Impairment through Efficient Convolutional fMRI and MRI Neural Network Topology Models. *IEEE Access: Practical Innovations, Open Solutions*, *7*, 155584–155600. https://doi.org/10.1109/ACCESS.2019.2949577

Sato, K., Niimi, Y., Mano, T., Iwata, A., & Iwatsubo, T. (2022). Automated Evaluation of Conventional Clock-Drawing Test Using Deep Neural Network: Potential as a Mass Screening Tool to Detect Individuals With Cognitive Decline. *Frontiers in Neurology*, *13*, 896403.https://doi.org/10.3389/fneur.2022.896403

Sirilertmekasakul, C., Rattanawong, W., Gongvatana, A., &Srikiatkhachorn, A. (2023). The Current State of Artificial Intelligence-Augmented Digitized Neurocognitive Screening Test. *Frontiers in Human Neuroscience*, *17*, 1133632. https://doi.org/10.3389/fnhum.2023.1133632

Tang, F., Uchendu, I., Wang, F., Dodge, H. H., & Zhou, J. (2020). Scalable Diagnostic Screening of Mild Cognitive Impairment using AI Dialogue Agent. *Scientific Reports*, *10*(1), 5732. https://doi.org/10.1038/s41598-020-61994-0

United Nations, Department of Economic and Social Affairs, Population Division (2019). *World Population Ageing 2019: Highlights* (ST/ESA/SER.A/430).

Veneziani, I., Marra, A., Formica, C., Grimaldi, A., Marino, S., Quartarone, A., &Maresca, G. (2024). Applications of Artificial Intelligence in the Neuropsychological Assessment of Dementia: A Systematic Review. *Journal of Personalized Medicine*, *14*(1), 113. https://doi.org/10.3390/jpm14010113

World Health Organization (2017). *Global action plan on the public health response to dementia 2017–2025*. Geneva: World Health Organization

Yim, D., Yeo, T. Y., & Park, M. H. (2020). Mild Cognitive Impairment, Dementia, and Cognitive Dysfunction Screening Using Machine Learning. *The Journal of International Medical Research*, *48*(7), 300060520936881. https://doi.org/10.1177/0300060520936881

10 Diet Management for Diabetes Patients Using AI

Seema P. Nehete

10.1 INTRODUCTION

Diabetes is a chronic illness that millions of people worldwide suffer from. It happens when the body finds it difficult to control blood sugar levels, which are essential for our cells to produce energy. Human body blood sugar level is strongly impacted by carbohydrates, although fat and proteins have less of an effect. Maintaining a regular carbohydrate intake during meals can assist with blood sugar regulation. The hormone insulin, which the pancreas produces and which helps the body to successfully regulate glucose levels, is essential for the human body. Complications with insulin synthesis, however, can cause aberrant blood sugar levels and diabetes. Diabetes falls into a lot of different categories, mostly type 1 and type 2 are known (American Diabetes Association, 2018). Type 1 is caused when there is no secretion of insulin in the human body. Type 2 is caused due to insulin resistance or insufficient insulin synthesis. Type 2 diabetes risk can be influenced by a number of factors, including sedentary lifestyle, poor nutrition, and genetic alterations. Genetic structure cannot be changed, but lifestyle and nutritional diet can control sugar levels in diabetes.

Since a balanced diet immediately affects blood sugar levels and general health, it is a key component of diabetes control. If diabetes patients use insulin, "carb counting" is very crucial since they will need to modify insulin dosage based on the amount of carbohydrates in their upcoming meal. Nevertheless, carb counting can assist diabetes patients in understanding how their blood sugar reacts to different carbohydrate levels during meals and snacks, even if they do not use insulin. By doing this, diabetes patients can prevent blood sugar levels from rising or falling too much. So the healthcare system is required, which will be helpful to individuals having assisted living with diabetes, to maintain a balanced diet rich in vegetables and legumes, lean protein sources, reduced-fat dairy products, and some high-fiber, low-GI carbs, cereals and fruit.

Every aspect of our lives is changing due to artificial intelligence and machine learning (AI/ML), and the healthcare system is no exception. India has a disproportionately high number of diabetes patients, which poses a unique set of challenges as well as a unique opportunity in terms of possible data availability. The idea and creation of virtual systems that can carry out activities routinely by exploiting human

DOI: 10.1201/9781003520184-13

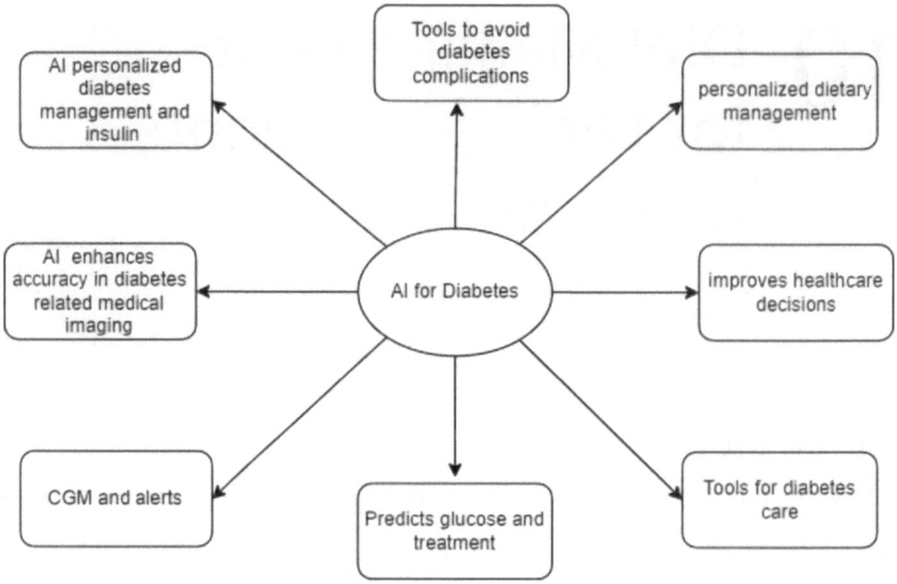

FIGURE 10.1 AI for diabetes patients.

intellect is known as AI. AI includes machine learning, which gives computers the capacity to automatically learn from and get better at tasks without being specifically programmed (Jiang et al., 2017; Kavakiotis et al., 2017). The use of AI and ML has the potential to significantly expand the accessibility and improve the effectiveness of diabetes care (Singla et al., 2019). AI and personalized nutrition have come together in recent years to form a novel discipline that can improve understanding of nutrition and general health of persons having assisted living. In this chapter, AI can provide personalized choices and similar for food intake through well-balanced diet to maintain sugar level, for such diabetes patients. Figure 10.1 shows how AI helps diabetes patients.

AI helps diabetes patients in all eight domains like dietry management, diabetes management and insuling, medical imaging, CGM, prediction of treatment on lower glucose level, tools to avoid complications, tools for dibetes care and healthcare decisions.

10.2 TRADITIONAL DIETARY GUIDELINES FOR DIABETES PATIENTS

A healthy diet may be created using a variety of strategies to maintain blood sugar levels within normal ranges. The following strategy, called the plate method (Saslow et al., 2017), is given generally to diabetes patients with the assistance of a nutritionist:

- Arrange non-starchy veggies, including tomatoes, spinach, and carrots, to cover half of your plate.

- Use a lean protein, such as chicken, lean pork, or tuna, to cover one quarter of your plate.
- Use a starchy vegetable, like green peas, or a carbohydrate, like brown rice, to fill the final quarter.
- Incorporate "good" fats in moderation, including those found in nuts or avocados.
- Include a dish of dairy or a piece of fruit, along with a glass of water, unsweetened tea, or coffee.
- Eating six little meals a day as opposed to three huge.

10.2.1 Importance of Carbohydrate Counting and Glycemic Index/Load

Carbohydrates have the most impact on blood sugar level since they convert to sugar. Diabetes patients need dieticians to learn how to calculate carbs in their intake to help regulate blood sugar. But it is not possible for every old age or disabled person to every time go to clinic and check glucose level to choose a balanced diet. Some diabetics choose their diets based on the glycemic index (Miller, 1994) particularly when it comes to carbs. Using this strategy, meals high in carbohydrates are ranked according to how they affect blood sugar levels. For instance, brown rice has more complex carbohydrates than white rice, which has a lower glycemic index. Researchers also found glycemic load, which records the kinds of carbohydrates included in food as well as the quantity in a dish. In essence, it illustrates the impact of a food portion on blood sugar levels. Numerous factors influence the glycemic load, such as food processing, fruit ripeness, meal preparation, and food storage duration.

10.2.2 Emphasis on Balanced Meals, Portion Control, and Meal Timing

Eating roughly the same quantity of meals at the same time every day is crucial. Fasts and feasts should be avoided since they are unhealthy alternatives to skipping meals or overindulging. A well-balanced diet can assist in controlling blood sugar levels and averting diabetic complications. Limiting the consumption of processed foods that are heavy in salt, added sugars, and saturated and trans fats is important. Eating the appropriate quantity of food at the appropriate times is another need of a balanced diet called portion management.

10.3 CHALLENGES IN TRADITIONAL APPROACHES

Traditional approaches have different limitations.

10.3.1 Limitations of Traditional One-Size-Fits-All Dietary Recommendations

Blood sugar increases more, the more carbohydrates are consumed. Dr. Somdat Mahabir of the NIH says, "The glycemic index really doesn't take into consideration how much you eat." Glycemic load and index are difficult to utilize because they are not listed on labels of food. However, labels do provide useful details such as calories, fiber, sugars, and total carbs for the complete food, not for the plate portion of the individual.

10.3.2 Variability in the Individual Response to Different Foods

Every person has a different reaction to the foods he eats, depending on his genetic composition, gut flora, and other variables (Mattioli et al., 2011). An individual's health outcomes, such as their susceptibility to illnesses, capacity to manage chronic disorders, and general well-being, are significantly influenced by this variability. Variations in diet and food reactions have been linked to an increased risk of chronic illnesses, including obesity, type 2 diabetes, cardiovascular disease, and several cancers. Developing customized nutrition strategies that are suited to each person's unique requirements might result from an understanding of how different people react to different dietary components.

10.4 INTEGRATION OF AI IN DIET MANAGEMENT

AI tools and algorithms can be used to recommend a personalized diet to diabetes patient of all ages. AI can help in monitoring continuous glucose levels of diabetes patients and then predict risk if glucose level increases by analyzing patterns and trends in diabetes data. To mitigate risk, AI can recommend food to the patients to lower their glucose levels. This chapter uses the PIMA Indian diabetes dataset available on the Kaggle website to demonstrate how AI algorithms are used to find patterns and trends.

10.4.1 Data-Driven Approach Using Patient Health Records, Biometrics, and Dietary Logs

For risk analysis, the suggested RNN model (Srinivasu et al., 2022) is assessed using tabular patient data from PIMA, where auxiliary memory elements like GRU and LSTM are used for improved prediction performance.

RNN is a deep-learning model trained to interpret and translate a sequential data input into a specific sequential data output is called a recurrent neural network (RNN) as shown in Figure 10.2. Data with complicated semantics and syntactic rules governing the relationships between sequential components, such as words, phrases, or time series data, is referred to as sequential data.

Neurons, which are collectively known as data-processing nodes, are the building blocks of RNNs. The input, output, and hidden layers of neurons are arranged in this way. The result is provided by the output layer, while the input layer receives the data to process. The hidden layer is where analysis, prediction, and data processing happens.

RNNs function by sequentially feeding the incoming input to the hidden layers one step at a time. They do, however, also feature a self-looping or recurrent workflow: a short-term memory component allows the hidden layer to recall and utilize past inputs to anticipate future events. To forecast the sequence, it makes use of both

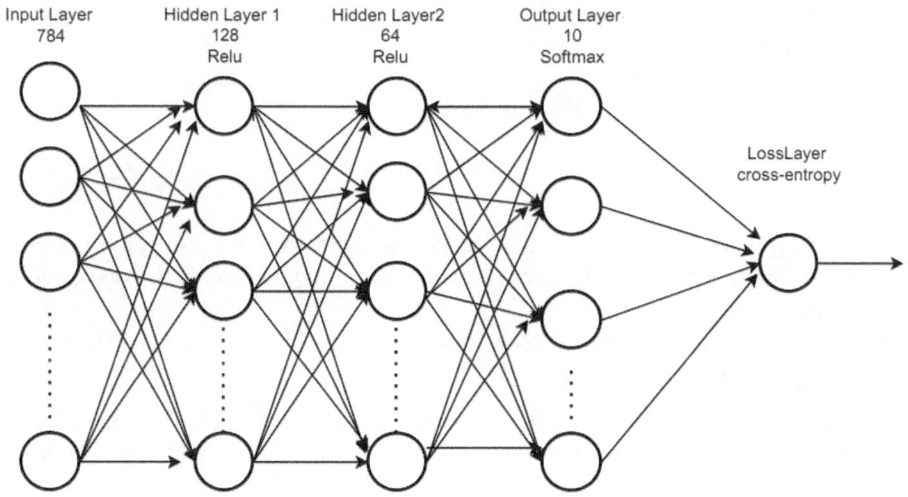

FIGURE 10.2 Working of a RNN.

the stored memory and the present input. There are two variants of RNN as long short term memory (LSTM) (Rahman et al., 2020) and gated recurrent unit (GRU) (Rochman et al., 2022).

LSTM: An RNN variation called extended short-term memory (LSTM) allows the model to extend its memory to support a longer timeframe. An RNN can only recall input from the recent past. It cannot enhance its prediction by incorporating inputs from multiple prior sequences.

GRU: Selective memory retention is made possible using an RNN called a gated recurrent unit (GRU). The hidden layer of the model, which has the ability to add and remove information from memory, receives an update and forgets the gate.

10.4.2 Machine-Learning Algorithms for Analyzing Dietary Patterns and Glucose Responses

YOLO (Chopra et al., 2022) can identify food items in the meal image of the patient and then calculate nutritional weightage of calories like fat, carbohydrates, and protein. YOLO stands for you look only once. It is to overlay on an input image with an *S X S* grid. Each grid cell produces two things:

(1) It produces a set of bounding boxes-B centered on a point inside the grid cell with associated confidence score-C that an object exists inside each bounding box and
(2) It also produces a class probabilities map for each grid cell, which essentially tells what object class is most likely to be in that cell given that an object in facts exists in that cell at all.

And finally it combines it to yield object detection. This abstracted framework works as follows:

Confidence score is given by following formula:

$$C = P_r(\text{obj}) \times \text{IoU}$$

where $P_r(\text{obj})$ is the probability of the object, IoU is intersection over union, which gives the difference between the ground truth and predicted box. If the object does not exist then $C = 0$.

For each grid cell it computes a set of output vectors. The first vector is the vector class probability $P_r(C_i)$.

It creates a set of bounding box B with parameters $[X, Y, \sqrt{w}, \sqrt{h}, C]$, where X and Y are the center position of the bounding box, $\sqrt{w}$ and $\sqrt{h}$ are the width and height of the bounding box.

These conditional class probabilities are tested by multiplying them by the confidence estimates for each individual box, yielding class-specific confidence scores for every box. These ratings indicate how well the box matches the object as well as the likelihood of that class as given below.

$$P_r(C_i/\text{obj}) \times P_r(\text{obj}) \times IoU = P_r(C_i) \times \text{IoU}$$

The final predictions are represented as below

$$S \times S \times (B \times 5 + C).$$

10.4.3 Real-Time Monitoring and Feedback Systems

For individuals, after monitoring their glucose level at particular times using wearable sensors and calculating meal nutritional values using YOLO, proposed systems will predict the risk for diabetes patients. If glucose level is high, it will alert patients about carbohydrate intake at particular meal and recommend food which will take care of their glucose level at that time. A glycemic response prediction framework is used with the following steps:

Information Gathering: Gather information on the makeup of meals, personal traits (such as age, weight, and degree of exercise), and data from continuous glucose monitoring (CGM).

Pre-processing Data: Pre-process and normalize the data, deal with missing values, and provide characteristics like the timing of meals, the composition of macronutrients, and the degree of physical activity.

Training of Models: Utilizing past data, train several models (such as random forest and LSTM) to identify trends in the relationship between glycemic reactions and meal composition. In order to assess model performance and prevent over fitting, use cross-validation.

Prediction in Real Time: To anticipate glycemic responses in real time depending on meal inputs, use the trained model.

Observation and Input: Real-time patient feedback should be provided, along with dietary recommendations based on expected glycemic responses. Monitor model performance and retrain it frequently to account for individual differences in metabolism.

10.5 AI TOOLS AND TECHNOLOGIES

An overview of AI-driven systems and applications for managing diabetes is as given below.

10.5.1 Examples of AI Algorithms Used in Predicting Glycemic Responses to Meals

For diabetes management and dietary plan optimization, it is critical to comprehend how different foods affect blood glucose levels and to anticipate the glycemic responses of meals. By assessing a range of factors, such as physical activity, unique metabolic reactions, food composition, and other specific health data, AI systems may produce accurate estimates. AI algorithms (Rigla et al., 2018) that are frequently employed in this sector.

10.6 ALGORITHMS FOR MACHINE LEARNING

These algorithms (Mahesh, 2020) are capable of seeing patterns in data and forecasting future events based on past performance.

10.6.1 Classification

Models of Regression: Use linear regression to find clear-cut relationships between food intake and glycemic response. Multiple regression accounts for higher-degree multiple features, capturing more complex connections.

- *Ensembles and Decision Trees*: Random forests is a collection of decision trees with the ability to manage feature interactions and non-linear connections. Gradient boosting machines (GBM) are models constructed one after the other, with each new model fixing mistakes from the prior one.
- *Support Vector Machines (SVM):* SVMs adapt inputs into high-dimensional spaces to describe complicated connections, making them useful for problems involving classification and regression.

Deep-Learning Techniques: In terms of forecasting glycemic reactions, deep-learning models, particularly those that use neural network have shown considerable potential.

- *Artificial Neural Network:* Through the use of many layers of neurons, artificial neural networks (ANN) are able to learn from data and represent intricate connections.

- *RNNs, or recurrent neural networks*: Sequential data is handled by LSTM and GRU networks, which makes them appropriate for time-series blood glucose level forecasts.
- *CNNs or convolutional neural networks:* CNNs may be modified to handle time-series data by capturing geographical dependencies in meal composition and glycemic reactions, even though they are mostly utilized in image processing.

Mixture Models: The strengths of each algorithm may be combined to increase forecast accuracy.

- *Ensemble Approaches:* Combining neural networks with other machine-learning models (such as random forests and GBM) to improve prediction performance.
- *Models of Deep Hybridom:* CNNs and RNNs may be integrated (e.g., CNN-RNN) to capture data's temporal and geographical patterns.

Customized Models for Prediction: Individual differences in glycemic reactions may be substantial and personalized models allow for this.

- *Cooperative Screening:* These algorithms anticipate glycemic reactions based on commonalities with data from other people, much as recommendation systems do.
- *Customized Models of Regression*: Regression models should be customized based on personal traits and past glycemic reactions.

Learning via Reinforcement: With this method, the environment (blood glucose readings, for example) provides feedback on the best eating practices to learn.

- *Q-Learning:* A kind of model-free reinforcement learning system that maximizes cumulative reward (e.g., stable blood glucose levels) by learning the value of actions in states.
- *Deep Learning with Reinforcement*: Combines reinforcement learning with deep learning (Liu et al., 2020) to handle huge state and action spaces, making it appropriate for situations involving sophisticated nutritional control.

10.6.2 Wearable Devices and Sensors for Continuous Glucose Monitoring (CGM) Linked with AI Systems

Parts of the CGM System Sensors: These sensors (Cappon et al., 2017), which are inserted beneath the skin, assess the amount of glucose in the interstitial fluid. Typical sensors come from Abbott (FreeStyle Libre), Medtronic, and Dexcom.

Transmitters: Connected to the sensor, transmitters communicate glucose readings to a mobile device or recipient.

Receivers/Smartphones: Present alarms, trends, and real-time glucose data. Smartphone apps are currently widely used by CGM systems for data administration and visualization.

10.7 BENEFITS OF AI IN DIET MANAGEMENT

Personalized Recommendations: AI systems can analyze enormous volumes of data, including a person's nutritional preferences, objectives, and medical history. This makes it possible to create diet programs that are unique to each person. AI-powered diet planning can offer tailored recommendations that are challenging to accomplish with conventional approaches by taking into account variables like allergies, food intolerances, and nutritional needs.

Effective and Time-Saving: Making meal plans, doing manual calculations, and looking up nutritional data are all part of traditional diet planning. These chores can be automated by AI-powered devices, saving time and effort for both patients and medical personnel. AI can swiftly analyze data and create optimized meal plans by utilizing machine-learning algorithms, taking into account a variety of dietary limitations and goals.

Constant Monitoring and Flexibility: AI-driven meal plans can offer feedback and monitoring in real time. Through the integration of wearable devices or apps, people can monitor their food consumption, physical activity, and other pertinent aspects. After this, AI systems can examine the data to offer insights and suggestions for modifications, ensuring that diet programs continue to be appropriate and flexible in the face of shifting conditions.

10.8 CASE STUDIES AND SUCCESS STORIES

The proposed system gives AI-driven diet management solution to diabetes patients for diet management. It takes glucose level reading of patient using wearable devices or sensors. This continuous glucose monitoring CGM is simulated using AI algorithm. Predicted simulated data is replaced by real-time glucose data after fetching form sensors. Using predicted and actual data patterns and temporal trends are found using RNN. According to this analysis of glucose level, balanced diet is recommended to the patient. Also the patient can upload real-time meal image to app and get the nutritional values in that. The proposed system uses the YOLO algorithm to detect different food items in the meal image and uses collaborative recommendation to calculate similarity between food items using their nutritional values. The proposed system is shown in Figure 10.3.

The solution works in the following steps.

(1) **CGM:** For diabetes patients continuous glucose monitoring is done at 15 minute intervals for three months with integration of wearable devices and sensors. It is used to find patterns in the data.

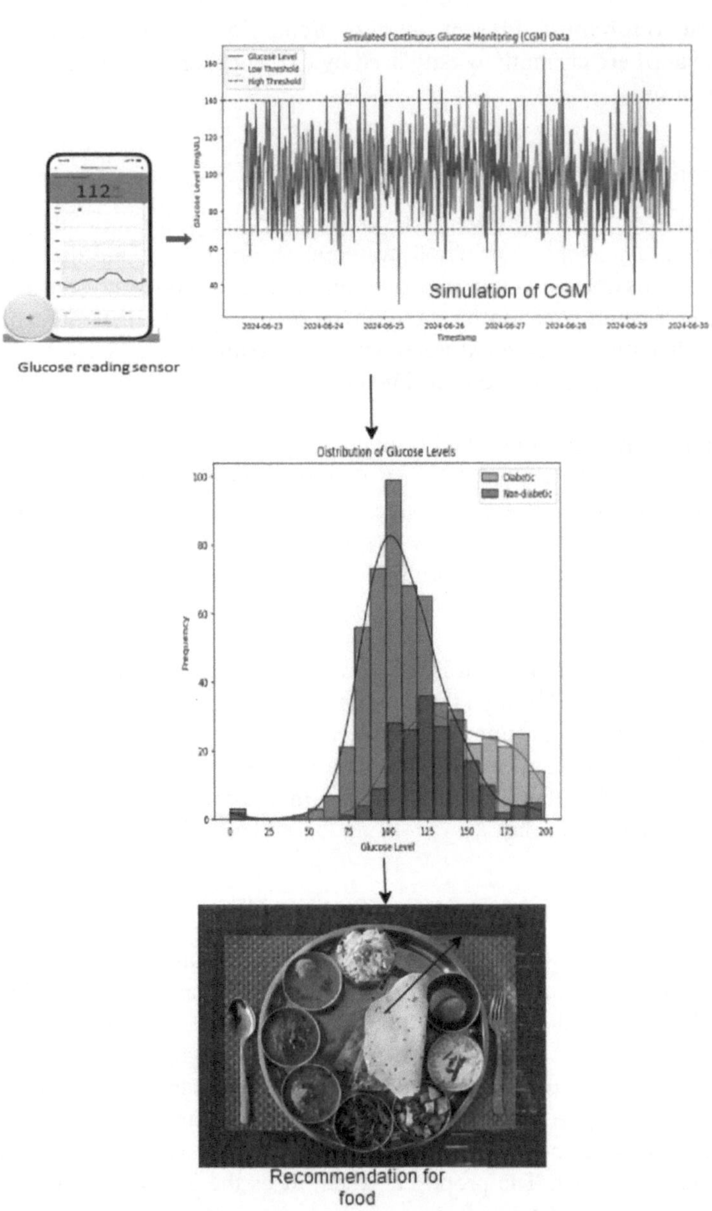

Total Carbohydrates: 40g (Rice) + 20g (Dal) + 15g (Vegetable Curry) + 10g (Paneer Dish) + 3g (Pickle) + 10g (Raita) + 20g (Chapati/Roti) + 5g (Papad) + 5g (Salad) + 30g (Sweet Dish) = 158g

FIGURE 10.3 Proposed system for diet management of diabetes patients.

(2) **Detecting Pattern/Analysis of Glucose Level:** To explain pattern detection in glucose level data, the standard PIMA Indian diabetes dataset available at Kaggle is used. This dataset is from the National Institute of Diabetes to predict diabetes. It contains various medical parameters, like pregnancies, glucose, blood pressure, BMI, insulin, age, skin thickness, diabetes pedigree function and one outcome of 768 patients. To improve prediction results, feature selection and weight optimizations are carried out over the PIMA dataset's features. The patterns and trends are analyzed using exploratory data analysis, correlation matrix, and feature importance. For the PIMA dataset, feature importance is shown in Figure 10.4 and correlation matrix is shown in Figure 10.5.

It clearly shows diabetes totally depends on glucose level of patients.

The relationship of all features with outcome can be seen from the above matrix. The relationship of glucose with other features is studied from the matrix and used for predicting risk of higher glucose level for patients. The current study's results are compared to those of other standard classification methods, including random forest, decision tree, K nearest neighborhood, adaboost, XGBoost and Support Vector Machine as shown in Figure 10.6.

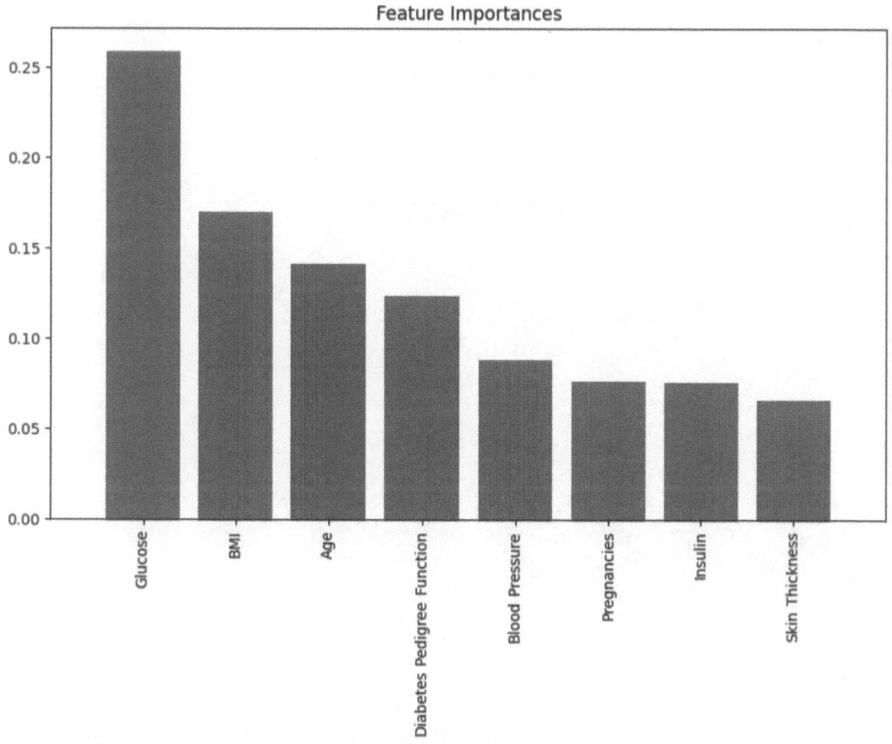

FIGURE 10.4 Feature importance of the PIMA diabetes dataset.

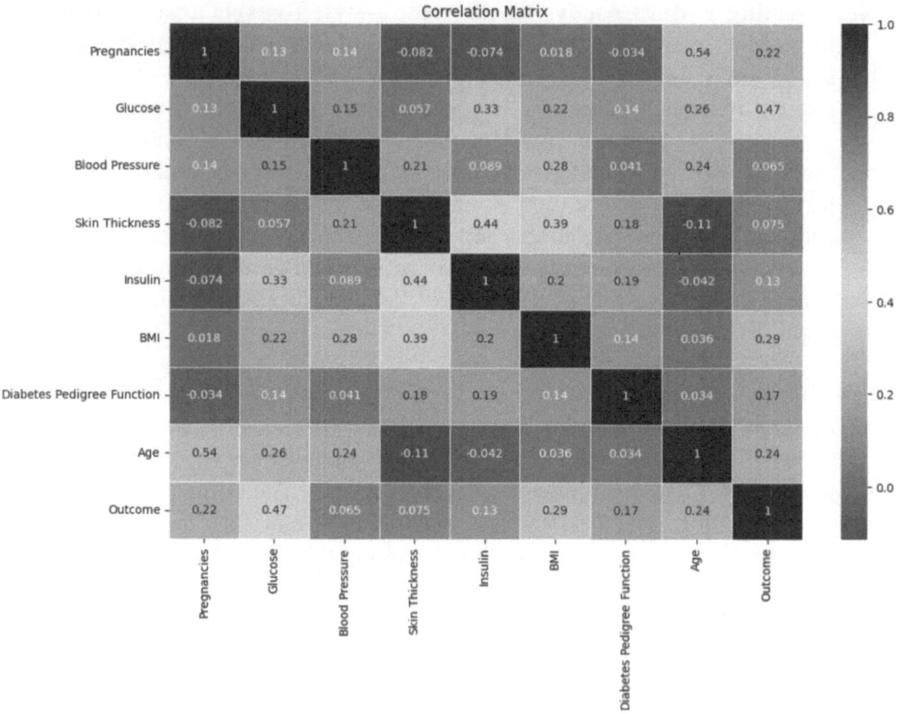

FIGURE 10.5 Corelation matrix for the PIMA dataset.

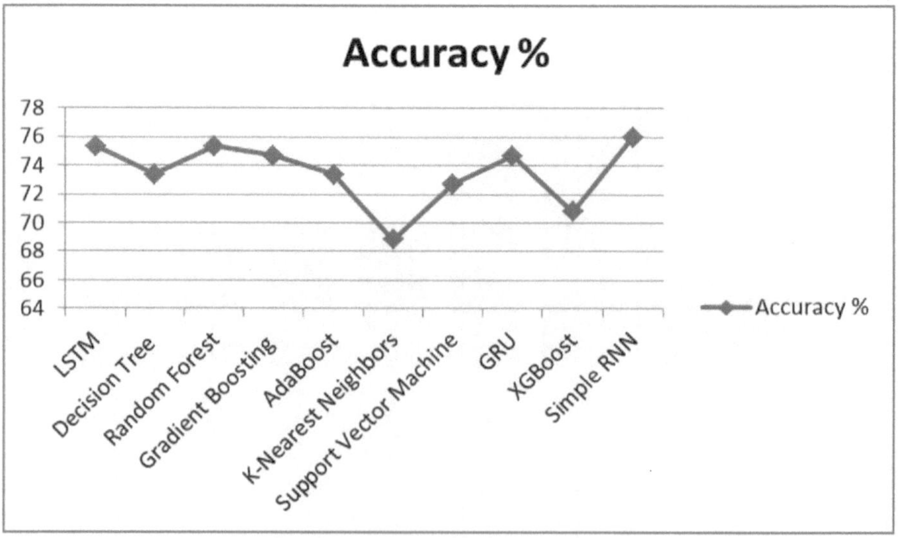

FIGURE 10.6 Comparison of accuracy of different classifiers for the PIMA dataset.

It can be seen from Figure 10.6 that simple RNN is better than LSTM and GRU.

If glucose level is below 70 it is considered as 'Low', if it is between 70 and 146 it is 'Normal' otherwise it is 'High'. The patterns are detected on real-time glucose data of patient.

(3) **Recommend Diet and Similar Food:** After getting an analysis of glucose levels, the proposed system recommends a balanced diet for maintaining carbs for glucose levels, as shown in Figure 10.3 of the proposed system for the individuals. As each food shows a different effect on every human body, diabetes patients can take meal images according to recommended diet and get confirmation of nutritional intake to maintain glucose level. The YOLO algorithm takes this food image and detect food items in that image. The proposed system recommends similar food to patients as in the image with required nutritional contents to maintain glucose level. Also, according to the recommended diet, the YOLO algorithm creates a meal image and suggests it to old age and disabled persons so that they can take the correct food.

10.8.1 Success Story

The proposed system is used for a 65-year-old female, Sunita. The real-time analysis of her glucose level in the morning during breakfast time is performed at 9.10am, the sugar level drops below 70 indicating low glucose and requires the patient to have nutritional fruit juice to maintain the glucose level. So at breakfast, Sunita is recommended fruit juice and her glucose level comes into the normal range after juice intake at 9.30am. Also, after examining Sunita's glucose data, the RNN model found patterns that suggested specific types of carbs were responsible for her glucose spikes. Sunita received a personalized diet plan recommendation from the system, which included low-glycemic-index items that helped stabilize her blood sugar levels. Also Sunita uploads photos of her meals and get comprehensive nutritional information.

10.8.2 Success Metrics

After a proper diet, the following results are reported for the above patient whose real-time glucose analysis is performed.

(1) **HbA1c Levels:**
Initial average HbA1c: 8.5%
Post-intervention average HbA1c: 6.7%

(2) **Medication Needs:**
Initial average daily insulin dose: 40 units
Post-intervention average daily insulin dose: 30 units

(3) **Quality of Life:**
Considerable gains in mood, energy, and everyday activities as measured by standardized questionnaires.

10.9 CONCLUSION

AI's revolutionary contribution to diabetes care is the provision of proactive, individualized, and effective solutions. This analysis shows how AI improves diabetes care using diet management, enhancing the precision and effectiveness of care. AI gives patients better self-management resources and expands knowledge of diabetes as a multifaceted illness. In conclusion AI-based glycemic response prediction to meals uses a variety of techniques, ranging from straightforward regression models to intricate deep-learning networks. In order to increase prediction accuracy and offer people controlling their blood glucose levels useful information, personalized diet is recommended. The RNN and YOLO provides accurate results as observed in the patient's results. The proposed system properly gives diet management to diabetes patients having assisted living. AI can recommend recipes, which will create balanced diets also in the future according to the requirement of the diabetes patient.

REFERENCES

American Diabetes Association. (2018). Classification and diagnosis of diabetes: standards of medical care in diabetes—2018. *Diabetes Care*, 41(Supplement_1), S13–S27.

Cappon, G., Acciaroli, G., Vettoretti, M., Facchinetti, A., & Sparacino, G. (2017). Wearable continuous glucose monitoring sensors: a revolution in diabetes treatment. *Electronics*, 6(3), 65.

Chopra, M., & Purwar, A. (2022). Food Image Recognition Using CNN, Faster R-CNN and YOLO. In *Applications of Artificial Intelligence, Big Data and Internet of Things in Sustainable Development* (pp. 81–89). CRC Press.

Jiang, F., Jiang, Y., Zhi, H., Dong, Y., Li, H., Ma, S., ... & Wang, Y. (2017). Artificial intelligence in healthcare: past, present and future. *Stroke and Vascular Neurology*, 2(4).

Kavakiotis, I., Tsave, O., Salifoglou, A., Maglaveras, N., Vlahavas, I., & Chouvarda, I. (2017). Machine learning and data mining methods in diabetes research. *Computational and Structural Biotechnology Journal*, 15, 104–116.

Liu, Z., Ji, L., Jiang, X., Zhao, W., Liao, X., Zhao, T., ... & Xie, G. (2020, November). A deep reinforcement learning approach for type 2 diabetes mellitus treatment. In *2020 IEEE International Conference on Healthcare Informatics (ICHI)* (pp. 1–9). IEEE.

Mahesh, B. (2020). Machine learning algorithms-a review. *International Journal of Science and Research (IJSR)*, 9(1), 381–386.

Mattioli, A. V., Pennella, S., Pedrazzi, P., & Farinetti, A. (2011). Gender differences in adherence to Mediterranean diet and risk of atrial fibrillation. *Journal of Hypertension and Cardiology*, 1(4), 4–13.

Miller, J. C. (1994). Importance of glycemic index in diabetes. *The American Journal of Clinical Nutrition*, 59(3), 747S–752S.

Rahman, M., Islam, D., Mukti, R. J., & Saha, I. (2020). A deep learning approach based on convolutional LSTM for detecting diabetes. *Computational Biology and Chemistry*, 88, 107329.

Rigla, M., García-Sáez, G., Pons, B., & Hernando, M. E. (2018). Artificial intelligence methodologies and their application to diabetes. *Journal of Diabetes Science and Technology*, 12(2), 303–310.

Rochman, E. M. S., Suprajitno, H., Rachmad, A., Nindyasari, R., & Rachman, F. H. (2022, October). Comparison of LSTM and GRU in Predicting the Number of Diabetic Patients.

In *2022 IEEE 8th Information Technology International Seminar (ITIS)* (pp. 145–149). IEEE.

Saslow, L. R., Mason, A. E., Kim, S., Goldman, V., Ploutz-Snyder, R., Bayandorian, H., ... & Moskowitz, J. T. (2017). An online intervention comparing a very low-carbohydrate ketogenic diet and lifestyle recommendations versus a plate method diet in overweight individuals with type 2 diabetes: a randomized controlled trial. *Journal of Medical Internet Research*, 19(2), e36.

Singla, R., Singla, A., Gupta, Y., & Kalra, S. (2019). Artificial intelligence/machine learning in diabetes care. *Indian Journal of Endocrinology and Metabolism*, 23(4), 495–497.

Srinivasu, P. N., Shafi, J., Krishna, T. B., Sujatha, C. N., Praveen, S. P., & Ijaz, M. F. (2022). Using recurrent neural networks for predicting type-2 diabetes from genomic and tabular data. *Diagnostics*, 12(12), 3067.

11 Optimizing Diabetes Classification

Hybrid FLANN Model with Evolutionary Optimization Techniques

P. Pujari

11.1 INTRODUCTION

The increase of blood sugar levels due to diabetes mellitus is a persistent metabolic disorder that results in very serious health issues at a later stage of life. The damaging effects of diabetes mellitus on the health of people, along with the escalating cost of healthcare and countries' economies, make it even more imperative to achieve accurate prediction and management. Diabetes does have life-threatening complications, for example, heart disease, kidney failure, blindness, and amputation, which all greatly reduce the quality of healthy life style. These complications have a lot of implications for healthcare and they put pressure on healthcare in terms of cost and availability of resources. The constant increase in these costs is a result of frequent consultations, prescription and consumption of drugs, and admission to hospitals. From the implications of diabetes, it is clear that there is a great danger, and there is a huge need to come up with early prediction as well as management for the disease. Therefore, there is a requirement of more robust techniques within the realm of healthcare analytics to overcome the issues associated with diabetes by detecting it at early stage. From the literature, machine learning and artificial intelligence are found to be more suitable tools in the field of healthcare analytics with potentials to enhance the process of disease detection. On the other hand, evolutionary techniques are found to be more suitable in the field of optimization providing the best solutions to a given problem. The objective of this chapter is to construct a hybrid model by utilizing FLANN as the fundamental classifier and employing the DE optimization technique for the prediction of diabetes. The FLANN is a specific type of neural network architecture that does not include any hidden layers and hence reduces the overall computational complexity of the system. On the other hand, the DE optimization technique is more suitable for adjusting the parameters of the base classifier. In this chapter, the dataset collected from Kaggle, which includes observations of patients with or without diabetes is used to train and gain insights from data. The weight parameters of the FLANN classifier are fine-tuned with the DE optimization

DOI: 10.1201/9781003520184-14

technique to increase the generalization capability of the proposed hybrid model advancing in the domain of diabetes prediction.

11.2 LITERATURE REVIEW

In the past, numerous literary works have been proposed for building of efficient models for the prediction of diabetes utilizing artificial intelligence techniques. Reza et al. (2024) suggested a model for diabetes prognosis using two stacking-based ensemble models. The suggested model is applied on the PIMA Indian diabetes dataset and local healthcare data. For improving the classification accuracy of the model, they used classical and deep-learning-based ensemble models where the results generated by numerous classification models were combined. An accuracy of 96.50% was accomplished by arranging a collection of three neural network designs in a stacked manner. Tuppad and Patil (2024) suggested a novel machine-learning approach using a hybrid filter-wrapper technique for the prediction of prediabetes and type II diabetes. Clustering method based on agglomerative and visualization techniques based on dendrogram were used for the analysis of features. In addition, for local and global explanation of features, an explainability technique based on a model-agnostic method called Shapley additive explanation (SHAP) is used. An accuracy of 98.8% was obtained for type II diabetes, and 90.11% was obtained for prediabetes. El-Sofany et al. (2024) developed a machine-learning technique through a mobile app for the prediction of diabetes in Saudi Arabia. They employed a range of machine-learning methods and attained an accuracy of 97.4% with the XGBoost algorithm and the SMOTE feature selection method. In addition, the XAI technique SHAP was used for the explanation of model prediction. To access the implemented model, a mobile application was developed for the end user. Lugner et al. (2024) proposed a model using the XG-Boost algorithm and SHAP for identifying the top ten predicting factors for the development of type II diabetes. The model was applied to the UK Biobank dataset and the performance ability of the model was measured using the ROC curve, sensitivity, and specificity. Maniruzzaman et al. (2020) proposed a technique, which integrated feature selection approach based on LR approach and random forest classifier for the categorization of diabetes patients. With the National Health and Nutrition Examination Survey dataset the suggested techniques produced an accuracy of 94.25%. El-Bashbishy and El-Bakry (2024) suggested a model based on the deep-learning approach. With the Mansoura University Children's Hospital Diabetes (MUCHD) dataset the suggested model attained a 99.8% accuracy. Soumya and Raja (2024) have integrated latent Dirichlet allocation (LDA) and the artificial neural networks (ANN) technique for the classification of diabetes. The bivariate filter feature extraction technique was used to select the best features for classification. On the combined datasets of the PIMA Indian and the North California State University (NCSU) dataset, an accuracy of 93% was achieved. With CNN a self-adaptive optimization algorithm was proposed for prediction of diabetes (Chinnababu and Jayachandra, 2024). The Pima Indian Diabetes dataset (PIDD), collected from Frankfurt Hospital, Germany, and North California State University (NCSU) was used for the application purpose. The feature extraction phase utilized a chi-square-based feature selection technique. The proposed model underwent evaluation on

PIDD and German datasets, achieving accuracies of 99.87% and 99.99%, respectively. Various machine-learning methods were employed to predict the occurrence of chronic diabetes illness (Saeed, 2023). The efficacy of the model was evaluated using the PIMA Indian Diabetes dataset (PIMA) and the Behavioral Risk Factor Surveillance System (BRFSS) diabetes dataset. The suggested model achieved an area under the curve (AUC) of 96% for the PIMA dataset and 99% for the BRFSS dataset. Phongying and Hiriote (2023) suggested random forest machine-learning approach prediction. The suggested model attained an accuracy of 97%. Ghodeswar and Keote (2024) developed a model using naive Bays, XG-Boost, and random forest machine-learning techniques and obtained satisfactory results with these models when applied to the diabetes dataset from Kaggle. The deep-learning techniques, CNN and LSTM, were used for the prognosis of diabetes (Moussati et al., 2024). The model attained an accuracy of 97%. An ensemble model was proposed utilizing a range of machine-learning classifiers like k-NN, SVM, DT, RF, AdaBoost, and GNB (Oladimeji, Oladimeji, & Oladimeji, 2024). An accuracy of 98.87% was achieved with the ensemble model. Abnoosian, Farnoosh, and Behzadi (2023) introduced an approach that utilized a weighted ensemble model for the prognosis of diabetes. Hyper parameter tuning involved the utilization of optimization techniques such as grid search and Bayesian optimization. The proposed model achieved an accuracy of 98.87% as compared to other base machine-learning models.

From the literature review, these recent efforts emphasize the dynamic nature of diabetes prediction. These studies are enhancing our understanding of the risk factors, temporal patterns, and predictive abilities related to diabetes through the use of machine learning. These researches provide valuable insights into various methodologies that contribute to more accurate and prompt prediction of diabetes, making them valuable tools for healthcare professionals and researchers in the field of healthcare analytics. FLANN has demonstrated successful utilization in several application domains, as indicated by the literature review (Zhao & Zhang, 2009; Majhi, Panda, & Sahoo, 2009; Patra & Kot, 2002; Patra, Pal, Chatterji, & Panda, 1999; Patra, Chin, Meher, & Chakraborty, 2008; Patra & Bos, 2000; Majhi, Panda, & Sahoo, 2009; Anish & Majhi, 2016) such as nonlinear communication channels, prediction of exchange rate, identification of nonlinear dynamic system, equalization of nonlinear communication channel in wireless system, design of pressure sensor, stock marketing, and many more. Conversely, the differential evolution (DE) optimization algorithm has numerous benefits. Due to DE's exceptional ability to detect global optimization problems, a wide range of applications can get advantages from its utilization (Storn & Price, 1997). Qin, Huang, and Suganthan (2009) found that DE is robust against noise in objective functions and can effectively handle challenges such as uneven search spaces and unknown attributes. DE is a more straightforward and precise optimization method compared to certain other methods, as it involves less control parameters. Additionally, DE is particularly well-suited for solving multi-objective problems (Rakshit and Konar, 2015). DE can be efficiently parallelized on high-performance computer systems, allowing for effective optimization. The versatility and effectiveness of the FLANN and DE optimization method are showcased in numerous disciplines, such as engineering, data science, and healthcare, through their applications and advantages. This chapter presents a hybridization strategy that utilizes FLANN as the underlying classifier, where the weight parameters of the FLANN model are fine-tuned using the DE optimization technique. The chapter is structured in the following manner: the overview of this chapter is described in Section 11.1. Section 11.2 provides a description of the associated literary work, while Section 11.3 elaborates on the proposed technique. The simulation, experimental work carried out, and the findings are outlined in Section 11.4. Section 11.5 provides an account of the conclusion part.

11.3 PROPOSED METHODOLOGY

The proposed methodology integrates the FLANN classifier with the DE evolutionary algorithm to develop a hybrid model where the weight parameters of the FLANN classifier are fine-tuned with the DE optimization technique. The hybrid model is applied to the diabetes dataset collected from the Kaggle website. The dataset contains features which are highly important in the prediction of diabetes and target indicating patient's diabetes condition, which may be diabetic, nondiabetic, or predict-diabetic. FLANN is used as a base classifier for the prediction of diabetes. A number of other evolutionary algorithms, like the genetics algorithm (GA), particle swarm optimization (PSO), DE, clonal selection algorithm (CSA), cat swarm algorithm (CSO), and ant colony optimization (ACO), are also used with the FLANN classifier to create the most resilient model for diabetes prediction. The outcomes of various hybrid models are contrasted to find the most efficient model.

11.3.1 FUNCTIONAL LINK ARTIFICIAL NEURAL NETWORK (FLANN)

One advantage of artificial neural networks is the solution that they solve highly nonlinear problems. In a multi-layer perceptron (MLP) as the number of hidden layers increases, it needs more time to adjust its weight vector, which increases the computational complexity of the neuron. Therefore, the FLANN model is selected for adoption in this chapter (Anish & Majhi, 2016). FLANN is a neural network architecture that does not have any hidden layers and is considered to be of higher quality or better than others. Due to the nonlinear expansion procedure, it provides a nonlinear decision boundary for robust decision control. In this study, trigonometric function is used to expand each input into five terms. The FLANN model's architecture is depicted in Figure 11.1 with trigonometric expansion. The trigonometric function expansion includes basic models and expressions based on sin and cosine expansions. Trigonometrically, each input is expanded into five terms, as shown below:

$$Z_i = \left[z_i \quad \sin(\pi z_i) \quad \cos(\pi z_i) \quad \sin(3\pi z_i) \quad \cos(3\pi z_i) \right] \quad \text{where } 0 \le i \le n \tag{1}$$

11.3.2 DIFFERENTIAL EVOLUTION

The hybrid model is formed with the integration of the FLANN classifier and DE optimization algorithm (Quaranta, Marano, Greco, and Monti, 2014). One of the advantages of the FLANN model is its lower computational complexity due to the

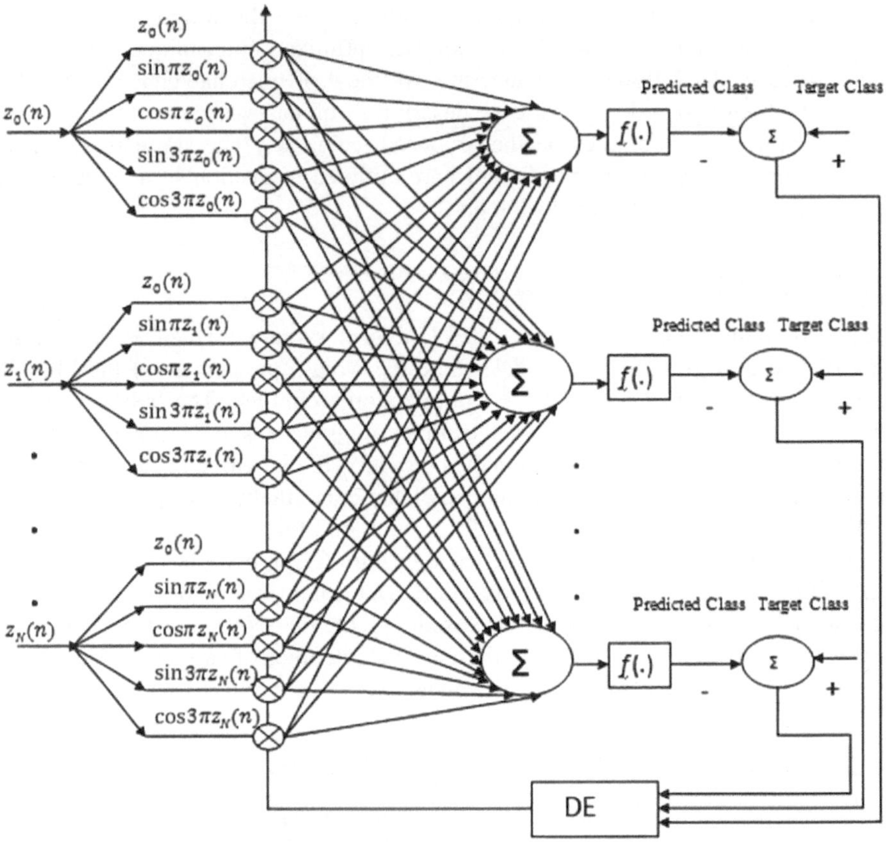

FIGURE 11.1 Architecture of the FLANN-based DE algorithm with trigonometric expansion.

nonexistence of hidden layers. For several nondifferentiable, noncontinuous, and nonlinear optimization problems, the DE algorithm is found to be more suitable. DE is a bio-inspired evolutionary algorithm that is adaptive and can deal with the problems of local minima over continuous space. It is free from gradient-based algorithm, which uses population-based bio-inspired techniques. It is widely used in disciplines, such as machine learning, engineering, scientific research, etc., because it helps to optimize particularly common and diverse tasks. Population growth is a viable solution propagated by DE often. In the DE optimization algorithm, each solution, or "individual" parameter, is represented as a vector. The three main steps in the algorithm are mutation, crossover, and selection. In the mutation step, new candidate solutions are formed by calculating the weighted disparity between two randomly chosen vectors and then adding it to the third vector. In crossover operation, a "trial vector" is generated by combining an existing individual from the population with the mutant vector according to a crossover factor, $Cross_r$. This step helps in exploring various areas of the solution space for an optimal solution. In the selection step, a comparison is made between the trial vector and the target vector. The trial vector is evaluated to find a better solution. Out of the two vectors, the vector that provides a better solution is considered for the next generation.

11.3.3 General Steps of the DE-Based Evolutionary Technique

General steps of the hybrid FLANN_DE model (Mohapatra and Patra, 2012) is as follows:

Step1: Randomly choose N_p number of individuals $\vec{Y}_{i,\text{gen}}$, which is the ith individual of gen^{th} generation.
Step 2: Let $f_i = f\left(\vec{Y}_{i,\text{gen}}\right)$ for $i = 1$ to N_p, here f_i is the fitness of ith individual at gen^{th} generation.
Step 3: Iterate through the following steps until a specified stopping criterion is met.
Step 4: For $i = 1$ to N_p iterate all the following steps.
Step 5: Between 1 to N_p $\left(\text{where } i \neq \text{rand}_0 \neq \text{rand}_1 \neq \text{rand}_2\right)$ select three indices randomly as $\text{rand}_0, \text{rand}_1, \text{rand}_2$.
Step 6: Then calculate the mutant vector using the following equation:

$$\vec{V}_{i,\text{gen}} = \vec{Y}_{\text{rand}_0,\text{gen}} + F\left(\vec{Y}_{\text{rand}_1,\text{gen}} - \vec{Y}_{\text{rand}_2,\text{gen}}\right) \tag{2}$$

Take the value of F within the range [0.0 to 1.0].

Step 7: For $j = 1$ to N reiterate the procedures from 8 to 9.
Step 8: Get two random numbers rand_j and j_{rand} where $\left(0 \leq \text{rand}_j < 1\right)$ and j_{rand} index is less than N and equal to or greater than 1, i.e., $(1 \leq r_{\text{rand}} < N)$.
Step 9: Evaluate the trial vector $\vec{U}_{i,\text{gen}}$. If $\text{rand}_j \leq \text{Cross}_r$ or $j = j_{\text{rand}}$ then

$$U_{j,i,\text{gen}} = V_{j,i,\text{gen}} \quad \text{else} \quad U_{j,i,\text{gen}} = Y_{j,i,\text{gen}} \tag{3}$$

Take the value of crossover factor Cross_r from 0.0 to 0.1.
Step 10: carry out selection as, if $f\left(\vec{U}_{i,\text{gen}}\right) \leq f_{i,\text{gen}}$ then $\vec{Y}_{i,\text{gen}+1} = \vec{U}_{i,\text{gen}}$ and

$$f_i = f\left(\vec{U}_{i,\text{gen}}\right) \quad \text{else} \quad \vec{Y}_{i,\text{gen}+1} = \vec{Y}_{i,\text{gen}} \tag{4}$$

Figure 11.2 shows the structural outline of the DE optimization technique.

11.3.4 Steps of the FLANN_DE Hybrid Model for Prediction of Diabetes

(a) Represent each individual in the population by N weight parameters in the FLANN architecture. Take population of M size and initialize the population

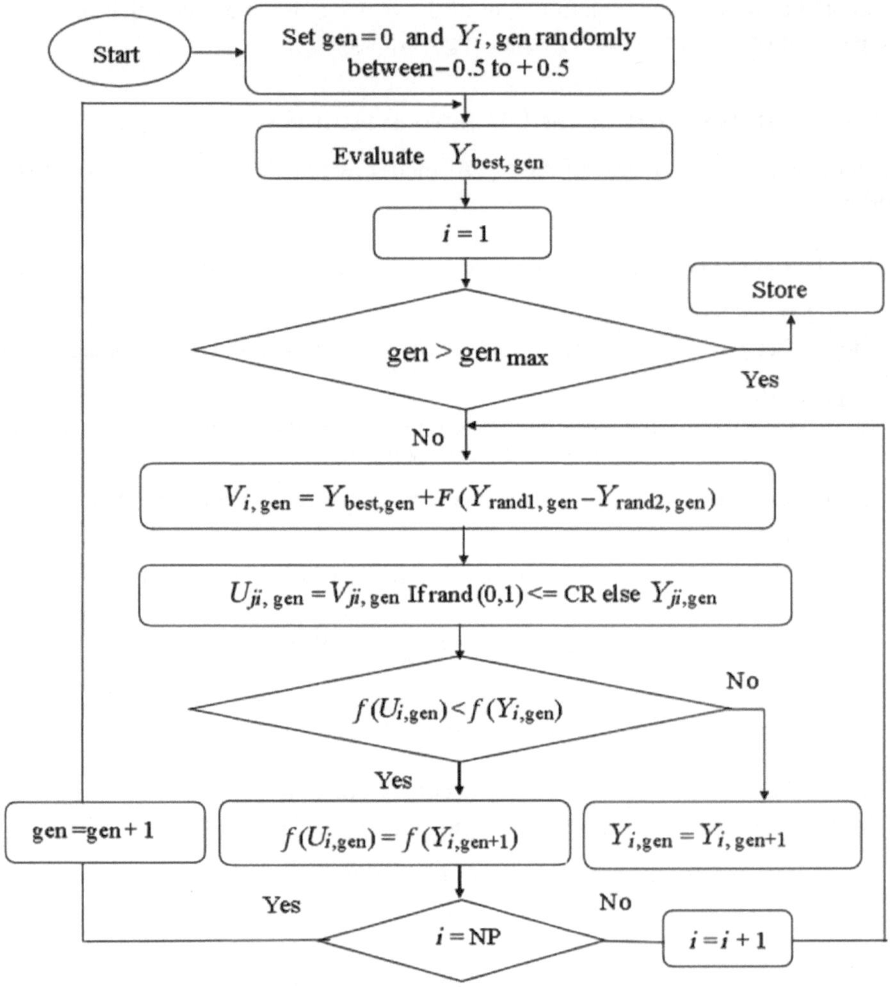

FIGURE 11.2 Structural outline of the differential evolution technique.

randomly where weights of the FLANN classifier are represented by the mth member of the population.

(b) Take K numbers of inputs from feature vector. Next, apply trigonometric expansion to each element of the inputs, resulting in five nonlinear values for each element.

(c) Determine the estimated outputs y_i using following equation:

$$y_i = \sum_{n=1}^{N} \text{weight}_n x_n \tag{5}$$

where x_n represents trigonometrically expanded input sample and weight$_n$ represents the weights of FLANN classifier.

(d) Generate K errors using following equation:

$$\text{error}_i(k) = d(k) - y_i(k) \quad \text{where} \quad k = 1 \; to \; K \tag{6}$$

where $\text{error}_i(k)$ is the i_{th} error, $d(k)$ is the desired error and $y_i(k)$ is the i_{th} predicted error.

(e) Compute the mean square error (MSE) of the ith member to find the fitness value using (7).

$$\text{MSE}(i) = \frac{\sum_{k=1}^{K} \text{error}_i^2}{K} \tag{7}$$

Above process is iterated for M number of times.

(f) Using the DE algorithm to minimize MSE.
(g) Using (2) to calculate the mutant vector.
(h) Using (3) to obtain trial vectors using crossover operation.
(i) According to the lowest MSE criteria, choose individuals for the next generation. For a desired number of generations, repeat the total process.
(j) When the classification model reaches to the minimum MSE (MMSE) and there is no change in MMSE value, stop the process of training. Now the weights obtained gives the best optimized solution for the FLANN classifier.

11.4 SIMULATION STUDY OF FLANN_DE MODEL

The suggested hybrid FLANN_DE model's performance is assessed by a simulation-based experiment carried out with python software. The proposed model is applied to the diabetes dataset from the Kaggle website. The dataset contains 1000 samples with three classes. The FLANN is selected as the adaptive recognition model, and the DE optimization approach is used to update its weights. 90% of the dataset is given for training and 10% for testing. In order to introduce nonlinearity into the recognition model, each input is expanded using trigonometric expansion to include five terms. The FLANN model utilizes the sigmoid activation function to introduce additional nonlinearity. Every input sample's error term is produced by finding the difference between the expected and estimated outputs. Next, MSE is calculated using the error terms. The MMSE is considered as the fitness value, which gradually decreases as the training process progresses. The parameters chosen in this simulation study are as follows: a population size of 40, a scale factor (F) value of 0.001, a cross over operator (Cr) value of 0.45, and 5000 number of generations are taken to fine tune the model. The proposed hybrid model is also contrasted with other FLANN-based evolutionary models like FLANN-based genetic algorithm (FLANN_GA), FLANN-based clonal selection algorithm (FLANN_CSA), FLANN-based particle swarm optimization (FLANN_PSO), and FLANN-based ant colony optimization (FLANN_ACO) models. Figure 11.3 shows the convergence graph of all hybrid models during the training process. From the graph, the FLANN_

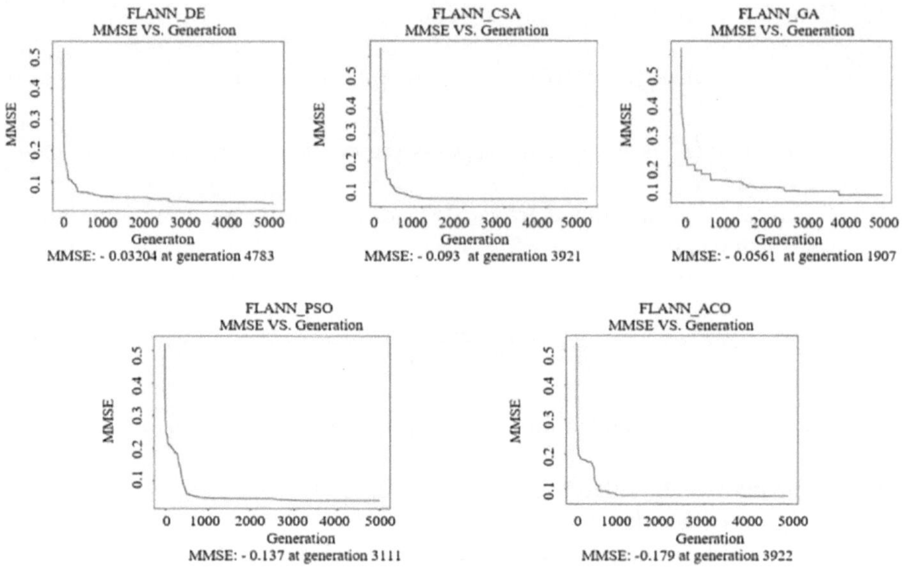

FIGURE 11.3 Convergence graph of different models during training.

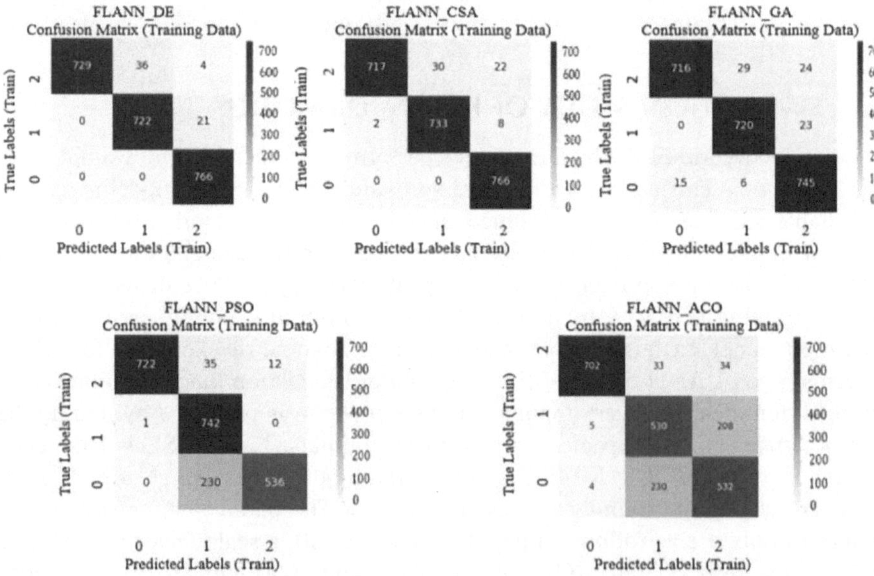

FIGURE 11.4 Confusion matrix of different hybrid models on training data.

DE model offers the best convergence among the hybrid models. Figure 11.4 and Figure 11.5 represents the confusion matrix of several hybrid models for the training and testing dataset, respectively. Table 11.1 represents the performance measures of all hybrid models. From experimental result, the suggested FLANN_DE model

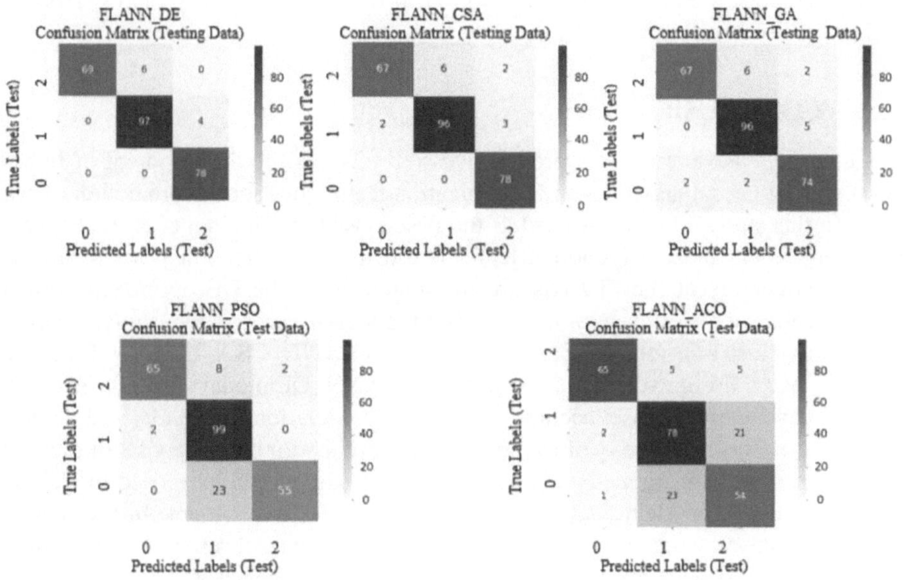

FIGURE 11.5 Confusion matrix of different hybrid models on test data.

TABLE 11.1
Various Performance Measures of Hybrid Models on Test Data

Hybrid Models	Accuracy	Precision	Recall	F1 Score
FLANN_DE	96.06 %	96.43 %	96.01 %	96.14 %
FLANN_CSA	94.88 %	95.06 %	94.79 %	94.84 %
FLANN_GA	93.30 %	93.58 %	93.08 %	93.26 %
FLANN_PSO	86.22 %	89.88 %	85.06 %	86.24 %
FLANN_ACO	77.55 %	78.21 %	77.55 %	77.80

performed better at predicting diabetes than the other FLANN-based evolutionary models. The hybrid model's efficacy is measured by using standard performance indicators like accuracy, precision, recall, and F1 score. From the experimental result it is found that the FLANN_DE hybrid model outperformed other models and achieved an accuracy of 96.06 %, precision of 96.43%, recall of 96.01%, and an F1 score of 96.14%. With an accuracy of 94.88%, precision of 95.06%, recall of 94.79%, and an F1 score of 94.84%, the FLANN_CSA model also performed well. The FLANN_GA model followed closely, with an accuracy of 93.30%, precision of 93.58%, recall of 93.08%, and an F1 score of 93.26%. Comparatively lower performance is achieved by FLANN_CSO hybrid model. Lowest performance is observed by the FLANN_ACO hybrid model. The experimental result highlights the effectiveness of different optimization techniques with FLANN as a classifier. Such findings show the engagement of optimization strategies in elevating the efficiency of the prediction models. Among all, the proposed FLANN_DE model performed well in the prediction of diabetes.

11.5 CONCLUSION

This comprehensive study is a progressive step towards the development of hybrid models using neural networks and optimization techniques for the prediction of diabetes. In this study, FLANN is used as the base classifier. The inputs of the FLANN classifier are expanded trigonometrically before the classification process and the weight parameters of the FLANN are fine-tuned using the DE optimization technique to enhance the efficacy of the suggested model. A comparative study is carried out among the hybrid models like FLANN_GA, FLANN_CSA, FLANN_PSO, and FLANN_ACO. From experimental study, the FLANN_DE model outperformed with an impressive testing dataset accuracy of 96.06 % in relation to other hybrid models. This work reveals the novelty of the suggested approach for the prognosis of diabetes in the field of healthcare analytics. In predictive modeling, the proposed model is a robust technique for identification precise diabetes risk assessment. In the field of healthcare analytics, the proposed work is highly beneficial for researchers to explore various hybridization techniques across different clinical scenarios.

REFERENCES

Abnoosian, K., Farnoosh, R., & Behzadi, M. H. (2023). Prediction of diabetes disease using an ensemble of machine learning multi-classifier models. *BMC Bioinformatics*, 24(1), 337. https://doi.org/10.1186/s12859-023-05465-z

Anish, C. M., & Majhi, B. (2016). Hybrid nonlinear adaptive scheme for stock market prediction using feedback FLANN and factor analysis. *Journal of the Korean Statistical Society*, 45(1), 64–76. https://doi.org/10.1016/j.jkss.2015.07.002

Chinnababu, S. K., & Jayachandra, A. (2024). Diabetes prediction and classification using self-adaptive evolutionary algorithm with convolutional neural network. *International Journal of Intelligent Engineering and Systems*, 17(3), 460–472. https://doi.org/10.22266/ijies2024.0630.36

El-Bashbishy, A. E.-S., & El-Bakry, H. M. (2024). Pediatric diabetes prediction using deep learning. *Scientific Reports*, 14(1), 2206. https://doi.org/10.1038/s41598-024-51438-4

El-Sofany, H., El-Seoud, S. A., Karam, O. H., El-Latif, Y. M. A., & Taj-Eddin, I. T. F. (2024). A proposed technique using machine learning for the prediction of diabetes disease through a mobile app. *International Journal of Intelligent Systems*, 2024, 1–13. https://doi.org/10.1155/2024/6688934

Ghodeswar, U., & Keote, M. (2024). Analysis of diabetic prediction and regression system using machine learning algorithms. *Journal of Electrical Systems*, 19(4), 750–762. https://doi.org/10.52783/jes.2999

Lugner, M., Rawshani, A., Helleryd, E., & Eliasson, B. (2024). Identifying top ten predictors of type 2 diabetes through machine learning analysis of UK Biobank data. *Scientific Reports*, 14(1), 2102. https://doi.org/10.1038/s41598-024-52023-5

Majhi, R., Panda, G., & Sahoo, G. (2009). Development and performance evaluation of FLANN based model for forecasting of stock markets. *Expert Systems with Applications*, 36(3), 6800–6808. https://doi.org/10.1016/j.eswa.2008.08.008

Majhi, R., Panda, G., & Sahoo, G. (2009). Efficient prediction of exchange rates with low complexity artificial neural network models. *Expert Systems with Applications*, 36(1), 181–189. https://doi.org/10.1016/j.eswa.2007.09.005

Maniruzzaman, M., Rahman, M. J., Ahammed, B., & Abedin, M. M. (2020). Classification and prediction of diabetes disease using machine learning paradigm. *Health Information Science and Systems*, 8(1), 7. https://doi.org/10.1007/s13755-019-0095-z

Mohapatra, P., & Patra, T. (2012). Indian stock market prediction using differential evolutionary neural network model. *International Journal of Engineering, Computing and Control Technologies*, 2, 159–166.

Moussati, A. E., Ayat, Y., Benzekri, W., Mir, I., Benzaouia, M., & Elaouni, A. (2024). Novel diabetes classification approach based on CNN-LSTM: Enhanced performance and accuracy. *Diagnostyka*, 1–15. https://doi.org/10.29354/diag/183633

Oladimeji, O. O., Oladimeji, A., & Oladimeji, O. (2024). Classification models for likelihood prediction of diabetes at early stage using feature selection. *Applied Computing and Informatics*, 20(3/4), 279–286. https://doi.org/10.1108/ACI-01-2021-0022

Patra, J. C., & Bos, A. (2000). Modelling of an intelligent pressure sensor using functional link artificial neural networks. *ISA Transactions*, 39(1), 15–17. https://hdl.handle.net/10356/94343

Patra, J. C., Chin, W. C., Meher, P. K., & Chakraborty, G. (2008). Legendre-FLANN based nonlinear channel equalization in wireless communication system. In *Proceedings of the IEEE International Conference on Systems, Man, and Cybernetics* (pp. 1826–1831). IEEE. https://doi.org/10.1109/ICSMC.2008.4811554

Patra, J. C., & Kot, A. C. (2002). Nonlinear dynamic system identification using Chebyshev functional link artificial neural networks. *IEEE Transactions on Systems, Man, and Cybernetics. Part B: Cybernetics*, 32(4), 505–511. https://doi.org/10.1109/TSMCB.2002.1018769

Patra, J. C., Pal, R. N., Chatterji, B. N., & Panda, G. (1999). Identification of nonlinear dynamic systems using functional link artificial neural networks. *IEEE Transactions on Systems, Man, and Cybernetics. Part B: Cybernetics*, 29(2), 254–262. https://doi.org/10.1109/3477.752797

Phongying, M., & Hiriote, S. (2023). Diabetes classification using machine learning techniques. *Computation*, 11(5), 96. https://doi.org/10.3390/computation11050096

Qin, A. K., Huang, V. L., & Suganthan, P. N. (2009). Differential evolution algorithm with strategy adaptation for global numerical optimization. *IEEE Transactions on Evolutionary Computation*, 13(2), 398–417. https://doi.org/10.1109/TEVC.2008.927706

Quaranta, G., Marano, G. C., Greco, R., & Monti, G. (2014). Parametric identification of seismic isolators using differential evolution and particle swarm optimization. *Applied Soft Computing*, 22, 458–464. https://doi.org/10.1016/j.asoc.2014.04.039

Rakshit, P., & Konar, A. (2015). Differential evolution for noisy multi-objective optimization. *Artificial Intelligence*, 227, 165–189. https://doi.org/10.1016/j.artint.2015.01.004

Reza, M. S., Amin, R., Yasmin, R., Kulsum, W., & Ruhi, S. (2024). Improving diabetes disease patients classification using stacking ensemble method with PIMA and local healthcare data. *Heliyon*, 10(2), e24536. https://doi.org/10.1016/j.heliyon.2024.e24536

Saeed, M. A. H. (2023). Diabetes type 2 classification using machine learning algorithms with up-sampling technique. *Journal of Electrical Systems and Information Technology*, 10(8). https://doi.org/10.1186/s43067-023-00074-5

Soumya, K. N., & Raja, P. K. N. (2024). Diabetes Mellitus disease prediction and classification using Latent Dirichlet Allocation and Artificial Neural Network classifier. *International Journal of Intelligent Systems and Applications in Engineering*, 12(10s), 98–106. Retrieved from https://ijisae.org/index.php/IJISAE/article/view/4353

Storn, R., & Price, K. (1997). Differential evolution – A simple and efficient heuristic for global optimization over continuous spaces. *Journal of Global Optimization*, 11(4), 341–359. https://doi.org/10.1023/A:1008202821328

Tuppad, A., & Patil, S. D. (2024). An efficient classification framework for Type 2 diabetes incorporating feature interactions. *Expert Systems with Applications*, 239, 122138. https://doi.org/10.1016/j.eswa.2023.122138

Zhao, H., & Zhang, J. (2009). Adaptively combined FIR and functional link artificial neural network equalizer for nonlinear communication channel. *IEEE Transactions on Neural Networks*, 20(4), 665–674. https://doi.org/10.1109/TNN.2008.2011481

12 Leveraging Technology for Healthcare Transformation

Telemedicine and Remote Health Monitoring

S.N. Kumar, Prabu Selvam, Jomin Joy, Nicole Rakov and Alan James

12.1 INTRODUCTION

Telemedicine utilizes information and communication technology to ensure efficient healthcare for the society. The easy accessibility, low cost, and ease of time management for patients are the key advantages of telemedicine, security and technology barriers are the challenges. Telemedicine is part of telehealth, a broader term encompassing various remote healthcare services. Remote patient monitoring (RPM) is a vital aspect of telemedicine, involving real-time collection and analysis of patient health data using wearable devices and sensors. RPM enhances chronic condition management and provides valuable insights into patients' well-being. It complements telemedicine by enabling continuous monitoring outside traditional clinical settings, improving patient outcomes, and reducing healthcare costs. It creates a revolution in the healthcare sector by providing services to remote locations and enhancing patient care under emergency conditions. The increased patient appointments, low cost, and timely attention are features, however, the internet facility is a challenge in many rural areas. Figure 12.1 represents the layout of telemedicine.
Telemedicine comprises the following:

- Real-time sessions that enable patients and healthcare professionals to interact virtually, enabling diagnosis, primary treatment planning, and follow-up care.
- Transmission of patient data with the aid of wearable sensors and devices in real-time mode enables the continuous monitoring of chronic disease.
- Transmission of healthcare data, such as scan images or lab test results, termed an asynchronous mode for evaluation and diagnosis by healthcare professionals.
- Utilization of smartphones and tablets for healthcare delivery, including medication reminders, symptom tracking, and access to educational resources.

DOI: 10.1201/9781003520184-15

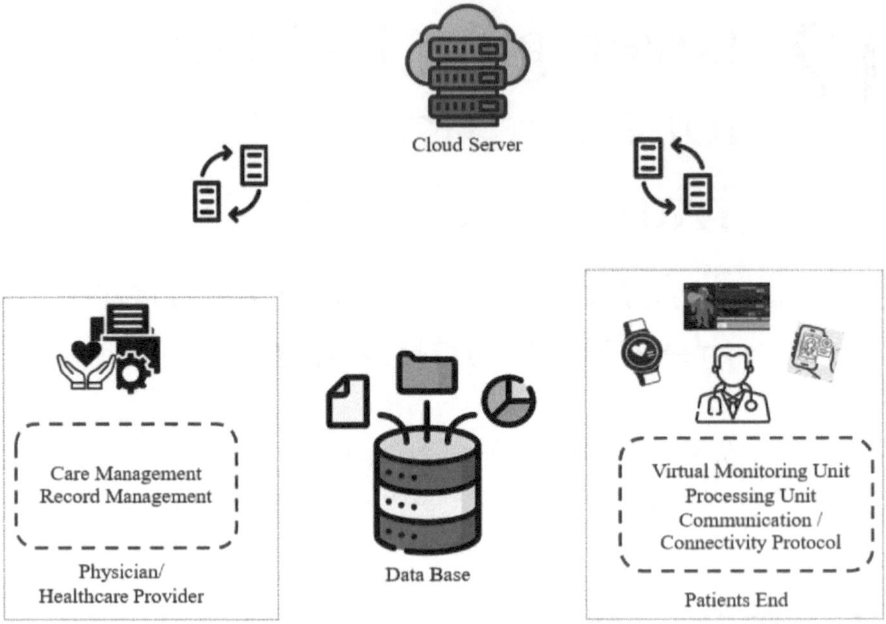

FIGURE 12.1 Layout of telemedicine.

12.2 THE EVOLUTION OF TELEMEDICINE

The development of telemedicine can be traced back historically, beginning with simple remote methods of communication and ending with the advanced digital healthcare technologies available today (Bashshur, 2009). The development of telemedicine originated in the early 1900s when radios were used to give medical advice to ships at sea. NASA and the U.S. Indian Health Service were among the first organizations to use technology for communication for distant medical consultations in the 1960s and 1970s. The establishment of telemedicine was greatly aided by the internet and advancements in telecommunications infrastructure. Improved effectiveness and efficiency in remote healthcare services have been rendered possible by mobile devices, high-speed internet, and modern medical software. Telemedicine has been developed along with its most ahead application in the medical field. This review offers a wide framework for evaluating the opportunities and challenges associated with the advent of e-medicine by presenting several telemedicine examples from a range of applications (Saechow et al., 2014). These examples give a glimpse into a home telemedicine system for diabetic care, a military teleradiology system, and teleconsultations utilized in neurosurgery and hemodialysis. A framework for comprehending the progression of telemedicine applications through four stages is presented, drawing on telemedicine's history, growth, and examples. The various stages consist of the following: (a) the advancement of fundamental technological skills; (b) the creation of pertinent applications; (c) the incorporation of technical applications into a complicated setting; and (d) the modification of the computing

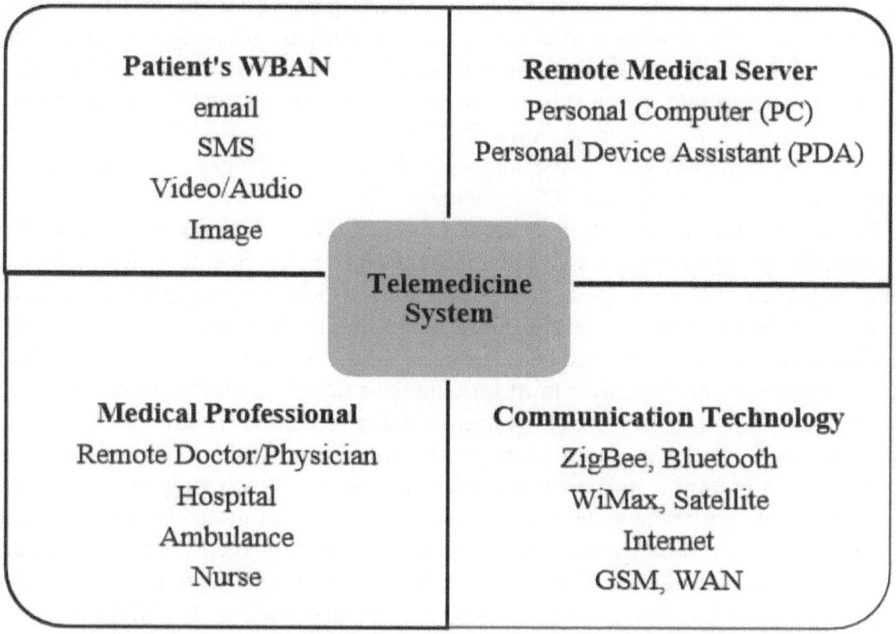

FIGURE 12.2 Components of telemedicine.

environment. As new technologies become available, new applications are realized, and these technologies are gradually incorporated into the field of medicine, and telemedicine applications are growing. Telemedicine emphasizes the significance of acknowledging the transition process and the opportunities it brings by providing answers to particular healthcare issues and expanding our understanding of where healthcare can be given (Mun, 1999). The components of telemedicine are depicted in Figure 12.2.

In Whitten et al. (2006), the authors provide a thorough examination of the creation of telemedicine in the US, emphasizing three important stages in the process: data transfer and storage, synchronous versus asynchronous modalities, and automating robotics and decision-making. It highlights how crucial it is for engineers, scholars of society, and medical professionals to work with transdisciplinary to solve obstacles and establish goals for the advancement of telemedicine in the future. To drive future telemedicine breakthroughs, the study proposes cooperation among engineers, social scientists, and medical experts and concludes by highlighting the roadblocks that telemedicine faces.

To improve patient care and access to medical resources, it highlights the necessity of developing an agenda for future telemedicine development and stresses the significance of fusing advances in technology with healthcare services (Whitten et al., 2006).

The investigation looks into the history, current circumstances, and possible future directions of wireless medical technology in the ever-changing field of medical technology. Starting with its historical origins and proceeding forward to its pivotal position in the provision of contemporary healthcare, an analysis of the revolutionary influence of telemedicine is conducted. The narrative examines emerging technologies reshaping the healthcare industry while navigating ethical dilemmas. It demonstrates how it can break down obstacles to accessibility and promote diversity. In Mallipeddi et al. (2017), the authors analyze the challenges and limitations of current medical technology and telemedicine.

The present stage of healthcare is more important due to the increasing popularity of telemedicine, which would have laid milestones for various practices. Telemedicine has achieved extensive acceptance by people due to technological advancements in the medical field inventions and practices. According to the emergency declared by the Centres for Medicare & Medicaid Services (CMS) on March 17, 2020, it is clear that telemedicine practices are a must for clinicians to offer patient care in hospitals, clinics, nursing homes, and other locations related to healthcare around the states. Moreover, new steps have been taken in place to ensure patient care privacy and safety. This minimum resource modality's ease makes it much simpler for doctors to communicate with others and provides an accurate substitute for patients who are not able to see doctors in person due to factors such as medical reasons or social intellections. Nonetheless, it is necessary to foster comfort and relationships between doctors and patients given the subjective nature of the practice. It is impossible to overestimate the future effects of telemedicine on healthcare settings, especially for hospice and assisted living homes where it has the potential to enhance senior citizen monitoring and treatment effectiveness. Contemporary developments like remote patient monitoring systems can serve as safety nets for patients in clinics, and increasing the availability of electronic health records (EHRs) will significantly increase the range of available treatments. However, community reimbursement and doctors' ability to continuously provide in-person services are prerequisites for the growth of telehealth. Doctors and other medical professionals also need to incorporate these new technologies into their practices while upholding patient autonomy and security principles (Paul, 1999).

During the COVID-19 pandemic, most medical areas saw an increase in the use of remote video consultations (VC) to reduce the risk of infections (Feldheim et al., 2023). Telemedicine in neuro-oncology does present some special opportunities and challenges. There currently needs to be more evidence-based insights available to assess and maybe modify existing concepts. To close this gap, we examined over 3,700 neuro-oncological consultations, of which more than 300 were performed as virtual consultations per patient request. This enabled us to identify how both groups of patients differ from one another. We also used an anonymous survey to look at the reasons given by patients, appropriate and inappropriate encounters, advantages and disadvantages of venture capital, and potential future directions. Patients who took part in virtual communities (VC) had worse clinical outcomes, higher malignancy grades, more glioblastoma diagnoses, and longer trip distances (all $p < 0.01$). Except for initial consultations, virtually every conversation in which patients opted to participate (>70%) was deemed to be a completely suitable substitute for in-person consultations. The majority of participants favored virtual consultation (VC) over phone consultation, however, they would rather switch between the two modalities.

Patients felt guaranteed with VC, and participants wanted to see more telemedicine modalities (such apps) used in neuro-oncology. In neuro-oncology, VC is a possible advantageous adjunct to patient therapy. Patients and communications, however, ought to be selected separately (Feldheim et al, 2023).

Numerous technology tools that enable patients to remotely access a wide range of care services are revolutionizing traditional healthcare through telemedicine. Telemedicine's growth is likely to reshape the field of healthcare in the EU in the years to come, primarily influencing how the health systems of the member states are structured and how much health protection is provided throughout the EU. Since there is now no EU legal framework for telemedicine, the purpose of this analysis is to examine the most pertinent acts that were recently published in the (traditional) healthcare sector and determine whether or not they are appropriate for use with telemedicine services. To preserve telemedicine's growth in everyday practice and to provide instructions, the necessity for a suitable regulatory system in the EU will be addressed throughout the conclusion (Botrugno, 2018).

The study (Pramanik et al., 2019) offers an architecture and protocols for employing wireless body area networks (WBAN) to enable remote health monitoring in e-healthcare, in the context of telemedicine. It addresses the design factors and difficulties in WBAN-based systems for remote health tracking and suggests a thorough architecture to deal with these difficulties. Enabling simultaneous data transfer, reception, and analysis of physiological parameters taking place, the overall system consists of sensor nodes, a WBAN controller, a healthcare provider server, and the patient's cell phone. The information sharing, data transfer, and security processes within the suggested architecture are also covered in the chapter. The applicability of the put-forward architecture and protocols for facilitating wireless health monitoring via WBANs is made crisp and clear by the implementation. Since the system uses the mobile phone of the patient to send data to the server it does not require additional aid for this process. Also, the protocols guarantee effective data aggression, significantly lowering the transmission overhead and making real-time health monitoring credible. In a nutshell, it is suggested that architecture and standards offer a compelling foundation for transitioning e-healthcare beyond telemedicine and toward WBAN-based remote health monitoring. The system tackles major design issues as well as obstacles, promoting optimal communication and data analysis, thereby elevating the general standard and accessibility of medical services. The successful use of the methodology indicates its efficacy and efficiency in providing remote health monitoring, which could eventually contribute to beneficial patient outcomes (Pramanik et al., 2019).

In Whitten (2010), the authors examine the vital components needed to establish a telemedicine program that will operate for a while to come. Stakeholder involvement in order monetary viability, regulatory compliance, technological systems, and provider and patient contentment comprise some of the crucial factors listed. This research work underscores the necessity of using a blended approach in both the preparation and execution of telemedicine services to guarantee their long-term survival and accomplishments. Effective telemedicine programs, according to the research, are built on sturdy technologies that offer dependable and secure communication. Popularity and use are dependent on involvement from stakeholder groups,

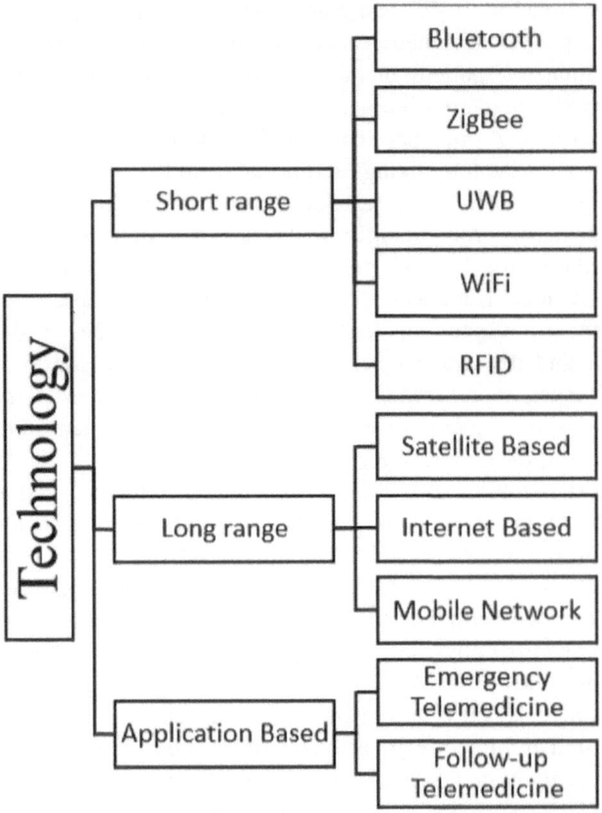

FIGURE 12.3 Telemedicine technological communication categorization.

specifically from healthcare providers and patients, and legal and ethical obstacles need to be resolved through regulatory compliance. Figure 12.3 depicts the technologies used in telemedicine.

The study investigates the body of present data to identify the elements which influence efficient telemedicine deployments (Broens et al., 2007). It analyses the conclusions of multiple research investigations that identify the essential variables underlying the long-term sustainability as well as the success of telemedicine initiatives. There are a number of reasons: user popularity, legal and regulatory structures, fiscal concerns, technological infrastructure, and administrative preparedness for each event. The intention is to provide an in-depth awareness of the crucial elements that contribute to rendering telemedicine operations success. Effective telemedicine implementation depends on numerous fundamental components. The easy access to trustworthy, high-quality technology is crucial above every other consideration. This includes having efficient computer apparatus, software, and networking services that promote safe and rapid interactions. Being adopted by users entails an agreement on behalf of patients as well as doctors to embrace telemedicine, which is a further important factor.

This popularity can be affected by the technology's ostensible effectiveness, ease of use, and confidence. Clear administrative and legislative frameworks that address challenges, including security, privacy, licensure, and remuneration, are required to direct the utilization of telemedicine. Sustainable financial models are a further aspect that should be taken into consideration. These forms of business should have sufficient financing, affordable cost strategies, and insurance procedures for reimbursement that ensure that they are financially viable. Lastly, for medical facilities to successfully utilize telemedicine, organizations must have the requisite people, and infrastructure, along with effective operations. A summary of the research is, that successful telemedicine placements require an amalgamation of technological, human, financial, regulatory, and cultural considerations. The ongoing performance and long-term sustainability of telemedicine operations depend upon many variables, including the preservation of trustworthy technology, growth of acceptance by patients, and development of transparent regulations. A variety of variables must be addressed for the effective running and continued viability of telemedicine courses, which includes the upkeep of reliable infrastructure, the encouragement of user acceptability, the construction of visible administrative and regulatory frameworks, getting hold of credible financial models, and the current state of healthcare businesses. By resolving these factors, telemedicine can dramatically enhance both the quality and accessibility of medical services provided by traditional healthcare delivery (Broens et al., 2007).

12.3 BENEFITS OF TELEMEDICINE AND REMOTE HEALTH MONITORING

The use of technology to give healthcare from a distance has been proven to be an effective way of overcoming certain barriers for people in rural and isolated places. There is a shortage of physicians, and telemedicine can fill in the gaps in the essential treatment that is provided to rural populations. With the advancement of wearable and portable embedded physiological and cognitive monitoring systems, medical professionals will be able to take care of patients without having to admit them to a hospital. Thus, this real-time monitoring could allow a team to handle patient issues before they require serious intervention at a hospital (Ee et al., 2011).

In rural areas or isolated communities, patients may benefit from hospital services since it allows them to get treatment from doctors who are far away. Consultations online help patients avoid the stress and inconvenience of in-person appointments by allowing them to receive consultations from home. One of the pluses of telemedicine is that patient's time and expense of travel can be reduced. Providing access to medical guidance and support to patients might save lives when an emergency arises (Imberti et al., 2021). The benefits of telemedicine are depicted in Figure 12.4.

Continuous health monitoring can be made possible through equipment like glucose meters, heart rate monitors, and blood pressure monitors. Patients can manage their health by having access to real-time data. The doctors can make sure that patients are recovering as per plan after surgery or hospitalization with the help of monitoring equipment. The merging of telemedicine and remote monitoring ensures supervision and medical guidance. During pandemics and natural calamities, health services were

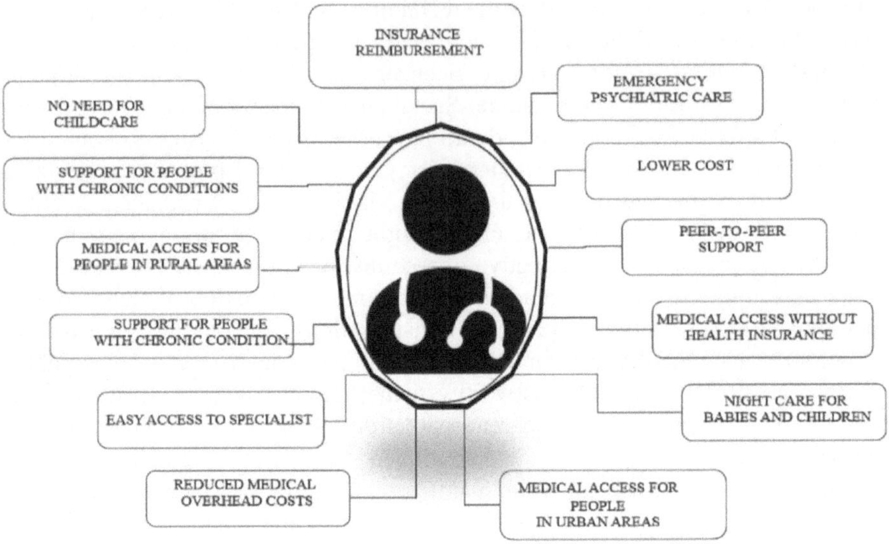

FIGURE 12.4 Benefits of telemedicine.

not interrupted without affecting conventional healthcare facilities with the help of telemedicine, thus improving patient satisfaction and health outcomes.

12.3.1 Challenges and Barriers to Adoption

There are several obstacles and hurdles to the broad use of telemedicine and remote health monitoring, even though they have many advantages. Financial, social, governmental, and technological aspects are among them. Resources are not typically allocated to assessment since it is rarely viewed as a necessary component of implementation. It is not always viable to collect baseline data in the future since resources are allocated after deployment. The process of collecting health information retrospectively poses several difficulties with the selection of relevant sources and methods of collection. These problems make evaluating many programs more difficult, and the particulars of telemedicine evaluation add even more challenges (Brear, 2006).

The lack of access to high-speed internet and advanced technologies in rural and underdeveloped areas impedes telemedicine adoption. The telecentre's broadband 3G connectivity has not been all that great. Remote monitoring and virtual consultations can be interfered with by technical difficulties, software defects, and network problems. The primary issue causing users to become frustrated with the system is the lengthy wait times for the patient's record to be downloaded or uploaded. Telehealth platforms can be difficult for older people or others who are not as tech-savvy to use efficiently. Compatibility concerns between healthcare systems and equipment might make it difficult to share data seamlessly (Goodridge & Marciniuk, 2016).

The time-consuming and inconsistent credentialing procedures might add to the administrative load. Strong security measures are necessary to shield patient data from cyberattacks, but putting them in place can be expensive and difficult. Large initial expenditures are needed to set up telemedicine infrastructure and buy remote monitoring equipment. Since they feel there will not be as much face-to-face engagement with telemedicine, some patients might prefer in-person appointments. By making sure that these issues are not available, remote health monitoring and telemedicine can benefit and make changes in remote areas.

To accommodate varied demographics, make sure telemedicine services are offered in a variety of languages. To better understand and meet the specific requirements of various patient groups, healthcare providers should receive cultural competency training. Gaining patient's faith in the telehealth system requires open communication about how their data will be used, stored, and safeguarded. Ensure that patient rights and confidentiality are always given priority by developing and abiding by ethical rules for the use of telehealth. Assess and revise ethical standards regularly to stay abreast of developing privacy issues and technology developments. Healthcare practitioners can increase trust in telemedicine and remote health monitoring by proactively addressing privacy, security, and equity concerns, ensuring that these technologies benefit all patients equally.

12.4 INFRASTRUCTURE REQUIREMENTS FOR TELEMEDICINE

The year 2020 saw a substantial surge in telemedicine use, driven by the pandemic. However, data from Medical Economics suggests that telemedicine is not a temporary trend but is expected to persist and expand. According to their findings (Andrei, 2024):

- 83% of patients intend to continue using telemedicine in the aftermath of the pandemic environment (Andrei, 2024).
- More than 50% of patients utilize telemedicine for initial consultations with new providers if it offers convenience (Andrei, 2024).
- 91% find telemedicine beneficial for managing drug replenishments, scheduling consultations, and maintaining overall fitness through remote consultations with their healthcare professionals (Andrei, 2024).
- 93% would leverage telemedicine to administer their prescriptions more efficiently (Andrei, 2024).

The rising popularity of telemedicine can be attributed to the increasing availability of tools that facilitate patient-provider connections (Zimiles, 2024). This section highlights some of the most essential and commonly used telemedicine and remote health monitoring equipment providers should adopt to ensure efficient and effective telemedicine services.

High-Speed Internet: The foremost requirement for ensuring seamless, uninterrupted telemedicine services is high-speed internet, which supports continuous data transmission. Clinics and patients should consult their internet providers to secure the bandwidth for effective communications.

High-Definition Webcams: Desktop computers can support higher-definition webcams, even though most laptops and portable smart devices have built-in cameras that are good for video discussions. Purchasing a high-quality webcam helps many healthcare practitioners avoid problems with connectivity and visual clarity.

Tablets: Physicians use ICT-based tablets for data storage and analysis. Electronic tablets minimize the use of paper and improve accuracy. Automatic software is also there for assisting physicians that help to zoom the medical scan images and even filtering algorithms arc also thcrc for improving the image quality.

12.5 TRAINING AND EDUCATION FOR HEALTHCARE PROVIDERS

Telemedicine involves special training for human personnel in handling telehealth technology to ensure efficient healthcare. In the current scenario, artificial intelligence-based training imparts more information through user interaction and visual aids.

Virtual Learning: It is imperative that trainees be given chances for research and be involved in virtual clinical work. It is recommended that virtual learning be included in several aspects of the medical school curriculum, including disaster preparedness, clinical process acquisition, mentorship programs, fellowship interviews, and disaster preparedness efforts. The quality of clinical practice must be evaluated about the effects of virtual learning. As a backup plan or to help with the integration of telehealth into clinical practice in the future, virtual case-based teaching can be added to health professions courses.

Simulation Training: Hospitals and medical facilities must use simulation training to increase health personnel's preparedness, efficacy, and confidence while handling novel and high-risk operations, such as wearing and doffing PPE. To improve teamwork and maximize the standard of patient care, multi-professional simulation training ought to be employed.

Program Evaluation and Improvement: An evaluation of the student's readiness for autonomous practice and, if needed, an extension of the training program are crucial stages. It is critical to set up appropriate policies and procedures for online meetings to enhance interpersonal communication, resolve technological issues, lessen awkward scheduling, decrease overlapping themes and skewed scientific content, and support health educators. Pupils get increasingly used to using internet resources.

12.6 INTEGRATION WITH EXISTING HEALTHCARE SYSTEMS

TeleHealth Integrations: The demand for telehealth solutions is rapidly increasing within today's medical technology infrastructure. It is possible to improve communication between patients and medical professionals by using telehealth services, such as video conferencing platforms, remote patient monitoring systems, and technologies for telemedicine. Telemedicine also allows medical practitioners to compile a documented list of prescriptions for their patients and transmit it directly to partnered pharmacies, reducing the risk of prescription abuse or mishandling. Moreover, it simplifies communication among different healthcare establishments.

Laboratory Information System Integrations: Laboratory data plays a vital role in the analysis of physiological parameters of the body. Especially blood sample analysis by automatic software enables fast response and quick decision-making.

Medical Billing Integration: Billing and reimbursement for procedures constitute a lengthy and complex task. Ensuring accurate calculation of every utility, resource, time, and service can prolong the medical billing process. Medical billing integrations significantly reduce the time required to process each patient's records while enabling easier access to information, such as Medicare insurance.

Remote Diagnosis and Treatment: Teleconsultations have played a significant role and have seen an increase following the outbreak of COVID-19 (Andrei, 2024). In terms of clinical diagnosis, numerous advances have been made since then, and the field continues to expand. Enhancements such as web-based teleconsultation systems for clinical diagnosis focus on delivering real-time services via the Internet to remote areas (Perdoncini et al., 2021), and the utilization of smartphone video calls for diagnosing oral lesions has led to earlier diagnoses (Ahir et al., 2019). The integration of IoT modules designed to aid in diagnosis is also on the rise and has shown promise as a tool for real-time and in-depth monitoring of patients by doctors (Hsu et al., 2008). This supports the necessity for frequent information exchange to provide an effective diagnosis remotely (Vladzymyrskyy, 2004). The employment of teleconsultation has demonstrated a reduction in the average duration of in-hospital treatment by 16%, indicating a more efficient treatment process (Padilha et al., 2024). Teleconsultations hold the potential to enhance access to specialized care, particularly for patients in remote locations or for those who encounter transportation challenges. By diminishing the necessity for patients to travel extensive distances for face-to-face appointments, teleconsultations can improve convenience and potentially foster greater patient involvement in their care (Bynum et al., 2011). Furthermore, they facilitate alterations in patient diagnoses and treatment plans, impact clinical outcomes, and contribute to the reduction of superfluous costs (Guaiana et al., 2021).

Telepsychiatry and Mental Health Services: Telecommunication technology enables mental health professionals to provide services to individuals who may have limited access to traditional in-person care due to geographical, logistical, or other barriers. It has also been shown to be effective in reducing the stigma associated with seeking help and offers benefits comparable to in-person sessions (Thomas et al., 2018). In the context of pediatric mental health emergencies, reports indicate satisfaction with the use of technology (Malhotra et al., 2013). However, there are challenges associated with teleconsultation, particularly in telepsychiatry. Generally, developed nations possess superior infrastructure and resources to support telepsychiatry initiatives, including financial support, training, and a regulatory framework. In these countries, telepsychiatry is often aimed at improving access to specialized mental health services in remote or underserved areas. Conversely, in developing nations, telepsychiatry plays a critical role in bridging the substantial gap in mental health services and reaching populations with limited access to care (Guaiana et al., 2021; Tumma et al., 2022).

Telestroke: The management of acute stroke in emergency departments through technological support has expanded, and its implementation has proven beneficial. However, it also suggests a high initial cost, which can pose a barrier (Busti et al., 2021). The scarcity of stroke specialists in certain regions underscores the need to reorganize medical educational models and foster an open-minded approach among stakeholders to effectively harness the benefits of digital health technologies (Mohamed et al., 2024). Telestroke has been deemed safe, with minimal and non-significant differences in long-term outcomes compared to conventional face-to-face treatment for acute ischemic stroke, establishing its value as a tool (Sharma et al., 2016). The adoption of a smartphone-based telestroke model has emerged as a cost-effective alternative to video-conferencing-based telestroke services. This model has demonstrated promising results in delivering timely treatment for acute ischemic stroke in underserved and resource-limited settings (Hubert et al., 2019). Improving stroke treatment and guaranteeing the safety and efficiency of telestroke networks necessitate periodic evaluations of pre-established indicators of quality. Monitoring progress, discovering areas for development, and confirming that the network complies with set standards are made easier by participating in quality improvement activities and evaluations. Telestroke networks can enhance patient outcomes, boost efficiency, and raise the standards for stroke treatment by using such techniques (Sharifi Kia et al., 2023). Obviously, this is the new version that retains the reference numbers yet has grammatical corrects and an academic tone.

Emergency Telemedicine: Emergency medicine has made a lot of improvements in the quality of healthcare particularly evidenced by the decreased number of patient transfer rates and reduced mortality rates throughout the world. However, the implementation of this technology encounters several challenges (O'Sullivan & Schneider, 2023; Zachrison et al., 2020). The cost of implementation is frequently cited as the most significant barrier to the adoption of emergency telemedicine (Salman et al., 2021). Technologies such as machine learning (ML) can be leveraged to enhance the performance of emergency telemedicine by providing an electronic emergency triage system to prioritize patients. The integration of machine learning represents a progressive step in the evolution of emergency telemedicine. Nonetheless, this technology may present certain limitations (Creber et al., 2023).

Telemonitoring of Chronic Conditions: Telemonitoring facilitates the remote management of chronic conditions and can be a cost-effective approach to delivering care for chronic diseases. Numerous studies have indicated positive outcomes from telemonitoring, with patients expressing a preference for the convenience it offers over attending regular clinic visits (Gordon, 2020). It contributes to an integrated care model by monitoring specific signs and symptoms and establishing a clinical workflow that serves as a tool for the frequent monitoring of patients with complex chronic conditions (Ekstedt et al., 2023). Additionally, it bridges the gap between patients and healthcare professionals, enhancing their availability to one another (Liljeroos & Arkkukangas, 2023). Remote monitoring also promotes the interdisciplinary collaboration of professionals and the tailoring of care. Nevertheless, the adoption of this technology presents challenges, particularly for older adults, as it necessitates a degree of digital literacy among patients (Li et al., 2021). The technology also impacts healthcare professionals, who may need to manage and interpret data from telemonitoring devices, communicate with patients remotely, and coordinate care based on the received information. Consequently, professionals will require training to effectively utilize telemonitoring technology and interpret the data collected. Adequate support systems, such as technical assistance and guidelines for telemonitoring practices, are crucial in assisting professionals to navigate this new modality of care (Wilson & Maeder, 2015).

12.7 CONCLUSION

In the following years, telemedicine evolved to become a vital part of healthcare access in this modern era given its increasing popularity. Telemedicine facilitates phone calls, video conferences, and text messages that can be used for patients to seek medical advice or a consultation from home, which keeps the visit count low at hospital premises (primarily case consultations), hence time-saving with less exposure to health risks. This has been further aided by the integration of more advanced, technology-enhancing tools in telemedicine wearable sensors. These sensors continuously monitor various vital signs and send the data to air via the cloud enabling real-time remote health monitoring. This allows healthcare providers to offer primary consultations in 75 minutes, which addresses the very demand both patients and doctors have for greater flexibility. Telemedicine has its benefits, but there are challenges in telehealth, particularly around data security and privacy. Security is the first when it comes to transferring sensitive medical records. Encryption and blockchain are both useful technologies to keep data safe, add a hyperlink in the word 'encryption' that is/are used for quite efficient protection of the lifted data so that it is exchanged securely.

12.8 FUTURE DIRECTION AND EMERGING TRENDS

Technological Innovation in Telemedicine: Technological advancements in telemedicine are revolutionizing the way healthcare is delivered, increasing its effectiveness, efficiency, and accessibility. One of the most significant medical advancements of the twenty-first century may be the employment of cutting-edge technology to provide healthcare remotely. Increased efficiency, better patient outcomes, and improved access are all being brought about by technological advancements in telemedicine. These technologies will become more and more important in providing high-quality, patient-centered care as they develop (Teyhen et al., 2014).

The industry is becoming more established due to the quick development of health-related technology, which also offers enormous potential to reduce and/or mitigate obstacles to reaching optimal performance, health, and well-being. High-quality video consultations and real-time data transmission from remote monitoring devices are made possible by the implementation of 5G networks, which increase internet connection speed and dependability (Wilson & Maeder, 2015).

Applications have high criticality, where specialized knowledge must be rendered quickly and be available at the point of treatment. Excessive volume, when it becomes more challenging to physically co-locate the patient and the data related to them, as well as the skills necessary to handle that data. Asynchronous telemedicine will remain in demand as a result of co-location that can take place both in space and time. This trend toward more efficient use of healthcare resources will be driven by mounting demand on health systems to provide high-quality treatment within stringent budgetary restrictions.

Telemedicine is presently operating in a more diverse information environment than in the 1990s. Ophthalmoscopes and other peripheral devices are frequently connected to telemedicine systems. Some camera-based systems are even utilizing several viewpoints, some of which are high resolution. During the telemedicine consultation, it may also be necessary to send a variety of multi-dimensional medical pictures (such as 3D CT or real-time ultrasound). An individual patient's data space goes beyond what is communicated during a telemedicine appointment. More generally, the adoption of novel care models has the potential to be aided and encouraged via telemedicine. Many of the impediments to telemedicine expansion stem from this domain rather than technology, which has, if anything, surpassed telemedicine applications (Field & Grigsby, 2002).

Novel technologies have auspicious prospects for mitigating this disparity and enhancing healthcare accessibility in isolated regions. How wearable technology, wearable health apps, wearable Internet of Things (IoT) devices, telemedicine, and artificial intelligence (AI) might improve access to healthcare. Legislators, medical professionals, and tech developers may work together to design more effective and easily accessible healthcare systems for rural communities by having a better knowledge of these new developments. Artificial intelligence-powered diagnostic instruments possess the ability to precisely identify ailments like infections, cancers, and fractures by analyzing medical pictures like MRIs and X-rays. Virtual reality platforms such as Limbix offer therapeutic environments that are immersive for mental health purposes, such as exposure therapy for PTSD and anxiety (Wahezi et al., 2021)

Policy and Regulatory Consideration: Technological advancements and the growing acceptability of telehealth as a standard healthcare delivery model are reflected in recent trends in policy and regulatory issues for telemedicine. Medicare and Medicaid telehealth coverage had notable increases during the COVID-19 epidemic. A wider acceptability of telehealth services is shown in the extension or permanentization of these improvements in some situations. A lot of private insurers have also modified their policies to provide more extensive coverage for telehealth services. A few jurisdictions have parity rules requiring insurers to pay for telehealth services at the same rate as in-person visits (Puentes et al., 2007). Technological advancements and the growing acceptability of telehealth as a standard healthcare delivery model are reflected in recent trends in policy and regulatory issues for telemedicine. Medicare and Medicaid telehealth coverage had notable increases during the COVID-19 epidemic. A wider acceptability of telehealth services is shown in the extension or permanentizing of these improvements in some situations. A lot of private insurers have also modified their policies to provide more extensive coverage for telehealth services. A few jurisdictions have parity rules requiring insurers to pay for telehealth treatments at the same rate as visits to the doctor.

Telemedicine Potential for Global Health Impact: The delivery of healthcare around the world could be drastically altered by recent advances in digital health and telemedicine trends. Access to specialized care that was previously unattainable is being made possible for underprivileged and rural populations by telemedicine. In isolated areas, this enhances results and lessens healthcare inequities. The management of chronic illnesses like diabetes, hypertension, and heart disease is greatly aided by wearable technology and remote monitoring systems. The accuracy of diagnoses is being improved by the application of AI and machine-learning technologies. For instance, compared to conventional approaches, AI can examine medical images to discover diseases like cancer earlier (Omboni et al., 2022)

International cooperation is being made easier by initiatives to standardize healthcare data and enhance system interoperability. This is essential for sharing medical research, monitoring and controlling pandemics, and enhancing patient care. Particularly in poor nations, mHealth apps are being utilized to spread health education and information. These applications give information about immunization regimens, illness prevention, and maternal health. Global health could be greatly impacted by the current trends in telemedicine and digital health. Through the utilization of these technologies, healthcare systems can attain more accessibility, equity, and efficiency, which will ultimately lead to an improvement in health outcomes for people globally. Patient outcomes are improved by this technology's capacity for ongoing observation and prompt intervention. The full promise of these technologies can only be realized with sustained investment, policy backing, and international cooperation. (Omboni et al., 2022).

REFERENCES

Ahir, Y., Rathkanthiwar, S. V., & Kale, Y. (2019). A review on teleconsultation and telediagnosis using IoT module. In *2019 International Conference on Communication and Signal Processing (ICCSP)* (pp. 0153–0156). IEEE. https://doi.org/10.1109/ICCSP.2019.8698073

Andrei, A. (2024). The future of telemedicine: Trends and patient insights post-pandemic. *Journal of Health Informatics*, 15(3), 123–135.

Bashshur, R. L., & Shannon, G. W. (2009). *History of telemedicine: Evolution, context, and transformation*. Mary Ann Liebert, Inc., Publishers.

Botrugno, C. (2018). Telemedicine in daily practice: Addressing legal challenges while waiting for an EU regulatory framework. *Health Policy and Technology*, 7(2), 131–136.

Brear, M. (2006, September). Evaluating telemedicine: Lessons and challenges. *Health Information Management Journal*, 35(2), 23–31.

Broens, T. H., Huis in't Veld, R. M., Vollenbroek-Hutten, M. M., Hermens, H. J., van Halteren, A. T., & Nieuwenhuis, L. J. (2007). Determinants of successful telemedicine implementations: A literature study. *Journal of Telemedicine and Telecare*, 13(6), 303–309.

Busti, C., Gamboni, A., Calabrò, G., Zampolini, M., Zedde, M., Caso, V., & Corea, F. (2021). Telestroke: Barriers to the transition. *Frontiers in Neurology*, 12. https://doi.org/10.3389/fneur.2021.689191

Bynum, A. B., Irwin, C. A., & Della Mea, V. (2011, May). Evaluation of the effect of consultant characteristics on telemedicine diagnosis and treatment. *International Journal of Telemedicine and Applications*, 2011, Article 701089. https://doi.org/10.1155/2011/701089

Creber, A., Leo, D. G., Buckley, B. J. R., et al. (2023). Use of telemonitoring in patient self-management of chronic disease: A qualitative meta-synthesis. *BMC Cardiovascular Disorders*, 23, 469. https://doi.org/10.1186/s12872-023-03486-3

EE, G. B. B. M., Farr, R., & Ben Raimer, M. D. (2011). Benefits of telemedicine in remote communities & use of mobile and wireless platforms in healthcare. UTMB Telemedicine and Center for Health Research and Policy.

Ekstedt, M., Nordheim, E. S., Hellström, A., et al. (2023). Patient safety and sense of security when telemonitoring chronic conditions at home: The views of patients and healthcare professionals – A qualitative study. *BMC Health Services Research*, 23, 581. https://doi.org/10.1186/s12913-023-09428-1

Feldheim, J., Schmidt, T., Oster, C., Feldheim, J., Stuschke, M., Stummer, W., Grauer, O., Scheffler, B., Hagemann, C., Sure, U., & Kleinschnitz, C. (2023). Telemedicine in neuro-oncology—An evaluation of remote consultations during the COVID-19 pandemic. *Cancers*, 15(16), 4054. https://doi.org/10.3390/cancers15164054

Field, M. J., & Grigsby, J. (2002, July). Telemedicine and remote patient monitoring. *JAMA*, 288(4), 423–425.

Goodridge, D., & Marciniuk, D. (2016, May). Rural and remote care: Overcoming the challenges of distance. *Chronic Respiratory Disease*, 13(2), 192–203.

Gordon, K., Steele Gray, C., Dainty, K. N., DeLacy, J., Ware, P., & Seto, E. (2020). Exploring an innovative care model and telemonitoring for the management of patients with complex chronic needs: Qualitative description study. *JMIR Nursing*, 3(1), e15691. https://doi.org/10.2196/15691

Guaiana, G., Mastrangelo, J., Hendrikx, S., et al. (2021). A systematic review of the use of telepsychiatry in depression. *Community Mental Health Journal*, 57, 93–100. https://doi.org/10.1007/s10597-020-00724-2

Hsu, Y.-C., Lin, P.-Y., Hsu, S. J., & Chan, C.-T. (2008). Design and implementation of a teleconsultation system for instant treatment. In *2008 2nd International Conference on Bioinformatics and Biomedical Engineering* (pp. 1355–1358). IEEE. https://doi.org/10.1109/ICBBE.2008.668

Hubert, G. J., Santo, G., Vanhooren, G., et al. (2019). Recommendations on telestroke in Europe. *European Stroke Journal*, 4(2), 101–109. https://doi.org/10.1177/2396987318806718

Imberti, J. F., Tosetti, A., Mei, D. A., Maisano, A., & Boriani, G. (2021, June). Remote monitoring and telemedicine in heart failure: Implementation and benefits. *Current Cardiology Reports*, 23(1), 1. https://doi.org/10.1007/s11886-021-01469-4

Li, J., Varnfield, M., Jayasena, R., & Celler, B. (2021). Home telemonitoring for chronic disease management: Perceptions of users and factors influencing adoption. *Health Informatics Journal*, 27(1). https://doi.org/10.1177/1460458221997893

Liljeroos, M., & Arkkukangas, M. (2023). Implementation of telemonitoring in health care: Facilitators and barriers for using eHealth for older adults with chronic conditions. *Risk Management and Healthcare Policy*, 16, 43–53. https://doi.org/10.2147/RMHP.S396495

Malhotra, S., Chakrabarti, S., & Shah, R. (2013, January–March). Telepsychiatry: Promise, potential, and challenges. *Indian Journal of Psychiatry*, 55(1), 3–11. https://doi.org/10.4103/0019-5545.105499

Mallipeddi, S. R., Goda, D. R., Yerram, S. R., Varghese, A., & Ande, J. R. (2017). Telemedicine and beyond: Navigating the frontier of medical technology. *Technology & Management Review*, 2(1), 37–50.

Mohamed, A., Elsherif, S., Legere, B., Fatima, N., Shuaib, A., & Saqqur, M. (2024). Is telestroke more effective than conventional treatment for acute ischemic stroke? A systematic review and meta-analysis of patient outcomes and thrombolysis rates. *International Journal of Stroke*, 19(3), 280–292. https://doi.org/10.1177/17474930231206066

Mun, S. K., & Turner, J. W. (1999). Telemedicine: Emerging e-medicine. *Annual Review of Biomedical Engineering*, 1(1), 589–610.

O'Sullivan, S., & Schneider, H. (2023). Comparing effects and application of telemedicine for different specialties in emergency medicine using the Emergency Talk Application (U-Sim ETA Trial). *Scientific Reports*, 13, 13332. https://doi.org/10.1038/s41598-023-40501-1

Omboni, S., Padwal, R. S., Alessa, T., Benczúr, B., Green, B. B., Hubbard, I., Kario, K., Khan, N. A., Konradi, A., Logan, A. G., & Lu, Y. (2022). The worldwide impact of telemedicine during COVID-19: Current evidence and recommendations for the future. *Connected Health*, 1, 7.

Padilha, F. V. de Q., et al. (2024). Analysis of the costs of teleconsultation for the treatment of diabetes mellitus in the SUS. *Revista de Saúde Pública*, 58. https://doi.org/10.11606/s1518-8787.2024058005433

Paul, D. L., Pearlson, K. E., & McDaniel, R. R. (1999). Assessing technological barriers to telemedicine: Technology-management implications. *IEEE Transactions on Engineering Management*, 46(3), 279–288.

Perdoncini, N. N., Schussel, J. L., Amenábar, J. M., & Torres-Pereira, C. C. (2021). Use of smartphone video calls in the diagnosis of oral lesions: Teleconsultations between a specialist and patients assisted by a general dentist. *The Journal of the American Dental Association*, 152(2), 127–135. https://doi.org/10.1016/j.adaj.2020.10.013

Pramanik, P. K., Nayyar, A., & Pareek, G. (2019). WBAN: Driving e-healthcare beyond telemedicine to remote health monitoring: Architecture and protocols. In J. D. Dewhurst (Ed.), *Telemedicine Technologies* (pp. 89–119). Academic Press.

Puentes, J., Bali, R. K., Wickramasinghe, N., & Naguib, R. N. (2007, January). Telemedicine trends and challenges: A technology management perspective. *International Journal of Biomedical Engineering and Technology*, 1(1), 59–72.

Saechow, S., Kamolphiwong, S., & Chandeeying, V. (2014). Web-based teleconsultation for clinical diagnosis. In *2014 International Conference on Electronics, Information and Communications (ICEIC)* (pp. 1–2). IEEE. https://doi.org/10.1109/ELINFOCOM.2014.6914423

Salman, O. H., Taha, Z., Alsabah, M. Q., Hussein, Y. S., Mohammed, A. S., & Aal-Nouman, M. (2021). A review on utilizing machine learning technology in the fields of electronic emergency triage and patient priority systems in telemedicine: Coherent taxonomy, motivations, open research challenges and recommendations for intelligent future work. *Computer Methods and Programs in Biomedicine*, 209, 106357. https://doi.org/10.1016/j.cmpb.2021.106357

Sharifi Kia, A., Rafizadeh, M., & Shahmoradi, L. (2023). Telemedicine in the emergency department: An overview of systematic reviews. *Journal of Public Health (Berl.)*, 31, 1193–1207. https://doi.org/10.1007/s10389-021-01684-x

Sharma, S., Padma, M. V., Bhardwaj, A., Sharma, A., Sawal, N., & Thakur, S. (2016, September–October). Telestroke in resource-poor developing country model. *Neurology India*, 64(5), 934–940. https://doi.org/10.4103/0028-3886.190243

Teyhen, D. S., Aldag, M., Edinborough, E., Ghannadian, J. D., Haught, A., Kinn, J., Kunkler, K. J., Levine, B., McClain, J., Neal, D., & Stewart, T. (2014, September). Leveraging technology: Creating and sustaining changes for health. *Telemedicine and e-Health*, 20(9), 835–849.

Thomas, J. F., et al. (2018, February). The use of telepsychiatry to provide cost-efficient care during pediatric mental health emergencies. *Psychiatric Services*, 69(2), 161–168. https://doi.org/10.1176/appi.ps.201700005

Tumma, A., Berzou, S., Jaques, K., Shah, D., Smith, A. C., & Thomas, E. E. (2022). Considerations for the implementation of a telestroke network: A systematic review. *Journal of Stroke and Cerebrovascular Diseases*, 31(1), 106171. https://doi.org/10.1016/j.jstrokecerebrovasdis.2021.106171

Vladzymyrskyy, A. V. (2004). The use of teleconsultations in the treatment of patients with multiple trauma. *European Journal of Trauma*, 30, 394–397. https://doi.org/10.1007/s00068-004-1346-4

Wahezi, S. E., Kohan, L. R., Spektor, B., Brancolini, S., Emerick, T., Fronterhouse, J. M., Luedi, M. M., Colon, M. A., Kitei, P. M., Anitescu, M., & Goeders, N. E. (2021, October). Telemedicine and current clinical practice trends in the COVID-19 pandemic. *Best Practice & Research Clinical Anaesthesiology*, 35(3), 307–319.

Whitten, P., & Sypher, B. D. (2006). Evolution of telemedicine from an applied communication perspective in the United States. *Telemedicine Journal & e-Health*, 12(5), 590–600.

Whitten, P., Holtz, B., & Nguyen, L. (2010). Keys to a successful and sustainable telemedicine program. *International Journal of Technology Assessment in Health Care*, 26(2), 211–216.

Wilson, L. S., & Maeder, A. J. (2015, October). Recent directions in telemedicine: Review of trends in research and practice. *Healthcare Informatics Research*, 21(4), 213–222.

Zachrison, K. S., Boggs, K. M., Hayden, E. M., Espinola, J. A., & Camargo, C. A. (2020). Understanding barriers to telemedicine implementation in rural emergency departments. *Annals of Emergency Medicine*, 75(3), 392–399. https://doi.org/10.1016/j.annemergmed.2019.06.026

Zimiles, A. (2024). Four new statistics that prove that telemedicine isn't just a pandemic fad. Medical Economics. Retrieved July 11, 2024, from www.medicaleconomics.com/view/four-new-statistics-that-prove-that-telemedicine-isn-t-just-a-pandemic-fad

13 Ethical Considerations of AI and Data Security in Assisted Living of this Era

Uchejeso Mark Obeta and Nkechinyere Linda Obeta

13.1 INTRODUCTION

The time of global healthcare is now and beyond with the aid of new technologies applicable in healthcare. This is because of global collaboration in healthcare with telemedicine, automation and robotics, machine learning, innovative computing, and several others (Etukudoh et al., 2023; Obeta et al., 2024). New technologies in healthcare have created a different real-time dashboard for real-time diagnosis, monitoring, and healthcare services. This has elevated AI across the board to the extent that several barriers of distances and difficulties in data sharing are currently eliminated (Baredo et al., 2020; Obeta et al., 2024).

Internet of Medical Laboratory Things (IoMLTs) or Internet of Medical Things (IoMTs) (Obeta et al., 2024) has been laced with a healthcare information management system and by extension information management in the medical laboratory science (Obeta et al., 2023). There is no doubt that these healthcare technologies and AI are challenged by data security. The new technologies target all healthcare spheres but most importantly the elderly, children, and disabled when ambient assisted living is concerned with the technologies.

This chapter shall explore AI and data security associated issues in ambient living of this era.

13.2 ARTIFICIAL INTELLIGENCE

Artificial intelligence (AI) is defined "as the capability of a computer program to perform tasks or reasoning processes that we usually associate to intelligence in a human being" (Rossi, 2016). With AI in healthcare where several data are generated, the ability of healthcare professionals to make a good decision on several patients and clients are with this technology assisted in various ways. The uncertainty or vagueness, or too much healthcare and laboratory data, AI have immensely helped

DOI: 10.1201/9781003520184-16

to analyze and take several helping decisions very timely to save the patients (Obeta et al., 2022).

AI brings to mind "augmented intelligence" where healthcare systems are built to enhance and improve healthcare professional skills, expertise, and professionalism rather than removing or replacing them. Also, "cognitive computing" is involved as a comprehensive set of capabilities that new technologies in healthcare laced with AI, decision technologies, language programs, machine learning, reasoning and speech, processing technologies, vision recognition and human interface technologies, distributed and high-performance computing, and new computing architectures and devices can be integrated to aid healthcare professionals to solve several practical problems, improve care productivity, quality improvement and foster new discoveries in healthcare practice (Rossi, 2016; Etukudoh et al., 2024).

13.3 HEALTHCARE DATA

Healthcare data is generated daily in every healthcare facility. Various departments generate data based on their contribution to patients' management. Numerous data has made data mining gain recognition in healthcare having recorded a huge success in business and marketing organizations. The use of data mining techniques for healthcare issues like brain tumors, cancer, hypertension, and several infectious diseases detection are on the increase with algorithms and machine-learning techniques (Obeta et al., 2022; Rehman et al., 2021).

Healthcare data mining is done in health with various clustering techniques leading to visualization and exploration, manipulation and modification, modeling and prediction, and accuracy assessment (Mittal et al., 2019).

The data mining in healthcare cannot be complete without mention of the aspect of medical laboratory services in healthcare services. The role of medical laboratory services in the clinical decisions for patients and other public health policies in general healthcare as a result of numerous data generated, contributes immensely to admission or discharge of a patient from any healthcare facility (Obeta et al 2022; Soni & Gandhi, 2014).

13.4 AI AND HEALTHCARE

Artificial intelligence (AI) has been seen in the promotion of innovation and improved techniques in overall healthcare and medical diagnostics, in particular. There is no doubt that manual processes of healthcare services can be time-consuming and prone to errors. The application of AI systems and methods such as machine vision and machine learning, can enhance healthcare services. In this new era of AI-supported processes and services in healthcare, the dynamic and constantly evolving systems are capable of analyzing data, learning from the generated information, and making predictions and decisions across the whole of healthcare (Obeta et al., 2024; Sisman & Basok, 2020).

The use of AI in healthcare assists physicians and other healthcare professionals in better clinical decision-making, thereby replacing some human judgment in many areas of healthcare, especially in diagnostic areas. AI also gives up-to-date medical information to both experienced and newly qualified experts. AI in healthcare aids early diagnosis and outcome prediction of the diagnosis and disease status and treatment options. AI reduce diagnostic and therapeutic errors. Above all, AI increases patient safety and the cost of healthcare, knowing very well that AI works extremely well in real-time healthcare services (Goyal et al., 2021).

AI in healthcare is challenged by development costs, integration issues, ethical issues, difficulty in changing aspects of medical and healthcare providers to adopt AI, the fear of human professionals, replacement and data privacy and security (Obeta et al., 2024).

13.5 BASIC PRINCIPLES OF ETHICS IN HEALTHCARE

The major principles of ethics in healthcare are autonomy, beneficence, non-maleficence, and justice, as presented well in Figure 13.1.

The ethical principles as applied in regular medical laboratory practice is not different from smart laboratory service, which starts from the pre-analytical phase, including patient's interaction with smart gadgets or professional laboratory staff, specimen or no specimen collection, receiving of sample and sample transport. The ethical issues of the analytical phase is related to actual testing and quality control while post-analytical phase ethical issues are related to issuance and reporting of smart laboratory results, keeping, storing, and maintaining healthcare records (Aggarwal et al., 2021; Gallicchio & Gallicchio, 2013).

Ethical principles identified in existing AI Guidelines according to Jobin et al.'s (2019) work presents transparency as the topmost, among freedom and autonomy,

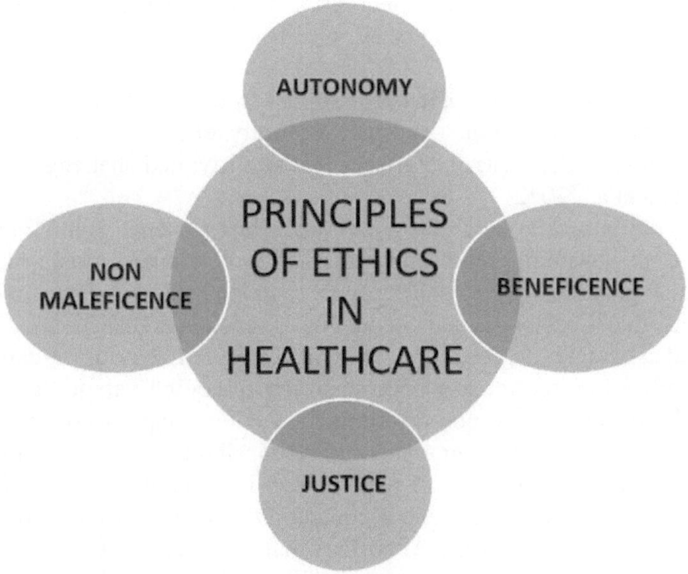

FIGURE 13.1 The AI-associated principles of ethics in healthcare.

justice and fairness, beneficence, non-maleficence, responsibility, trust, sustainability, privacy, dignity, and solidarity.

Transparency is achieved by increasing disclosure of information strategies by those developing or deploying AI in healthcare, which should be done in non-technical terms and is very auditable to participants and patients. Justice, fairness, and equity are well preserved by promoting the standard of justice, explicit normative encoding, or transparency through making information available for public awareness based on existing rights with regulation and as well as with testing and monitoring the available healthcare data. Adequate strengthening of available guidelines and the rule of law with systemic changes and support from various governmental action. For non-maleficence, harm is prevented using adequate guidelines focused on strategies employed during AI research, design, deployment, and development. This is followed by active cooperation among all healthcare professionals and stakeholders that use AI. Freedom and autonomy is achieved through transparency education or giving notice and consent and by actively avoiding collection and sharing of data without informed consent. The beneficence highlights the benefit of AI to healthcare clients and patients for the benefit of everyone not minding the health status while ensuring adequate human rights protection especially when some are affected (Jobin et al., 2019).

AI ethical debate is on the increase as to "what constitutes ethical AI?" and "which ethical requirements, technical standards and best practices are needed for ethical realization of AI?"

13.6 ETHICAL ISSUES WITH AI, NEW TECHNOLOGIES AND APPLICATIONS IN HEALTHCARE

There are many ethical and social matters that arises with new assistive technologies, automations, applications, tele-healthcare, healthcare data usage, and AI as applied in healthcare.

The ethical issues border on data bias, fairness, and equity; reliability and safety, malicious use of AI, transparency and accountability, effects on patients; effects on healthcare professionals; trust; data privacy and security; and challenges for governance (Petersson et al., 2022).

In consideration of accountability in AI healthcare systems from an ethical perspective, the responsibility and obligation of professionals, organizations, and systems is to explain and justify their decisions, actions, and outcomes in healthcare practice. The ethical perspective of accountability ensures transparency where there is a clear understanding of decision-making processes and algorithms; explainability where the ability to interpret and understand the reasoning behind healthcare services' decisions; fairness and non-discrimination in ensuring that smart systems do not perpetuate biases or discrimination; and responsibility for accountability of the impact of healthcare on individuals and society, in general. In all, accountability provides traceability, auditability, and accountability mechanisms. Notably, accountability in healthcare systems using AI ensures that there are consequences for unethical or illegal actions, promoting trust, reliability, and responsible development and deployment of these systems (Parikh et al., 2019).

The confidentiality in AI healthcare systems from an ethical perspective is the obligation to protect personal and sensitive information from unauthorized access, disclosure, or use. The ethical perspective cannot be complete without trust and privacy, which is in tandem with respecting individuals' autonomy and privacy expectations; secrecy and discretion in protecting sensitive information from unauthorized disclosure and protection of personal autonomy in ensuring individuals' control over their personal information. Confidentiality in ethics involves data minimization, data access control, encryption and security measures in place, anonymization and pseudonymization of data, and transparency and notice in use of data. Breaches of confidentiality in healthcare operating with AI and new healthcare technologies can lead to legal and ethical consequences, including fines, damages, and reputational harm. Therefore, ensuring confidentiality is essential for maintaining trust and respecting individuals' privacy and personal autonomy (Naik et al., 2022).

Data privacy in AI healthcare systems from an ethical point of view tells the rights and obligations related to the data collection, processing, storage, processing, and protection. The ethical perspective further emphasizes the respect for autonomy where individuals are recognized to take control over their personal information; privacy as a human right is acknowledged with a great deal of transparency and accountability in ensuring clear data handling practices and accountability for all data breaches. Ethical issues on privacy cannot be exhausted without data minimization, purpose limitation, data protection by design and default data subject rights and cross-border data transfers protection. Breaches of data privacy in healthcare especially with AI can lead to legal and ethical consequences, including fines, damages, reputational harm, and loss of trust. Therefore, prioritizing data privacy is essential for respecting individuals' autonomy, dignity, and human rights, especially in healthcare and medical laboratory information (Etukudoh et al., 2023).

The fairness in approach in AI healthcare systems from an ethical side is the principle of ensuring that individuals are treated justly and without bias, discrimination, or prejudice in such a service. An ethical view point on fairness presents justice and impartiality where fair treatment and equal opportunities for all is ensured; non-discrimination through avoiding biases and discrimination in all laboratory services; and transparency and explainability of all procedures and results towards better decision-making processes on clients. With fairness, there is avoidance of biases in data collection, processing, and analysis; algorithmic auditing regularly, fairness metrics; inclusive design that consider diverse perspectives and needs of patients and human oversight to detect and correct potential biases. Any breaches of fairness in a given AI healthcare organization can lead to legal and ethical consequences, including discrimination, perpetuation of biases, and erosion of trust. Therefore, prioritizing fairness is essential for ensuring just and equitable treatment of individuals in healthcare (Marshan, 2021).

The governance in healthcare operated with AI and new healthcare technologies from an ethical understanding entails all concerning rules, practices, and decision-making processes that ensure accountability, transparency, and responsibility in development, deployment, and use of new technology systems. They are associated with stakeholder involvement, value alignment with human values and ethical principles and transparency and explainability of all decision-making processes and algorithms.

In governance frameworks, risk management, compliance monitoring, ethical review processes, and accountability mechanisms are established for procedural reporting, investigating, and addressing errors or misconduct especially on the part of healthcare professionals. Effective governance in healthcare ensures trust, reliability, and responsible innovation, mitigating potential legal and ethical consequences, such as non-compliance, biases, and social harm (Farahans et al., 2018).

The liability in an AI healthcare system can ethically be described as responsibility and accountability for damages or harm caused by the system's actions or decisions in the form of healthcare decisions and outcome. This includes responsibility for harm in ensuring accountability for harm caused by healthcare practice, an instance of medical laboratory results; duty of care to prevent harm or injury in the healthcare service; transparency and explainability of any injury and decision-making about it; and accountability mechanisms for reporting, investigating, and addressing errors or misconduct. It is important to know that liability deals with direct causation and quantifiable damages, standard of care, and best practices for smart system development and deployment, compliance with regulations, liability allocation among stakeholders, including manufacturers, professional, operators, and users; insurance and risk management strategies in any hospital or healthcare centers using AI. Effective liability frameworks in smart laboratory systems ensure accountability, trust, and responsible innovation, mitigating potential legal and ethical consequences, such as harm to individuals, reputational damage, and financial losses (Martinez-Martin et al., 2021).

For accuracy in AI healthcare systems in ethical consideration ensuring that the system's results/outputs, decisions, or recommendations are reliable, trustworthy, and free from errors or biases. There should be truthfulness by providing accurate and reliable information, reliable and accurate performance, and transparency in methodology and result outputs, and accountability of all errors or inaccuracies in healthcare system result outputs. Accuracy ensures data quality in the accuracy, complete, and unbiased data, algorithms that minimize errors and biases, testing and validating smart devices, continuous monitoring and clear explanations for smart system decisions and results/outputs. Inaccurate laboratory result of AI healthcare systems can lead to legal and ethical consequences, including damages, reputational harm, and erosion of trust. Therefore, prioritizing accuracy is essential for ensuring reliable, trustworthy, and responsible healthcare services and practice (Martinez-Martin et al., 2021).

Security is one of the ethical issues of concern in smart laboratory systems, which refers to the responsibility to guard some sensitive information, data, and assets from unauthorized contact, access, disclosure, use, modification, disruption, or destruction. The ethical perspective displays confidentiality thereby protecting sensitive information and maintaining trust; integrity with data accuracy and preventing unauthorized modification; availability of system data when needed; authenticity as verified by the identity of users and devices and non-repudiation by ensuring accountability for actions and decisions. The healthcare services especially where AI usage is applicable has become a target for cybercriminals worldwide therefore, strong cybersecurity is vital to the use of technology in healthcare to identify, protect, and prevent common attack vectors. Cybersecurity challenges and privacy-related issues is depending on the specific layer of concern should consider the fact that privacy comes from a holistic and comprehensive security while security comes from the need to maintain privacy. The confidentiality and protection of healthcare information or patients' data from unwanted and unauthorized contact access, right to control access to such data is best described as security and privacy (Thilakarathne, 2020).

Inclusion in healthcare systems in the ethical arena is to ensure that these systems are accessible, usable, and equitable for all healthcare interested individuals, regardless of their simplicity or usage. Ethical presentation caters for universal design by ensuring that the systems are accessible and usable by everyone across the globe; equity and fairness such that they do not perpetuate biases or discrimination; transparency and explainability; and taking responsibility for ensuring inclusivity and addressing issues.

The ethical problems while considering the basic principles of ethics cannot permit the medical laboratory professionals to insist on carrying out a particular testing on a client when the subject objects to the procedure due to autonomy and also could not wait for an unconscious subject to carry out a laboratory procedure due to fairness and justice. The ethical problems in smart medical laboratory services still exists in the form of risk from device information leakage, risk from social network, and ambiguities in the laws associated with the medical laboratory regulations and practice. There is also a risk from smart or wearable devices in healthcare based on information leakage in consideration that the subject operator or under monitor is independent, and links can reveal user information or data recorded. This may cause loss or error in the information transfer process thereby affecting the final service quality. This depends on the smart devices in use for the laboratory whether installed at the subject's home, or worn on any part of the body for real-time body data collection but no extent of data protection put in place. There is another risk from the social network as strong social networks is capable of making security and privacy more challenging in personal data collection and exposure. The young people's social networking devices need more solutions (Denecke et al., 2015).

In some cases, we can see ambiguities in the laws surrounding the medical laboratory activities associated with smart laboratories. Globally, there are some laws about information security, however, many laws and regulations on ethical issues with regards to smart healthcare are ambiguous especially with responsibilities and boundaries. In the analysis of ethical problems associated with smart medical laboratories, ethical issues among different populations and in public health are to be re-examined.

Ethical issues in different populations in the smart medical laboratory service should ideally be protecting the elderly, children, and disabled population who needs smart systems most. In legal perspectives, the authorizations for carrying out medical laboratory procedures on those categories of people are mostly by guardians. The use of smart devices for the medical laboratory on the people and the release of such results should be adequately protected. Chung et al. (2016) raised a concern of how people could see the reputation of such people as it affects their normal social interaction. Smart medical devices may likely embarrass the users sometimes, such that the smart systems may force users to permit access and processing of data.

The ethical problems with regards to different groups of people, countries, and regions may differ in relation to smart medical laboratory services and medical services in general. The ethical problem of smart devices in one country may differ from the other or may not exist at all.

The application of AI healthcare may involve social issues, while it can be a problem solving service in another area while solving the problem of an uneven distribution of medical resources. It may be cheaper in one region but expensive in another due to applicable technological platforms. It is understandable that a person without a smartphone or computer cannot easily use any online medical laboratory platforms. Healthcare laced with AI may reduce hospital visits and financial burden but this may not be fairly and justly distributed among the people because of financial capacities using the cases of the cost of telemedicine as an instance (Henderson et al., 2013) and indirectly distinguishes the boundaries between the poor and the rich, countries or regions in their disparities.

Healthcare practice with AI is associated with public health and the ethical issues cannot be excluded. The public health plays around with numerous data generated from public health laboratories. For public health decisions, to make a decision without using the correct data is unethical practice associated with data torture, bias, and manipulation of data. Data is a valuable tool in public health laboratories and other healthcare facilities and in the hands of researchers and public health medical staff.

13.7 ETHICAL IMPLICATIONS AND HEALTHCARE DATA SECURITY AND PRIVACY

Patient privacy is a very important part of an ethical imperative and a crucial aspect of data protection in healthcare. This is because AI employs many new and digital technologies to improve patients' healthcare service, thereby making data privacy of high essence. Healthcare data security and privacy is of high essence. It is the responsibility of healthcare professionals to handle patients' information with care, trust and integrity. In consideration of the patient autonomy, any further use of the patients' data needs patient approval. The patients' privacy and confidentiality when utilizing their data for any healthcare studies or innovative research should be approved. No wonder the transparent communication as a way of better informed consent from patients is key to enable them to participate in decisions concerning their data usage (Margam, 2023).

13.8 GLOBAL IMPACT OF ETHICAL AND SECURITY ISSUES IN HEALTH DATA

There are several initiatives on ethical issues of AI in general or in healthcare in particular as we move across the globe. The WHO had a consultative meeting on AI and healthcare in the year 2019, which proceeded the European Group on Ethics in Science and New Technologies Conference resolution in 2018 that led to the "Guidelines for Trustworthy AI issued by European Commission" in 2018. There was the United Kingdom Government Centre for data ethics and Innovation in 2018. Also, is Asilomar AI principles, which was developed in 2017. The IEEE had a Global

Initiative on the Ethics of Autonomous and Intelligent Systems in the year 2016. Others are Ada Lovelace Institute of Nuffield Foundation on AI, Partnership on AI between Amazon, Apple, DeepMind, IBM, Facebook, Microsoft and Google, House of Lords committee on AI, and Global regulation and control of AI (WHO, 2017).

The core ethical principles in AI centered on the design/development, use and deployment of AI systems in such a way autonomy of every individual is adhered to as the ethical principles with respect for human subjects while preventing harm, fairness, and explicability. The AI in healthcare vendors and users should appreciate the ethical issues of AI to address the potential strains and tensions between the displayed principles.

Whether in healthcare or social issues, there should be special attention to situations involving more vulnerable groups like persons with disabilities, children, and other disadvantaged individuals who are at risk of exclusion in AI programmed systems. The AI benefits to healthcare, individuals and society are enormous but certain risks associated with it which may have a negative impact, should be checked very often to ensure that ethical principles are followed judiciously (Obeta et al., 2024).

13.9 ASSOCIATED ETHICO-SOCIAL CASES IN AI AND DATA SECURITY WITH AMBIENT ASSISTED LIVING

The elderly, disabled, children, and the less privileged population stand out for ambient assisted living that can be trusted for AI. In ambient leaving, the AI deployment should ensure that all stages of production and use of AI applications and systems meets the key requirements for trustworthiness such as oversight and human agency, safety and technical robustness, data governance and privacy, transparency, non-discrimination and fairness, diversity, societal and environmental well-being and accountability (Martinez-Martin et al., 2021). There should be consideration of technical and non-technical matters towards ensuring that the implementation meets the expected requirements.

There are several cases surrounding how AI can shortchange people for others and in some cases result in bias-related decisions. In the UK, a case for using AI to downgrade some students during enrollment was noted as the algorithm favored students from affluent areas and private schools, while high-achievers from free and state-schools were left out. The AI algorithm used in recruitment by Amazon developed a bias to prefer men over women because of working with features associated with men for up to 10 years. In the US, a Police AI tool for criminal acts showed bias for the Blacks. The Google facial recognition software AI showed bias against African-Americans where it classified them as "gorillas." Microsoft AI in 2014 exhibited racist and sexist behaviors on Twitter among the users. In the Argentinian Ministry of Early Childhood, Microsoft AI had bias in predicting teenage pregnancy based on analyzing data with age, ethnicity, country of origin and disability (USAID, 2023).

It is most likely that regular use of a particular data for healthcare analysis and diagnosis would make AI give a similar or biased result in healthcare. This issue should be addressed in healthcare as AI use in healthcare has become a necessity.

13.10 CONCLUSION

AI in ambient living has come to stay. Though it is challenged by ethical and data security issues such as autonomy, beneficence, justice, and non-maleficence on one part and data safety – data bias, fairness, and equity, transparency and accountability – on the other part. These issues affect the patients' trust, including healthcare professionals' credibility for ability to keep data security and privacy based on the malicious application and use of AI.

The same new technologies provides several ways to handle ethical and social issues. AI and data sharing in healthcare and assisted living can serve as a cross border issues and therefore, can affect the global community. This calls for a global approach through a global regulatory body approach especially by the WHO.

This chapter calls for a global regulatory framework for the regulation of healthcare technologies and data security taskforce. All national and international guidelines should therefore be reviewed towards a global healthcare regulator as this would reduce cross-border barriers and capital flight as experienced in Africa.

REFERENCES

Aggarwal, N., Kare, P.K., Datta, S.K. (2021). Ethics in Laboratory Medicine: An Overview of Considerations for Ethical Issues. In Thomas F. Heston, & Sujoy Ray (Eds.), *Bioethics in Medicine and Society.* InTechOpen. http://dx.doi.org/10.5772/intechopen.96122

Barredo, A. A., Díaz-Rodríguez, N., Del, S. J., Bennetot, A., Tabik, S. (2020). Explainable Artificial Intelligence (XAI): Concepts, Taxonomies, Opportunities and Challenges Toward Responsible AI. *Information Fusion,* 58, 82–115. https://bit.ly/2TLdMfX

Chung, J., Demiris, G., Thompson, H. J. (2016). Ethical Considerations Regarding the Use of Smart Home Technologies for Older Adults: An Integrative Review. *Annual Review of Nursing Research*, 34(1), 155–181.

Denecke, K., Bamidis, P., Bond, C., Gabarron, E., Househ, M., Lau, A. Y. S., Mayer, M. A., Merolli, M., Hansen, M. (2015). Ethical Issues of Social Media Usage in Healthcare. *Year book for Medical Informatics*, 10, 137–147. http://dx.doi.org/10.15265/IY-2015-001

Etukudoh, N.S., Esame, N.V., Obeta, U.M., Ejinaka, O.R. (2023). Automation and Robotics Improves Quality Healthcare in the Era of Digital Medical Laboratory. In A. Khang, V. Abdulyev, O. Hrybuk, A.A. Shukla (Eds.) *Computer Vision and AI Integrated IoT Technologies in the Medical Ecosystem*. CRC Press. Pg. 419–434.

Etukudoh, N.S., Obeta, U.M., Ejinaka, O.R., Etim, U.G. (2024). An Innovative Cloud Computing in Medical Laboratory Data Storage and Analytics. In A. Khang (Ed.) *Medical Robotics and AI-Assisted Diagnostics for a High–Tech Healthcare Industry.* IGI Global Press. Pg. 357–377.

Farahani, B., Firouzi, F., Chang, V., Badaroglu, M., Constant, N., Mankodiya, K. (2018). Towards Fogdriven IoT eHealth: Promises and Challenges of IoT in Medicine and Healthcare. *Future Generation Computer Systems*, 78, 659–676.

Gallicchio, V.S., Gallicchio, L.M. (2013). Ethics and Quality Assurance in Biomedical Laboratory Science. *International Journal of Biomedical Laboratory Science*, 2, 4.

Goyal, L.M., Saba, T., Rehman, A., Larabi, S. (2021). *Artificial Intelligence and Internet of Things: Applications in Smart Healthcare.* CRC Press.

Henderson, C., Beecham, J., Knapp, M. (2013). The Costs of Telecare and Telehealth. In A. Burns & L. A. Curtis (Eds.) *Unit Costs of Health and Social Care*. Personal Social Science Research Unit, University of Kent. Pg. 26–31.

Jobin, A., Ienca, M., Vayena, E. (2019). Artificial Intelligence: The Global Landscape of Ethics Guidelines. Preprint paper Madiega, T., VanDePol, A.L. (2022). Artificial intelligence act and regulatory sandboxes. European Parliamentary Research Service, PE 733.544

Marshan, A. (2021). Artificial Intelligence: Explainability, Ethical Issues and Bias. *Ann Robot Automation*, 5(1), 034–037. https://dx.doi.org/10.17352/ara.000011

Margam, R. (2023). Ethics and Data Privacy: The Backbone of Trustworthy Healthcare Practices. *Socio-Economic and Humanistic Aspects for Township and Industry*, 1(2), 232–236. https://doi.org/10.59535/sehati.v1i2.115

Martinez-Martin, N., Luo, Z., Kaushal, A., Adeli, E., Haque, A., Kelly, S.S., Wieten, S., Cho, M.K., Magnus, D., Fei-Fei, L., Schulman K., Milstein, A. (2021). Ethical Issues in Using Ambient Intelligence in Health-Care Settings. *Lancet Digit Health*, 3, e115–23. https://doi.org/10.1016/S2589-7500(20)30275-2

Mittal, M., Goyal, L.M., Hemanth, D.J., Sethi, J.K. (2019). Clustering Approaches for High-Dimensional Databases: A Review. *WIREs Data Mining Knowledge Discovery,* 9, e1300. https://doi.org/10.1002/widm.1300

Naik, N., Hameed, B.M.Z., Shetty, D.K., Swain, D., Shah, M., Paul, R., Aggarwal, K., Ibrahim, S., Patil, V., Smriti, K., Shetty, S., Rai, B.P., Chlosta, P., Somani, B.K, (2022). Legal and Ethical Consideration in Artificial Intelligence in Healthcare: Who Takes Responsibility? *Frontier Surgery*, 9, 862322. https://doi.org/10.3389/fsurg.2022.862322

Obeta, U.M., Lawrence, A., Etukudoh, N.S., Ejinaka, O.R., Ibanga, I. (2024). Internet of Medical Laboratory Things (IoMLTs) in the High-Tech Healthcare Industry. In A. Khang (Ed.) *Driving Medical Diagnostics through AI-Powered Technologies and Applications.* IGI Global Press. Pg. 222–237. https://doi.org/10.4018/979-8-3693-3679-3.ch014

Obeta, U.M., Etukudoh, N.S., Ejinaka, O.R., Odono, A.E. (2024). Medical Laboratory Artificial Intelligence: The Applicability in Nigerian Medical Laboratories. In D. Pradhan, P.K. Sahu, H.M. Tun, & P. Chatterjee (Eds.) *Artificial and Cognitive Computing for Sustainable Healthcare Systems in Smart Cities*. ISTE/Willey. Pg. 25–46.

Obeta, U.M., Njar, V.E., Etukudoh, N.S., Obiora, O.R. (2023). Applications of Information Management Systems (IMSML) in Medical Laboratories. In A. Khang (Eds.) *AI and IoT-Based Technologies for Precision Medicine.* IGI Global. Pg.447–463. https://doi.org/10.4018/979-8-3693-0876-9.ch026

Obeta, U.M., Ejinaka, O.R., Etukudoh, N.S. (2022). Data Mining in Medical Laboratory Service Improves Disease Surveillance and Quality Healthcare. In T. Saba et al. (Eds.) *Prognostic Models in Healthcare: AI and Statistical Approaches*, Studies in Big Data 109. Springer. Pg. 459–481. https://doi.org/10.1007/978-981-19-2057-8_17

Parikh, R.B., Teeple, S., Navathe, A.S. (2019). Addressing Bias in Artificial Intelligence in Health Care. *JAMA,* 322, 2377. https://doi.org/10.1001/jama.2019.18058

Petersson, L., Larsson, I., Nygren, J.M., Nilsen, P., Neher, M., Reed, J.E., Tyskbo, D., Svedberg, P. (2022). Challenges to Implementing Artificial Intelligence in Healthcare: A Qualitative Interview Study with Healthcare Leaders in Sweden. *BMC Health Services Research,* 22, 850. https://doi.org/10.1186/s12913-022-08215-8

Rehman, A., Haseeb, K., Saba, T., Lloret, J., Tariq, U. (2021). Secured Big Data Analytics for Decision-Oriented Medical System Using Internet of Things. *Electronics*, 10, 1273. https://doi.org/10.3390/electronics10111273

Rossi, F. (2016). *Artificial Intelligence: Potential Benefits and Ethical Considerations*. Legal Affairs Briefing European Union.

Thilakarathne, N.N. (2020). Security and Privacy Issues in IOT Environment. *International Journal of Engineering and Management Research*, 10(01), 26–29. https://doi.org/10.31033/ijemr.10.1.5.

Soni, N., Gandhi, C. (2014). Application of Data Mining to Health Care. *International Journal of Computer Science and its Applications*, 36(10), 245–248.

USAID. (2023). *Artificial Intelligence (AI) Ethics Guide*.

WHO. (2017). *WHO Guidelines on Ethical Issues in Public Health Surveillance*. World Health Organization.

14 The Impact of Telemedicine Technologies on Brain Small Vessel Disease and Ethical Concerns

Gopi Battineni, Sharmin Chougule, Nalini Chintalapudi, Giovanna Ricci and Francesco Amenta

14.1 INTRODUCTION

Brain small vessel disease (SVD) is a group of disorders that primarily affect the small blood vessels that supply the white matter and deep structures of the brain (Williamson & Kilo, 1980). Neurological manifestations of these diseases include cognitive decline, stroke, and vascular dementia. The small blood vessels in the brain gradually become damaged due to chronic hypertension and diabetes, reducing blood flow and oxygen supply (Mestre et al., 2017). A person with SVD will experience small, silent infarcts in the brain, leading to the death of brain cells. It is important to control and manage brain SVD since it has a substantial impact on public health.

The presence of SVD has been linked to an increased risk of stroke and poor cognitive function. White matter hyperintensities and lacunar infarcts, both of which are prevalent in the elderly, are closely associated with cognitive decline and other neurological disorders (Minagar et al., 2010; Williamson & Kilo, 1980; Zhang et al., 2020a). In Figure 14.1, age-related changes in white matter are shown in mild, moderate, and severe cases (Inzitari et al., 2009). In order to prevent disease progression and reduce complications, early detection and timely intervention are essential. Telemedicine technologies have emerged as powerful tools to provide patients with remote monitoring and access to specialized healthcare professionals as a result. By providing prompt diagnosis, customized treatment plans, and continuous disease management, patients receive improved outcomes.

For individuals with SVDs, telemedicine technologies have revolutionized healthcare delivery (Walsh & Markus, 2019). Video conferencing, remote monitoring devices, mobile applications, and electronic health records (EHRs) are just a few of the tools and platforms that these technologies encompass. The use of video

DOI: 10.1201/9781003520184-17

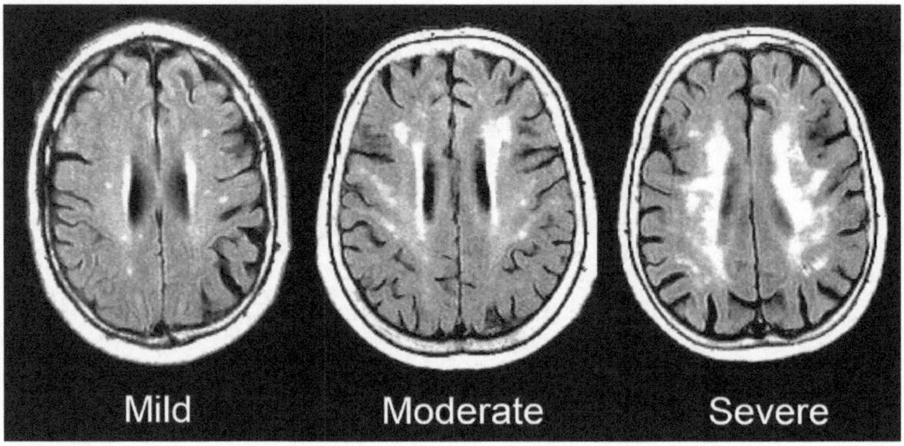

FIGURE 14.1 Small vessel disease progression on MRI (Inzitari et al., 2009).

conferencing now makes it possible for patients to have consultations with healthcare professionals, eliminating the need for in-person visits. Remote monitoring devices allow healthcare providers to monitor the vital signs and symptoms of patients continuously (Huang et al., 2015a). Personalized care plans can be provided to improve communication between patient-healthcare professionals through use of mobile applications. Sharing medical information seamlessly among healthcare providers facilitates collaboration and reduces errors in medicine through EHR. These technologies can be used to manage brain SVD more efficiently and effectively, which will result in enhanced access to healthcare (Ben-Assuli, 2022; Mestre et al., 2017).

Controlling brain SVDs can be achieved through the use of telemedicine technologies (Huang et al., 2015b; Walsh & Markus, 2019). Serious complications like strokes and cognitive decline can often arise from these disorders. Experts who can accurately diagnose and treat these conditions can provide patients with specialty care and consultations through telemedicine. Healthcare professionals can track patients' vital signs and adjust their treatment plans accordingly by utilizing remote monitoring devices like wearable sensors and blood pressure monitors (Ben-Assuli, 2022; Technology Assessment: Early Sense for Monitoring Vital Signs in Hospitalized Patients [Internet] – PubMed, n.d.; Walsh & Markus, 2019; Zhang et al., 2020b). This not only enhances patient outcomes, but also lessens the stress on healthcare facilities and enhances access to care for rural and underserved communities. Telemedicine technologies have greatly enhanced healthcare delivery, providing innovative solutions for overcoming geographical barriers and enhancing access to medical services. In cerebral amyloid angiopathy (CAA), amyloid-beta protein deposits within small arteries and capillaries of the cortex and leptomeninges (Wardlaw et al., 2019; Wightman et al., 2019). Haemorrhages, micro infarctions, and cognitive impairment can be linked to CAA lesions. Cognitive impairment can be attributed to hypoperfusion resulting from aortic stenosis and small vessel remodeling. In addition, SDD commonly has leukoaraiosis, which is also known as white matter hyperintensities and is linked to cognitive decline and an increased risk of stroke. Effective approaches to control and manage these conditions must be taken into consideration when learning about SVD of the brain.

For the development and progression of SVD, many risk factors have been identified, including hypertension, diabetes, hyperlipidaemia, smoking, and advanced age (Markus & Erik de Leeuw, 2023; Staals et al., 2014). The normal functioning of small arteries is impeded by hypertension as a result of endothelial dysfunction. The accumulation of risk factors over time leads to pathological changes, such as arteriosclerosis and cerebral small vessel damage, contributing to various neurological symptoms and cognitive decline. Mild to severe symptoms may occur in patients with SVD of the brain. Cognitive impairment, mood changes, motor dysfunction, and recurrent strokes are all common signs (Hamilton, Cox, Ballerini, et al., 2021; Hamilton, Cox, Okely, et al., 2021). In addition to affecting patients' quality of life, these symptoms can also result in long-term disability. SVD complications include ischemic lesions and hyperintensities of the white matter. Early detection and intervention of SVD can be enhanced by telemedicine technologies, leading to more timely treatment and improved patient outcomes.

To manage symptoms and risk factors of SVD of the brain, there are currently some treatment options available (Gao et al., 2022; Raghunath et al., 2019). An example of an antiplatelet agent is aspirin, which reduces the risk of stroke and blood clotting while optimizing vascular health. Blood pressure and cholesterol medications are also prescribed to optimize vascular health. It is important, however, to find more effective therapies for SVD that target its underlying mechanisms. Because these treatments do not reverse the damage caused by SVD and are limited in their ability to prevent disease progression, more effective therapies are needed. Healthcare professionals are able to monitor patients remotely in real time without requiring physical contact with them with telemedicine technologies, such as remote patient monitoring and teleconsultation. SVD patients have particularly benefitted from this, since it has made it possible to detect any changes in their condition early and intervene immediately if necessary. As a result of telemedicine technologies, individuals in remote areas, who would otherwise have limited access to specialized care, can now receive healthcare. In combination, these technologies will reduce the number of hospitalizations and healthcare costs associated with SVD, which will improve patient outcomes.

The objective of this chapter is to examine the significance of telemedicine technologies in regulating brain SVD by investigating the advantages and disadvantages of telemedicine-based treatments, as well as current research and advancements in the field. To aid in the diagnosis and prognosis of SVD, we are exploring how virtual reality (VR) and machine-learning (ML) algorithms can be integrated into telemedicine platforms. Medical imaging data, like magnetic resonance imaging (MRI) and computed tomography (CT), is utilized by these technologies to detect small vessel lesions, quantify disease severity, and predict patient outcomes. Data privacy and security, reimbursement policies, and technology requirements all play a role in the implementation of telemedicine technologies in SVD management. To address these challenges and ensure widespread adoption of telemedicine solutions, healthcare providers, policymakers, and technology developers need to collaborate. Through remote monitoring, teleconsultation, and advanced imaging analysis, SVD management can be improved through telemedicine. This chapter discusses how telemedicine can be used to control and manage brain SVD.

14.2 USE OF TELEMEDICINE TO CONTROL BRAIN SVD

14.2.1 Diagnosis

Technology has proven beneficial in providing timely treatment to patients with SVD and has emerged as a promising tool for controlling brain SVD. The advancement of telemedicine technologies has made remote consultations with healthcare professionals possible (Amadi-Obi et al., 2014; Schwamm et al., 2009). Patients can communicate with remote specialists in real time, sharing their images and test results, allowing for more efficient and accurate diagnosis and treatment. The use of telemedicine applications also allows healthcare providers to monitor their patients' progress continuously, allowing them to make necessary adjustments without having to visit patients often. In addition to reducing patient burden, SVD management is improved in general as a result. In addition to helping manage brain SVD remotely, telemedicine offers the advantage of monitoring patients' health status remotely using digital devices and sensors. By using the devices, healthcare providers can monitor patients' blood pressure, heart rate, and medication compliance without having to visit them personally, allowing them to stay on top of their progress. By utilizing this technology, brain SVD patients can be identified and managed in a timely manner in case of any changes in their health. Therefore, it is crucial that we collect and monitor data remotely in order to effectively manage this disease.

Figure 14.2 illustrates the implementation of a telemedicine framework in SVD control using teleconsultation and remote diagnostics. By using these technologies, healthcare providers can communicate remotely with patients, assess their conditions, and diagnose them accurately. By doing so, physical visits to healthcare facilities are eliminated, as well as healthcare costs and burdens are reduced. As a result of

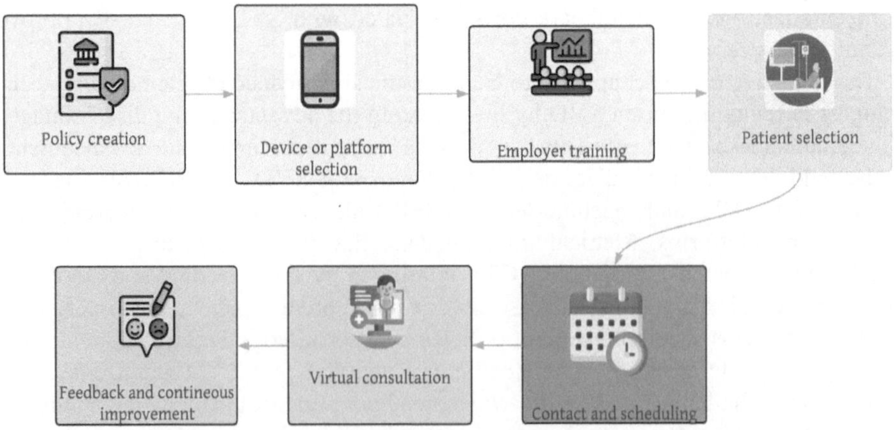

FIGURE 14.2 Telemedicine framework in the control of SVD.

teleconsultation and remote diagnostics, brain SVD is more likely to be detected early and treated promptly, improving patient outcomes and reducing complications. By implementing these technologies in healthcare settings, this prevalent condition can be managed and controlled much more effectively.

In healthcare, ML has been a significant application for automated disease detection and predictive analytics analysis (Javaid et al., 2022). A ML algorithm can analyze a large amount of data rapidly, enabling early diagnosis and detection of disease. With ML, clinicians can detect and analyze subtle manifestations of brain SVD automatically, improving patient outcomes and making accurate diagnoses. Healthcare providers are able to assess and manage SVD patients' conditions using remote monitoring devices and teleconsultations, reducing complications and ensuring timely interventions. Telemedicine also allows healthcare professionals to communicate and collaborate seamlessly, allowing them to exchange clinical information and make informed decisions regarding patient care. While further research is needed to fully understand how telemedicine can be used to control brain SVD, the results obtained so far indicate the transformative impact it can have on patient outcomes.

14.2.2 Remote Monitoring of SVD

Patients with SVD of the brain can greatly benefit from remote medication management and adherence monitoring. By using telemedicine technologies, healthcare providers can monitor patients' medication intake and ensure adherence to their treatment plans remotely. As a result, disease management can be improved and medication doses adjusted as needed, leading to better patient outcomes and timely intervention. It is also a convenient and cost-effective solution for patients and healthcare providers alike due to the lack of frequent hospital visits caused by remote medication management. In the management of brain SVD, virtual rehab and therapy sessions are emerging as promising alternatives. These sessions are delivered remotely using telemedicine technologies. Rather than having to travel, patients can access these sessions from the comfort of their own homes. Patients can benefit from targeted interventions and enhanced quality of life by achieving virtual rehabilitation and therapy sessions tailored to meet their specific needs.

It has become increasingly apparent that telemonitoring vital signs and disease progression can be effective in managing brain SVD in recent years. With this technology, healthcare providers can assess and monitor patients' vital signs remotely, including blood pressure, heart rate, oxygen levels, and disease progression. By continuously collecting and analyzing these data, healthcare professionals can improve patient outcomes by intervening and adjusting treatment plans in a timely manner. Additionally, telemonitoring reduces the frequency of hospital visits, which means both patients and healthcare systems benefit from more convenient, cost-effective solutions. In addition, telemedicine technologies have proven effective in treating and controlling SVD of the brain (Chirra et al., 2019). There are several diseases associated with cognitive decline and increasing disability in the aging population, including lacunar infarcts and hyperintensities of the white matter. Telemedicine is a powerful tool for identifying SVD early and implementing effective interventions through remote monitoring and assessment. The use of telemedicine allows healthcare providers and patients to communicate in real time, which reduces hospitalization and allows for timely adjustments to treatment plans. Improved outcomes could be achieved by patients with brain SVD thanks to this technology.

14.2.3 The Advantages of Telemedicine in SVD Control

There are benefits and challenges associated with the use of telemedicine in brain SVD. One of the main benefits is better access to specialized care, especially for rural or remote patients. As a result of telemedicine, hospital visits can be reduced, resulting in cost savings for both patients and healthcare systems. In addition, remote monitoring and timely interventions can enhance disease management efficiency through telemedicine. To ensure the success of telemedicine in controlling brain SVD, healthcare providers, patients, and/or their caregivers must be adequately trained, as well as the limitations of technology, privacy, and security concerns. For patients suffering from brain SVD, telemedicine technologies have significantly increased access to specialized care and expertise (Haleem et al., 2021). Through telemedicine platforms, patients in remote areas are able to consult with experts in neurology and neurosurgery without traveling far. By improving access, patients are able to receive the care and expertise they need, resulting in earlier diagnosis and better treatment. Additionally, telemedicine promotes collaboration among medical professionals and improves patient outcomes by facilitating the sharing of knowledge and expertise.

In contrast, telemedicine technologies can contribute to reduced healthcare expenses by controlling brain SVD in an efficient and cost-effective manner. Teleconsultations offer an alternative to in-person consultations that often require travel expenses, by allowing patients to communicate with healthcare professionals and receive prompt medical advice. As a result of telemedicine, SVD can also be detected and treated earlier, resulting in lower healthcare costs associated with complications and hospitalizations. Telemedicine technologies can lead to significant savings for both patients and healthcare providers.

14.3 ETHICAL CONCERNS RELATED TO BRAIN SVD AND TELEMEDICINE

Telemedicine has become a powerful tool for providing medical services and consultations. In the context of neurological diseases, telemedicine technologies offer the opportunity for early diagnosis, continuous care, and personalized treatment planning. The role of telemedicine in neurology care reflects its ability to overcome geographic limitations and improve patient access to speciality care. This section explores the data privacy, network requirements, artificial intelligence (AI) acts, etc., related with brain SVD and telemedicine.

14.3.1 Navigating Data Privacy and Security in Telemedicine

Telemedicine has provided a crucial solution for healthcare delivery through remote access to medical services. Maintaining the privacy and security of patient data is still of paramount importance. In this increasingly connected landscape, the healthcare industry is required to tackle these challenges while protecting sensitive patient information.

The General Data Protection Regulation (GDPR) in the European context establishes a comprehensive legal framework for data protection (Hussein et al., 2022). Upon processing data of EU individuals, telemedicine platforms operating outside the EU are subject to the GDPR's extraterritorial reach. Telemedicine platforms around the world face significant challenges as they deal with data of EU citizens when operating outside of Europe. This GDPR aspect ensures that European data subjects' rights are respected regardless of the location of the data processor.

The GDPR governs any telemedicine platform in Europe that collects, processes, and stores personal data. It is important for telemedicine platforms to adhere to data protection principles by processing data lawfully, obtaining informed consent, minimizing data, limiting its purpose, and being transparent in their operations. To maintain telemedicine services' trust, safeguard patient data, and avoid potential legal repercussions, it is argued that adhering to these data protection principles is crucial (Fields, 2020). Telemedicine platforms must make sure that data subjects are capable of exercising their rights under the GDPR, which include the ability to access, rectify, and delete their data. The importance of facilitating the exercise of data subjects' rights under the GDPR is precisely emphasized in (Article 12 GDPR – GDPRhub, n.d.). Data subjects are required to have access to their personal information and mechanisms for rectification, erasure, restriction of processing, and object processing on telemedicine platforms as a means of ensuring better control of their data. In another study, it was found that complying with GDPR is crucial for telemedicine platforms to maintain patient trust and avoid significant fines and penalties for non-compliance (Ricci et al., 2023). Telemedicine providers' reputational damage and legal consequences may result if they do not adhere to GDPR's provisions.

Telemedicine technologies have significant considerations regarding the ethical and legal implications of remote patient care. Concerns about patient autonomy, privacy, and informed consent arise from an ethical perspective. The question of whether patients can make well-informed decisions and their privacy is adequately protected is raised when it comes to remote patient care. In addition, the legal consequences of telemedicine technologies include concerns about liability and malpractice, as well as licensure in diverse jurisdictions. The efficient implementation and widespread use of telemedicine technologies to manage and control brain SVD relies on the ethical and legal frameworks being in place to govern remote patient care. Patient data security is ensured by integrating technologies that enhance privacy, such as encryption, access controls, and zero-trust security models, which enforce strict authentication before data access to prevent unauthorized access to medical records. According to a systematic review of legal and ethical aspects of telemedicine platforms, implementing privacy by design principles leads to increased patient trust and responsible data handling (Nittari et al., 2020). While challenges exist, effective solutions for safeguarding patient privacy and advancing telemedicine services can be found through multidisciplinary approaches and frameworks like privacy-enhanced telemedicine (PET) (Tan et al., 2022). Advanced encryption techniques, decentralized data storage, and granular access controls are among the features that this framework incorporates. It is demonstrated that PET can safeguard patient data while preserving telemedicine services' efficiency and effectiveness through simulations and data sensitivity analysis (Jordan et al., 2022).

To ensure adequate protection, data transfers outside the European Economic Area require special care. Standard contractual clauses (SCCs) or binding corporate rules (BCRs) are necessary for telemedicine platforms to enable lawful data transfer. According to these safeguards, patient's personal data are claimed to be protected when shared with entities outside the European Economic Area (EEA). To use telemedicine platforms, it is necessary to obtain valid and informed patient consent. It is important for patients to be informed about the processing of their personal data, and consent must be freely given, specific, and unambiguous. Telemedicine platforms were examined in a report for the challenges they face in implementing GDPR requirements during COVID pandemic (Solimini et al., 2021). It was found that many platforms had trouble establishing procedures for obtaining informed consent from patients in a telehealth setting. The research highlights the importance of having clear and user-friendly consent mechanisms in telemedicine. To ensure that consent is dynamic and revocable per GDPR guidelines, it is suggested to develop user-friendly patient portals or dashboards where users can manage data-sharing preferences. To enable patients to exercise their rights effectively, telemedicine platforms should have mechanisms for recording and managing consent.

Telemedicine platforms are obligated to implement rigorous security measures for personal data to protect patient information. Secure communication channels, encrypted data storage, access controls, automated compliance monitoring, data integrity checks, and regular security audits and assessments are just some of the things that need to be done. A strong security posture can only be achieved through compliance with industry standards, like ISO 27001. Telemedicine platforms must provide GDPR's breach notification, which includes Article 33, in the event of a data breach. Within a reasonable time and without delay, affected data subjects and the appropriate supervisory authorities need to be informed. Effective communication and minimization of breaches can be achieved by establishing contingency or incident response plans for telemedicine platforms. To successfully adopt telemedicine, it is necessary to have proper infrastructure in place and adhere to regulatory considerations. Addressing infrastructure requirements and regulatory considerations is crucial for the successful deployment of telemedicine in Europe. Ensure seamless and secure telemedicine services by ensuring robust broadband connectivity, appropriate hardware and software, mobile compatibility, and strong network security measures. Telemedicine platforms are able to effectively traverse the European landscape and provide safe, secure, and high-quality healthcare services based on compliance with GDPR, medical device regulations, and country-specific policies and guidelines. Investing in telemedicine infrastructure has become a priority for researchers and policymakers alike as it promotes equitable access to healthcare and improves patient outcomes in the rapidly evolving landscape of remote medical care. To ensure patient privacy, security, and quality of care, it is necessary to adhere to GDPR, telemedicine-specific guidelines, medical device regulations, cross-border data transfers, and other regulatory aspects. Telemedicine platforms are responsible for implementing practices that guarantee reliable consent, patient data control, compliance with licensing requirements, and compliance with varying reimbursement policies across European countries. Telemedicine platforms can provide patients with secure and high-quality healthcare services by effectively navigating the legal landscape and addressing these regulatory considerations.

14.3.2 Network Requirements Supporting Compliance with the Law

Telemedicine platforms require high-speed and uninterrupted internet connection to facilitate real-time communication and data transfer between healthcare providers and patients. In order to ensure seamless telemedicine services, it is necessary to have adequate broadband infrastructure in all areas, regardless of whether they are rural, semi-urban, urban, or even metropolitan. Additionally, the proper hardware and software components are necessary for telemedicine platforms. Telemedicine providers should utilize secure videoconferencing, data storage servers, remote monitoring devices, and user-friendly software for stakeholders. This ensures compliance with GDPR rights. To prevent data duplication, decentralized data-sharing models can be integrated, while AI-driven automation can flag discrepancies and enhance diagnostic accuracy. In a study, it was found that efficient telemedicine platforms rely on key components, as well as comprehensible software interfaces, to improve the user experience for stakeholders (Beheshti et al., 2022). Telemedicine platforms should strive to be compatible with mobile devices as smartphones and tablets become more common. The increase in user-friendliness for patients will be beneficial. Researchers evaluated usability to assess the impact of mobile compatibility on patient engagement, and they discovered that mobile compatibility improved patient satisfaction and access to telemedicine (Kruse et al., 2017). To ensure data protection on the network, dynamic encryption protocols (in line with GDPR) and network security measures, such as firewalls and proper detection systems for external interferences, are necessary. The transmission of data was discussed in relation to the aforementioned concerns (Javaid et al., 2023).

Addressing infrastructure requirements and regulatory considerations is crucial for the successful deployment of telemedicine in Europe. The success of telemedicine services rests on the ability to have robust broadband connectivity, the right hardware and software, mobile compatibility, and strong network security measures. Telemedicine platforms can deliver safe, secure, and high-quality healthcare services across Europe by complying with GDPR, medical device regulations, and country-specific policies and guidelines. Telemedicine platforms have to follow procedures that guarantee valid consent, patient data control, compliance with licensing requirements, and comply with varying reimbursement policies in European countries. Telemedicine platforms can navigate the legal landscape with the help of regulatory considerations and provide secure and high-quality healthcare services to patients.

14.3.3 Scratching the surface of the AI Act and the Data Act

There are additional regulatory layers that telemedicine platforms must consider to ensure compliance and safeguard patient data in addition to GDPR – referring to recently proposed AI Act (AI Act Implementation: Timelines & Next Steps | EU Artificial Intelligence Act, n.d.) and Data Act (Data Act – Publications Office of the EU, n.d.) in Europe. The AI Act, introduced by the European Commission, seeks to create a comprehensive regulatory framework for AI, emphasizing human oversight, transparency, and accountability. To meet the stringent requirements of the AI Act, telemedicine platforms that use AI for diagnostics, treatment recommendations, or patient monitoring need to classify and implement their AI systems. To build patient trust and uphold ethical standards, it is necessary to conduct risk assessments, implement data governance, and ensure transparency in AI-driven decisions, while also complying with the law. Additionally, clear liability agreements between telemedicine platforms and healthcare providers should specify responsibility for AI-generated misdiagnoses and treatment recommendations.

The Data Act emphasizes the need for interoperability and fair data usage practices, while focusing on data sharing and access. The goal of telemedicine platforms is to ensure that patient data is securely and efficiently shared across different healthcare providers and systems, resulting in a more integrated and responsive healthcare environment. Article 36 of the Data Act is a one-of-a-kind provision that outlines safe termination in data sharing agreements. It uniquely addresses the role of smart contracts in data governance and compliance within the European legislative framework. To comply with the Data Act, the telemedicine providers can start by cataloging patient data flows to ensure compliance with the Data Act's access and portability requirements, while strengthening interoperability through secure data-sharing protocols and blockchain validation to prevent duplication errors. To mitigate risks like misuse of patient data, data validation and automate access controls is useful, ensuring only authorized professionals retrieve sensitive information. Telemedicine providers may adopt standardized data formats like FHIR and HL7 to ensure smooth cross-platform communication. This can be implemented along with secure APIs for real-time patient data sharing to maintain GDPR's encryption standards.

According to Mazzini & Scalzo (2022), the regulatory framework for medical devices, which often relies on software, has been a key inspiration for the AI Act and has been successfully tested over the past 15 years. The AI Act's risk-classified methodology is a reflection of this approach, which prioritizes internal market goals over protecting fundamental rights (An EU Artificial Intelligence Act for Fundamental Rights A Civil Society Statement, n.d.). The AI Act combines health and safety imperatives with market access considerations, unlike the GDPR and the Digital Services Act, which focus on data privacy (Gregorio, 2022; Pałka, 2020; Regulation - 2022/2065 - EN - DSA - EUR-Lex, n.d.). The Technical Requirements of the Act aim to ensure that AI systems comply with market entry procedures, aligning with the EU's expertise in product safety regulation. This framework is designed to capitalize on the EU's extensive experience and institutional capabilities in product safety, with the goal of harmonizing AI regulation across Member States. The emphasis on market access may cause problems, as it may overlook the importance of addressing AI-specific risks and fundamental rights protections. The AI Act's aim is to balance innovation and safety by incorporating elements from the medical device regulatory framework, utilizing proven methodologies while navigating the unique challenges presented by AI technologies.

Telemedicine platforms must ensure regulatory compliance by integrating compliance under the AI Act and Data Act with the existing GDPR and other consumer protection laws, including those mentioned in this article. This involves taking rigorous steps to protect data, deploying AI transparently, and ensuring interoperability and patient control over data. Telemedicine can provide high-quality, secure, and equitable healthcare services throughout Europe by evolving and effectively addressing both current and future regulatory landscapes.

14.4 FROM THE PRESENT TO THE FUTURE

The evolution of telemedicine has the potential to revolutionize the way healthcare is delivered through emerging trends and advancements in technology. Data privacy and security concerns have become a critical focal point alongside these advancements. The healthcare industry has undergone a revolution due to the advancements in telemedicine technologies, particularly in neurology (Thimbleby, 2013). Mobile devices, such as smartphones, tablets, and wearables, are now providing remote monitoring and diagnosis for patients with SVD of the brain. By integrating advanced imaging techniques and AI algorithms, telemedicine technologies can detect these diseases accurately and timely, leading to early intervention and personalized treatment plans. Telemedicine also allows healthcare professionals to reach patients in remote areas, enhancing the accessibility and efficiency of healthcare services, ultimately leading to better patient outcomes.

Telemedicine's potential in effectively controlling and managing brain SVD has been demonstrated in several case studies and success stories in recent years. Patients with SVD have seen a significant reduction in hospital admissions and improved patient outcomes due to the use of telemedicine in remote monitoring and treatment (Heinzelmann et al., 2005). Remote imaging and video consultations, among other telemedicine interventions, have enabled timely diagnosis and treatment of SVD, thus reducing the risk of complications and progression of the disease. Evidence suggests that telemedicine has a positive impact on controlling SVD and that it is important to implement this technology further to improve healthcare outcomes for this patient population (Losorelli et al., 2021).

In the last few years, there have been numerous real-world examples of telemedicine implementation, particularly in the field of brain SVD control. A stroke telemedicine program at the Medical University of South Carolina provides specialized stroke care via telemedicine to rural areas, where access to neurologists is limited (Al Kasab et al., 2017). Similarly, the VR Tele stroke program at the Department of Veterans Affairs connects stroke specialists with patients in rural communities, ensuring early diagnosis and treatment (Telestroke Training Key in Caring for Veterans – Office of Academic Affiliations, n.d.). Telemedicine can be utilized to provide specialized healthcare services to underserved populations, as demonstrated by these real-life examples. The implementation of telemedicine technologies in controlling brain SVD has led to positive outcomes and improvements in the outcomes for patients. The advancements have made it possible to detect and diagnose diseases earlier, resulting in timely interventions and better treatment outcomes. Telemedicine has made it easier for healthcare providers and specialists to coordinate, leading to improved care and patient management. Remote monitoring and teleconsultation have made it easier for patients to access healthcare services, especially in rural areas where specialists are scarce. Telemedicine technologies have proved their worth in expanding access and improving the quality of care for patients with brain SVD (Silva et al., 2012).

Valuable insights and lessons for future practice have been gained from the implementation of telemedicine technologies in brain SVD control. Remote diagnosis and monitoring have been demonstrated to be effective and feasible, which allows for prompt and accurate interpretation of imaging studies. Additionally, it has demonstrated that teleconsultation and multidisciplinary collaboration can provide comprehensive and holistic care to patients. Furthermore, the use of telemedicine technologies has highlighted the significance of patient education and empowerment, which enable self-management and early diagnosis of symptoms. To improve patient outcomes and manage brain SVD, it is imperative to further explore and refine telemedicine strategies moving forward. Telemedicine technologies have the potential to control brain SVD with promising results. The potential for early detection and intervention is significant due to the advances in telehealth platforms, remote patient monitoring, and diagnostic tools. The accuracy and efficiency of diagnosing and monitoring these conditions can be greatly increased by integrating ML algorithms. To manage SVD effectively, large-scale randomized controlled trials are recommended for future research to evaluate their effectiveness and cost-effectiveness. Additionally, it is important to work towards eliminating barriers and concerns related to privacy, security, and telehealth service accessibility for all individuals, especially the elderly and those in underserved communities.

Wearable devices and the Internet of Things (IoT) can be integrated with telemedicine technologies. The use of IoT architecture leads to more thorough and accurate monitoring of patients with SVD of the brain. Continuously measuring vital signs and collecting valuable data is possible with wearable devices like fitness trackers, smartwatches, and blood pressure monitoring cuffs. Healthcare providers can provide prompt intervention, when necessary, when real-time data is remotely accessed by integrating these devices with telemedicine systems. In addition, the IoT architecture facilitates seamless integration and communication between different medical devices, allowing for more effective management of SVD, facilitating patient information sharing, and facilitating healthcare professional collaboration. Through connected medical wearables and devices, Internet of Medical Things (IoMT) allows for continuous data collection. Remote patient monitoring allows healthcare providers to receive continuous data to enable proactive interventions and personalized care. However, data privacy and security can also be a challenge when using IoMT. To ensure patient confidentiality and compliance with the GDPR, IoMT devices need to be authenticated, access controls enabled, and their data encrypted.

Several regulatory considerations and policy changes must be addressed in order to effectively implement telemedicine technologies for controlling brain SVD. Protecting patient privacy and ensuring the security of medical data is a crucial regulatory consideration. To ensure patient trust and data security, it is crucial to comply with applicable regulations and implement encryption and data protection measures. Policies must be set up to regulate reimbursement of telemedicine services, and healthcare providers must be licensed to practice telemedicine across state lines. Effective and seamless deployment of telemedicine for controlling SVD of the brain can be achieved by addressing regulatory considerations and enacting necessary policy changes. Moreover, telemedicine technologies have demonstrated their potential in controlling brain SVD. For patients in remote or underserved areas, traditional methods of diagnosis and treatment may be challenging due to the requirement of in-person assessments and interventions.

Telemedicine is a solution that allows for remote monitoring, consultations, and personalized care without the necessity of physical presence. The potential of these advancements in telemedicine is significant for improving healthcare access for individuals with SVD and enhancing the overall management of these conditions. ML algorithms and VR programs are being increasingly integrated into telemedicine platforms to assist in diagnosis, treatment planning, and patient monitoring. VR technologies are not limited to processing vast amounts of medical data; they also provide immersive experiences for patient education, training, and surgical planning. Healthcare professionals can visualize complex medical scenarios and increase patient engagement through these technologies.

14.5 CONCLUSIONS

The focus of this chapter is on the utilization of telemedicine technologies in managing and controlling brain SVD. The main topics discussed are the definition and prevalence of SVD, the limitations of traditional diagnosis and treatment methods, and how telemedicine could revolutionize healthcare delivery for SVD patients. Telemedicine can facilitate early detection, accurate diagnosis, remote monitoring, and personalized treatment plans for SVD patients, which can improve their overall outcomes and reduce healthcare costs. To successfully implement telemedicine in SVD management, it is important to address challenges such as data security and limited access to technology. SVD of the brain can be effectively managed and controlled through the use of telemedicine technologies. Telemedicine has the potential to improve patient outcomes and reduce the burden on healthcare systems by enabling remote monitoring, early detection, and timely intervention. In addition, telemedicine allows patients in rural or underserved areas to receive specialist care, thus bridging the healthcare gap. To fully appreciate the potential of telemedicine in this area, it is necessary to address challenges related to privacy concerns, lack of reimbursement policies, and technological limitations. In order to optimize telemedicine's role in managing brain SVD, it is necessary to conduct more research and collaborate among healthcare providers, policymakers, and technology developers.

Furthermore, the significance of telemedicine in managing SVD cannot be neglected. Healthcare providers have the ability to remotely monitor patients' conditions and provide real-time consultations by using telemedicine technologies. The risk of complications related to SVD can be minimized by early detection and intervention. Telemedicine eliminates geographical barriers, making it possible for people in remote areas to receive healthcare. Furthermore, it makes it easier for patients to learn and encourages their involvement in disease management. Controlling SVD and improving patient outcomes is made possible by telemedicine. In order to fully comprehend the potential applications and effectiveness of telemedicine technologies in controlling brain SVD, more research and implementation is required. The focus of future research should be on conducting clinical trials and longitudinal studies to examine the long-term effects of telemedicine interventions for this specific patient population. It is important to examine the obstacles and hindrances that prevent the widespread use of telemedicine technologies, such as legal and regulatory issues, reimbursement policies, and technological limitations. By dealing with these issues, healthcare professionals can determine the most effective methods for integrating telemedicine into routine clinical practice and improve the care provided for individuals with SVD of the brain.

REFERENCES

AI Act Implementation: Timelines & Next steps I EU Artificial Intelligence Act. (n.d.). Retrieved July 15, 2024, from https://artificialintelligenceact.eu/ai-act-implementation-next-steps/

Al Kasab, S., Adams, R. J., Debenham, E., Jones, D. J., & Holmstedt, C. A. (2017). Medical University of South Carolina Telestroke: a telemedicine facilitated network for stroke treatment in South Carolina-a progress report. *Telemedicine Journal and E-Health: The Official Journal of the American Telemedicine Association*, 23(8), 674–677. https://doi.org/10.1089/TMJ.2016.0229

Amadi-Obi, A., Gilligan, P., Owens, N., & O'Donnell, C. (2014). Telemedicine in pre-hospital care: a review of telemedicine applications in the pre-hospital environment. *International Journal of Emergency Medicine*, 7(1). https://doi.org/10.1186/S12245-014-0029-0

An EU Artificial Intelligence Act for Fundamental Rights A Civil Society Statement. (n.d.).

Article 12 GDPR – GDPRhub. (n.d.). Retrieved July 15, 2024, from https://gdprhub.eu/Article_12_GDPR

Beheshti, L., Kalankesh, L. R., DOSHMANGIR, L., & Farahbakhsh, M. (2022). Telehealth in primary health care: A scoping review of the literature. *Perspectives in Health Information Management*, 19(1), 1n.

Ben-Assuli, O. (2022). Measuring the cost-effectiveness of using telehealth for diabetes management: a narrative review of methods and findings. *International Journal of Medical Informatics*, 163. https://doi.org/10.1016/J.IJMEDINF.2022.104764

Chirra, M., Marsili, L., Wattley, L., Sokol, L. L., Keeling, E., Maule, S., Sobrero, G., Artusi, C. A., Romagnolo, A., Zibetti, M., Lopiano, L., Espay, A. J., Obeidat, A. Z., & Merola, A. (2019). Telemedicine in neurological disorders: opportunities and challenges. *Telemedicine Journal and E-Health: The Official Journal of the American Telemedicine Association*, 25(7), 541–550. https://doi.org/10.1089/TMJ.2018.0101

Data Act – Publications Office of the EU. (n.d.). Retrieved July 15, 2024, from https://op.europa.eu/en/publication-detail/-/publication/9f840928-aa62-11ec-83e1-01aa75ed71a1/language-en

Fields, B. G. (2020). Regulatory, legal, and ethical considerations of telemedicine. *Sleep Medicine Clinics*, 15(3), 409–416. https://doi.org/10.1016/J.JSMC.2020.06.004

Gao, C., Nie, M., Huang, J., Tian, Y., Wang, D., Zhang, J., & Jiang, R. (2022). Pharmacotherapy for mild traumatic brain injury: an overview of the current treatment options. *Expert Opinion on Pharmacotherapy*, 23(7), 805–813. https://doi.org/10.1080/14656566.2022.2054328

Gregorio, G. De. (2022). *Digital Constitutionalism in Europe: Reframing Rights and Powers in the Algorithmic Society*. Cambridge University Press. https://doi.org/10.1017/9781009071215

Haleem, A., Javaid, M., Singh, R. P., & Suman, R. (2021). Telemedicine for healthcare: capabilities, features, barriers, and applications. *Sensors International*, 2. https://doi.org/10.1016/J.SINTL.2021.100117

Hamilton, O. K. L., Cox, S. R., Ballerini, L., Bastin, M. E., Corley, J., Gow, A. J., Muñoz Maniega, S., Redmond, P., Valdés Hernández, M. del C., Wardlaw, J. M., & Deary, I. J. (2021). Associations between total MRI-visible small vessel disease burden and domain-specific cognitive abilities in a community-dwelling older-age cohort. *Neurobiology of Aging*, 105, 25–34. https://doi.org/10.1016/J.NEUROBIOLAGING.2021.04.007

Hamilton, O. K. L., Cox, S. R., Okely, J. A., Conte, F., Ballerini, L., Bastin, M. E., Corley, J., Taylor, A. M., Page, D., Gow, A. J., Muñoz Maniega, S., Redmond, P., Valdés-Hernández, M. del C., Wardlaw, J. M., & Deary, I. J. (2021). Cerebral small vessel disease burden and longitudinal cognitive decline from age 73 to 82: the Lothian Birth Cohort 1936. *Translational Psychiatry*, 11(1). https://doi.org/10.1038/S41398-021-01495-4

Heinzelmann, P. J., Lugn, N. E., & Kvedar, J. C. (2005). Telemedicine in the future. *Journal of Telemedicine and Telecare*, 11(8), 384–390. https://doi.org/10.1177/1357633X0501100802

Huang, Z., Tao, H., Meng, Q., & Jing, L. (2015a). Management of endocrine disease: effects of telecare intervention on glycemic control in type 2 diabetes: a systematic review and meta-analysis of randomized controlled trials. *European Journal of Endocrinology*, 172(3), R93–R101. https://doi.org/10.1530/EJE-14-0441

Huang, Z., Tao, H., Meng, Q., & Jing, L. (2015b). Management of endocrine disease. effects of telecare intervention on glycemic control in type 2 diabetes: a systematic review and meta-analysis of randomized controlled trials. *European Journal of Endocrinology*, 172(3), R93–R101. https://doi.org/10.1530/EJE-14-0441

Hussein, R., Wurhofer, D., Strumegger, E. M., Stainer-Hochgatterer, A., Kulnik, S. T., Crutzen, R., & Niebauer, J. (2022). General Data Protection Regulation (GDPR) Toolkit for digital health. *Studies in Health Technology and Informatics*, 290, 222–226. https://doi.org/10.3233/SHTI220066

Inzitari, D., Pracucci, G., Poggesi, A., Carlucci, G., Barkhof, F., Chabriat, H., Erkinjuntti, T., Fazekas, F., Ferro, J. M., Hennerici, M., Langhorne, P., O'Brien, J., Scheltens, P., Visser, M. C., Wahlund, L. O., Waldemar, G., Wallin, A., & Pantoni, L. (2009). Changes in white matter as determinant of global functional decline in older independent outpatients: three year follow-up of LADIS (leukoaraiosis and disability) study cohort. *BMJ*, 339(7715), 279–282. https://doi.org/10.1136/BMJ.B2477

Javaid, M., Haleem, A., Pratap Singh, R., Suman, R., & Rab, S. (2022). Significance of machine learning in healthcare: features, pillars and applications. *International Journal of Intelligent Networks*, 3, 58–73. https://doi.org/10.1016/J.IJIN.2022.05.002

Javaid, M., Haleem, A., Singh, R. P., & Suman, R. (2023). Towards insighting cybersecurity for healthcare domains: a comprehensive review of recent practices and trends. *Cyber Security and Applications*, 1, 100016. https://doi.org/10.1016/J.CSA.2023.100016

Jordan, S., Fontaine, C., & Hendricks-Sturrup, R. (2022). Selecting privacy-enhancing technologies for managing health data use. *Frontiers in Public Health*, 10, 814163. https://doi.org/10.3389/FPUBH.2022.814163/BIBTEX

Kruse, C. S., Krowski, N., Rodriguez, B., Tran, L., Vela, J., & Brooks, M. (2017). Telehealth and patient satisfaction: a systematic review and narrative analysis. *BMJ Open*, 7(8). https://doi.org/10.1136/BMJOPEN-2017-016242

Losorelli, S. D., Vendra, V., Hildrew, D. M., Woodson, E. A., Brenner, M. J., & Sirjani, D. B. (2021). The future of telemedicine: revolutionizing health care or flash in the pan?

Otolaryngology--Head and Neck Surgery: Official Journal of American Academy of Otolaryngology-Head and Neck Surgery, 165(2), 239–243. https://doi.org/10.1177/0194599820983330

Markus, H. S., & Erik de Leeuw, F. (2023). Cerebral small vessel disease: recent advances and future directions. *International Journal of Stroke: Official Journal of the International Stroke Society*, 18(1), 4–14. https://doi.org/10.1177/17474930221144911

Mazzini, G., & Scalzo, S. (2022). The proposal for the artificial intelligence act: considerations around some key concepts. *SSRN Electronic Journal*. https://doi.org/10.2139/SSRN.4098809

Mestre, H., Kostrikov, S., Mehta, R. I., & Nedergaard, M. (2017). Perivascular spaces, glymphatic dysfunction, and small vessel disease. *Clinical Science (London, England: 1979)*, 131(17), 2257–2274. https://doi.org/10.1042/CS20160381

Minagar, A., Fowler, M., Harris, M. K., & Jaffe, S. L. (2010). Neurologic presentations of systemic vasculitides. *Neurologic Clinics*, 28(1), 171–184. https://doi.org/10.1016/J.NCL.2009.09.015

Nittari, G., Khuman, R., Baldoni, S., Pallotta, G., Battineni, G., Sirignano, A., Amenta, F., & Ricci, G. (2020). Telemedicine practice: review of the current ethical and legal challenges. *Telemedicine and E-Health*. https://doi.org/10.1089/tmj.2019.0158

Pałka, P. (2020). Data Management Law for the 2020s: the lost origins and the new needs. *Buffalo Law Review*, 68(2), 559–640.

Raghunath, A., Desai, K., & Ahluwalia, M. S. (2019). Current treatment options for breast cancer brain metastases. *Current Treatment Options in Oncology*, 20(3). https://doi.org/10.1007/S11864-019-0618-5

Regulation – 2022/2065 - EN - DSA - EUR-Lex. (n.d.). Retrieved July 15, 2024, from https://eur-lex.europa.eu/eli/reg/2022/2065/oj

Ricci, G., Caraffa, A. M., & Gibelli, F. (2023). Telemedicine as a strategic tool to enhance the effectiveness of care processes: technological and regulatory evolution over the past two decades. *Healthcare*, 11(5), 734. https://doi.org/10.3390/HEALTHCARE11050734

Schwamm, L. H., Holloway, R. G., Amarenco, P., Audebert, H. J., Bakas, T., Chumbler, N. R., Handschu, R., Jauch, E. C., Knight IV, W. A., Levine, S. R., Mayberg, M., Meyer, B. C., Meyers, P. M., Skalabrin, E., & Wechsler, L. R. (2009). A review of the evidence for the use of telemedicine within stroke systems of care: a scientific statement from the American Heart Association/American Stroke Association. *Stroke*, 40(7), 2616–2634. https://doi.org/10.1161/STROKEAHA.109.192360

Silva, G. S., Farrell, S., Shandra, E., Viswanathan, A., & Schwamm, L. H. (2012). The status of telestroke in the united states: a survey of currently active stroke telemedicine programs. *Stroke*, 43(8), 2078–2085. https://doi.org/10.1161/STROKEAHA.111.645861/SUPPL_FILE/STR202178-SUPPLEMENTALMATERIAL.PDF

Solimini, R., Busardò, F. P., Gibelli, F., Sirignano, A., & Ricci, G. (2021). Ethical and legal challenges of telemedicine in the era of the COVID-19 pandemic. *Medicina (Kaunas, Lithuania)*, 57(12). https://doi.org/10.3390/MEDICINA57121314

Staals, J., Makin, S. D. J., Doubal, F. N., Dennis, M. S., & Wardlaw, J. M. (2014). Stroke subtype, vascular risk factors, and total MRI brain small-vessel disease burden. *Neurology*, 83(14), 1228–1234. https://doi.org/10.1212/WNL.0000000000000837

Tan, K.-L., Chi, C.-H., & Lam, K.-Y. (2022). How Privacy-Enhanced Technologies (Pets) are transforming digital healthcare delivery. *American Scientific Research Journal for Engineering, Technology, and Sciences*, 90(1), 351–361.

Technology Assessment: Early Sense for Monitoring Vital Signs in Hospitalized Patients [Internet] – PubMed. (n.d.). Retrieved July 15, 2024, from https://pubmed.ncbi.nlm.nih.gov/27606394/

Telestroke training key in caring for Veterans – Office of Academic Affiliations. (n.d.). Retrieved July 15, 2024, from www.va.gov/OAA/features/Telestroke_training_key_in_caring_for_Veterans.asp

Thimbleby, H. (2013). Technology and the future of healthcare. *Journal of Public Health Research*, 2(3), jphr.2013.e28. https://doi.org/10.4081/JPHR.2013.E28

Walsh, J., & Markus, H. S. (2019). Telemedicine for follow-up of rare neurological disease: development and evaluation in cerebral autosomal dominant arteriopathy with subcortical infarcts and leukoencephalopathy. *Stroke*, 50(3), 750–753. https://doi.org/10.1161/STROKEAHA.118.023779/SUPPL_FILE/STR_STROKE-2018-023779D_SUPP1.PDF

Wardlaw, J. M., Smith, C., & Dichgans, M. (2019). Small vessel disease: mechanisms and clinical implications. *The Lancet Neurology*, 18(7), 684–696. https://doi.org/10.1016/S1474-4422(19)30079-1

Wightman, A., Barlis, P., MacBain, M., Hodgson, L., Cheng, L., Gocuk, S., Hayat, U., Chow, D., Tacey, M., Hutchinson, A., Colville, D., Lamoureux, E., & Savige, J. (2019). Small vessel disease and intracoronary plaque composition: a single centre cross-sectional observational study. *Scientific Reports*, 9(1). https://doi.org/10.1038/S41598-019-39989-3

Williamson, J. R., & Kilo, C. (1980). Small-vessel disease: diabetic microangiopathy. *Angiology*, 31(7), 448–454. https://doi.org/10.1177/000331978003100702

Zhang, C. lin, Hong, C. dong, Wang, H. ling, Chen, A. qi, Zhou, Y. fan, Wan, Y., Li, Y. nan, & Hu, B. (2020a). The role of semaphorins in small vessels of the eye and brain. *Pharmacological Research*, 160. https://doi.org/10.1016/J.PHRS.2020.105044

Zhang, C. lin, Hong, C. dong, Wang, H. ling, Chen, A. qi, Zhou, Y. fan, Wan, Y., Li, Y. nan, & Hu, B. (2020b). The role of semaphorins in small vessels of the eye and brain. *Pharmacological Research*, 160. https://doi.org/10.1016/J.PHRS.2020.105044

Section IV

Natural Language Processing (NLP) for Assisted Living in Healthcare 5.0

15 NLP Techniques and Applications in Healthcare Systems

Atul Kumar

15.1 INTRODUCTION

NLP is the domain of computing systems that deals with natural language. It consists of the formation of patterns and algorithms that provide them with the ability to understand, analyze, and synthesize human language. Other applications of NLP are text classification, sentiment analysis, machine translation, question answering, health, and information extraction from unstructured data such as emails, tweets, and documents. The application domain of NLP finds its padre in the fifties as a subfield of linguistics and artificial intelligence, with the objective to translate human writing and speaking. First, it began with limited functionalities, such as word and phrase translations, checking grammars (Nadkarni et al., 2011), then moved towards providing broader services that would include summarization, information retrieval, sentiment analysis, chatbots, predictive analytics, and others. The field has rapidly expanded, with millions of persons actively researching its applications (Grosz, 1982).

However, the growing interest in research in the field of healthcare has also caused the development of NLP. The pipeline developments that would enable comprehensiveness at large scale of clinical notes could improve the different aspects of the comprehensive healthcare delivery process; quality assurance, the resources, and billing from details obtained from the analysis of EHRs to practice. This is because with the adoption of ICT in the healthcare sector there has been the introduction of technologies such as EMR and EHR hence improving the management of healthcare organizations. These solutions enable people to get the required medical data as soon as possible and with less cost and mistakes, protect the data's confidentiality and allow to save a lot of health-related information. Nonetheless, most of the information is in textual form and in natural language in most documents, which are difficult for an electronic system to interpret. Therefore, solutions in terms of NLP approaches were applied to extract the needed information from the narrative texts, and the structured data was incorporated into the decision-making.

DOI: 10.1201/9781003520184-19

15.2 RELATED WORK

In this section, we will highlight researches made in the field of healthcare using NLP. Moreover, Tyagi and Bhushan (2023) investigated the role of natural language processing (NLP) in Healthcare 4.0, noting its effectiveness in mining useful data from unstructured information. The paper provided an overview of the state-of-the-art in NLP in the healthcare domain. It stressed their capacity to address the current data-related challenges and improve the quality of patient care. According to Kumar and Gond, NLP in healthcare redefined the EHR system and contributed to faster diagnosis besides enhancing patient care during the COVID-19 pandemic. It supports CDSS, VR, and speech recognition tools, enhancing the documentation process as well as automatically identifying patients for clinical trials. Some of these are vision therapy and disease identification for Alzheimer's are expected to introduce a radical shift within the clinic. Some of the areas that healthcare institutions apply AI and NLP include payment reconciliation, chart analysis, and general improvement of the healthcare system. Basyal et al. (2020) presented a comprehensive state-of-the-art analysis on NLP and how it contributes to knowledge generation, documentation, dissemination, and utilization in the health sector. They described NLP techniques that can support knowledge management extraction and capture in healthcare contexts. Besides, they provided a conceptual model of the knowledge extraction process using NLP. Last but not the least, they enumerated challenges, future research initiatives, and prospective areas of healthcare NLP investigation. In their article, Friedman and Elhadad (2013) also talked about the necessity of NLP, possibilities of its application in biomedical and healthcare fields, types of knowledge incorporated in this field, and the primary methods used.

Abualigah et al. (2019) supplied methods and techniques for reading the usage of sensory analysis within the healthcare enterprise. Locke et al. (2021) discussed NLP strategies and herbal language expertise for appropriate responses. It supports unfastened textual content searches in medical information for predictive and triage gear. NLP is also said to enhance the prediction of patient mortality in intensive care and differentiate pre-treatment data, while chatbots provide patient-facing assistance through auditory questions and by raising appropriate responses (Garg and Gupta, 2024). In Natural Language Processing (NLP) in Hospital Health Care, we studied progress and setbacks in detail. This includes various NLP applications, such as clinical document classification, named workgroup validation, information extraction, clinical discussion process, and clinical decision support. These applications have provided great improvements in clinical documentation, patient care, and analytical outcomes. Nawab et al. (2020) produced tables containing commonly appearing nouns, adjectives, and bigrams. The comments that had these common characteristics were carefully examined in order to identify the factors that contribute to poor patient feedback. They then utilized this positive and negative feedback as training data for a neural network that classifies sentences from hybrid reviews. Attar and Komal (2022) investigated various applications that go as far as using scattered patient records to be rearranged into EHRs and processing data related to COVID-19 to improve crisis management. The review by Al-Garadi et al. (2022) on the application of natural language processing strategies over different scopes of the COVID-19 pandemic. The authors presented the argument for the advancements, underlined the possible prospects, and pointed to the difficulties. Their findings would seem to provide important recommendations for change within systems of health and social responses, improved preparedness for pandemics, and hence more. In this study, the researchers have compared the effectiveness of a few machine-learning techniques within the healthcare field to handle the problems in plain text data conversion and heterogeneity with the help of natural language processing. Their performance on diagnosis tasks was compared, and as a result, it is recommended to use TRSVM on smaller high-dimensional datasets, while TWNFI is recommended on bigger datasets due to its higher scalability and performance. The effectiveness and role of artificial intelligence in the health sector, as assessed in a current study by Kuwaiti et al. (2023), are of large magnitude. The referred areas of the study or AI implementation were medical imaging, virtual care, research, patient engagement, rehabilitation, and administrative activities. Ahmed et al.'s study (2023) detailed how natural language processing was going to change clinical decision support systems in health. NLP methods for information extraction include named entity recognition and relation extraction over unstructured text data sources, such as electronic health records and medical literature, extracting key clinical information that is helpful in diagnosis, treatment, and administrative activities.

15.3 WORKING OF NLP IN HEALTHCARE

NLP is a branch of AI that specializes in the connection among computers and human language. In the sphere of healthcare, NLP proves to be fantastically treasured because it allows the extraction of pertinent statistics from unstructured textual data like scientific notes, scientific literature, and patient facts. Figure 15.1 illustrates the functioning of healthcare in NLP.

Figure 15.1 illustrates the numerous steps involved in making use of NLP inside the area of healthcare.

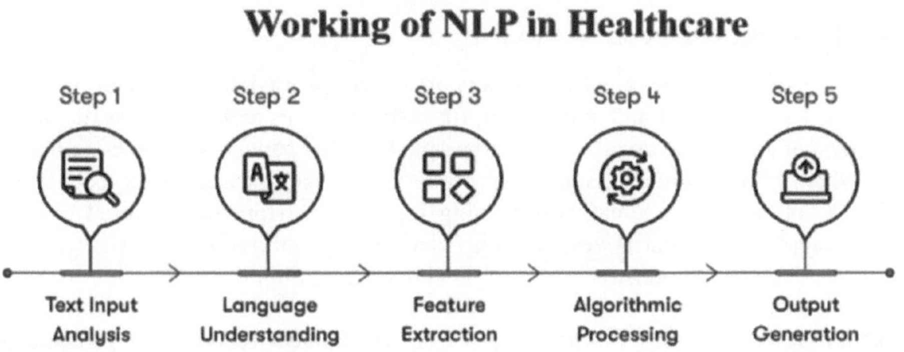

FIGURE 15.1 Steps of NLP in healthcare.

Analysis of the Textual Content Input: NLP evolved via studying large volumes of text facts, frequently along with clinical notes, affected person facts, and clinical literature. Tokenization breaks down the text into smaller components, like phrases or phrases, creating a structured foundation for analysis.

Understanding the Language: NLP uses best practices to understand relationships between words and captures nuances of language. Named entity recognition (NER) can identify and classify unique entities such as diseases, drugs, and procedures, facilitating a better understanding of the textual content

Extracting Features: Relevant scientific phrases are extracted from the textual content for analysis. This phase is important in making ready the information for further processing.

Algorithmic Processing: Machine getting to know algorithms are skilled on a numerous range of healthcare datasets and eventually applied. These algorithms make use of extracted features to correctly expect and categorize data.

Generating Output: The final end result is practical insights or prepared statistics received from the original unstructured text, which can consist of whatever from diagnostic codes to treatment hints.

15.4 NLP IN HEALTHCARE APPLICATIONS

NLP is a powerful technique that has several applications in healthcare, including improving patient care, streamlining processes, and propelling research forward. More so, to carry out this goal, NLP assists in extracting insights from the unstructured text leading to improved diagnosis accuracy tailored treatments and better result outcomes. From clinical documentation and decision assistance to patient monitoring, it touches every level of healthcare delivery. Several examples of such significant applications are the following:

15.4.1 Clinical Documentation

Clinical documentation refers to the way in which all medical data relevant for a given case are recorded and maintained, for instance, signs and symptoms diagnosis treatment and outcome details. In the past, much of this paperwork was done manually, which may be time-consuming or prone to mistakes as well. NLP technology offers a solution by automatically parsing information from unstructured clinical notes, transcriptions, narratives, etc., into electronic health record systems (EHRs). Figure 15.2 below demonstrates how clinical documentation functions.

Text Analysis: NLP algorithms analyze free text clinical records like physician's notes, discharge summaries, consultation reports, etc. Such records often provide a great deal of valuable information about a patient's medical history, current state, and treatment plan.

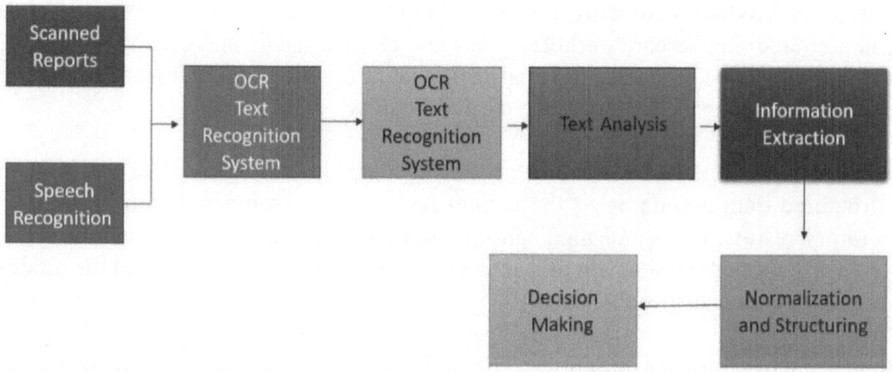

FIGURE 15.2 Workflow of clinical documentation.

Information Extraction: NLP identifies and extracts some textual features such as the patient's details, complaints, diagnosis, medications, lab results, and procedures. It can assist in finding out temporal associations of events, when the symptoms were observed or the treatment was administered.

Normalization and Structuring: After that, the data extracted is normalized and structured so that it can be implemented in EHRs conveniently using NLP tools. This could include ensuring there is uniformity in the documentation language, translating the different concepts to recognized codes as the ICD-10 diagnosis codes, SNOMED CT, and categorizing the data into domains of the EHR.

Integration with EHR Systems: The NLP-derived structured data can easily be integrated to the current EHR systems so as to provide the patient a complete and updated record. This saves time as it reduces the likelihood of transcribing errors while at the same time providing doctors the required time to attend to their patients.

Improving Clinical Workflow: NLP in the clinical setup enhances the clinical workflows by taking over the documentation process. Healthcare workers can access the information of their patients faster than before, hence broadening their decision-making base and thus increasing the chances of treating the patients.

Improving Data Analytics and Research: Structured data generated by NLP can be employed in data analysis, quality improvement initiatives, and research studies. A massive dataset is a valuable tool for exploring various patterns, trends, and insights that may be valuable in clinical practice and medical practice.

15.4.2 Clinical Decision Support

This is a very complex NLP-driven tool that helps health personnel to make sound decisions, since it allows the review of literature, patient data, and guidelines. This is how it works (Kumar and Gond, 2023).

Analysis of Medical Literature: NLP aids in the retrieval of knowledge from loads of data embodying research articles, journals, clinical trials, and case reports. This information may be regarding the treatment plan, drug–drug interaction, and possible adverse effects, versus the most recent research data.

Analysis of Patient Records: NLP works not only on structured data but also on unstructured data pertaining to the patient record. This includes the clinical notes, laboratory results, history of medication, and diagnostic reports. This harbors valuable information about the patient's antecedents and present condition and the modes of therapy at one's disposal.

Integration of Clinical Guidelines: The NLP can also analyze the clinical guidelines and protocols and can even come up with recommendations concerning certain medical diseases or even procedures. Such guidelines may concern diagnosis, treatments, medications, and therapy protocols concerning further management of the patient's condition.

Drug Interactions: This is possible with medication lists and patient data available. NLP can detect potential drug–drug interactions, allergies, and contraindications. This way, it becomes possible to alert treating health practitioners in time to avoid prescription of drugs with dangerous interaction or side-blow effects.

Therapy Recommendations: Depending on the patient's case history, symptoms, and diagnosis, NLP could recommend the type of therapy or action needed. This includes evidence-based treatment that is supported by guidelines and referencing medical literature.

Relevant Research Findings and Alert Clinicians: This NLP keeps combing for updated findings and clinical advancements and conveys relevant information to healthcare practitioners, which may alter the treatment of a patient. For instance, if some new research has pointed to revising the treatment methods for a certain illness, NLP can alert doctors and inform them about the new approach.

15.4.3 Clinical Coding

It involves classifying the diagnosis, treatment, and medication that are used by patients with relevant codes. In this case, NLP application is quite important, since it provides an automated method for managing the process with improving the overall accuracy. Among EMR data sources, NLP algorithms identify clinical documentation, including physician's progress notes, discharge summaries, and procedural reports. By utilizing lexical normalizations and identifying the semantic patterns in the narratives, NLP can identify diagnoses, procedures, and medications mentioned in the unstructured clinical notes. Then, it translates these notions into the uniform code systems, the most common of which includes ICD-10 for disease diagnosis, CPT for procedures, and RxNorm for medications. The current automatic coding system erases the need of the healthcare workers to code manually, thus making a difference in the issue of errors and the consistency of coding. Moreover, NLP may continually update its knowledge on code sets and clinical advising, meeting compliance and reimbursement standards. In conclusion, clinical coding that is backed by natural language processing enhances billing efficiency, augments revenue cycle adoption, and escalates the performance of healthcare organizations economically.

15.4.4 Health Monitoring and Surveillance

It is also beneficial for reporting trends in public health, identifying diseases or reporting the incidence of infectious diseases with the help of an assessment of various textual resources, such as social media, article news and other information on the Internet. Of course, there are AI algorithms in NLP that can search the unstructured text and find the valuable information about the symptoms, some kinds of illnesses, regions, or any other significant signals. NLP can discover new health issues based on the patterns and tone of related conversations, observe the increase of few diseases or symptoms in certain regions and find out unanticipated peaks that may indicate an epidemic. Through this, the disease spread can be prevented by allowing the authorities to attend to the problem as it unfolds, allocating resources efficiently, and conducting measures as they are needed. In addition, NLP can offer useful information pertaining to cognition, perception, and behavior of the population regarding particular health matters, which helps in delivering health-specific communication initiatives and campaigns with an emphasis on primary prevention and early disease identification.

As illustrated in Figure 15.3, disease symptoms are inputted in the smartphone application and based on these symptoms, a trained machine-learning algorithm makes a diagnosis on the condition. After that, the doctor suggests a plan of action based on the assessment outcome.

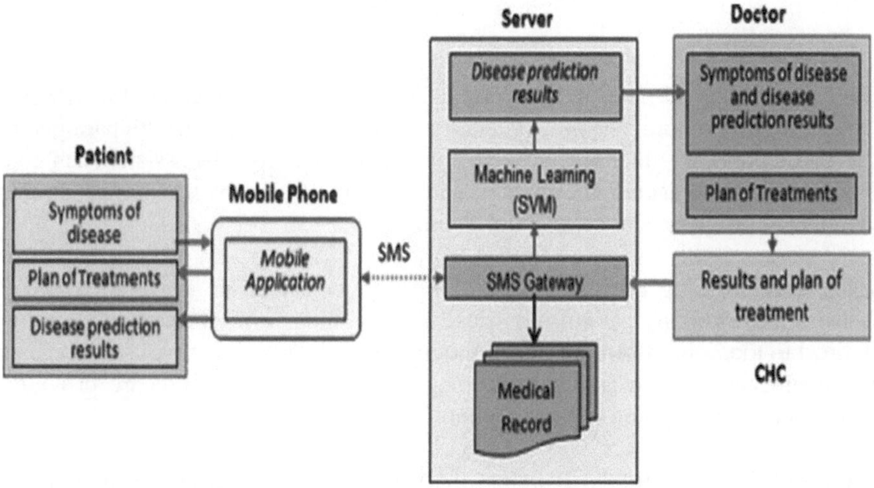

FIGURE 15.3 Workflow of health and monitoring system.

15.4.5 Patient Support and Education

The support of patients and their education is a crucial component of the healthcare process, and NLP helps to create advanced technologies like chatbots and virtual assistants for improved patient satisfaction and engagement. NLP-based chatbots and virtual assistants can engage patients through questions, answers, and information about medications, appointments, and other chronic diseases.

Answer Questions: Patients can ask questions about their health conditions, prescribed drugs and dosages, therapies, and remedies. To such queries, the algorithms of NLP respond with proper and relevant replies that are derived from accurate medical information and protocols.

Drug Enquiry: Some of the direct questions in this regard include dosage, probable drug side effects and other questions the patient would like to ask concerning their medicines. Through the use of NLP-assisted assistants, one can put an exact medicine detail for a particular patient in order to adhere to the doctor's prescription.

Appointment Reminders: It can remind people of any upcoming commitments beforehand; it can also ensure that patients comply with their prescribed therapy. Thus, appointment reminders may be tailored per patient request, coming as either an SMS, e-mail, or an online chat.

Provide Support for Chronic Conditions: Patients who are suffering from chronic diseases need the services since chronicity is an indicator that they must have follow-ups in taking care of and treating their diseases. NLP-powered assistants can offer information about treatment, living standards, and health advice when it comes to a certain disease such as diabetes, hypertension, or asthma, to mention a few (Poniszewska-Marańda et al., 2023). They can also assist in compliance of dosages and reporting of symptoms, thus empowering patients to have control over their well-being between physician visits.

Health Monitoring: At times, NLP promoted assistants can be integrated with wearable technologies or mobile health applications to monitor patient's health parameters such as blood pressure, glucose levels, etc., or physical activity. The assistant can give feedback on these measures, motivation, and escalation of problems where patients and healthcare providers may encounter them.

Triaging and Guiding Patients: This is why systems that are powered by NLP could help in prioritizing patient inquiries based on their level of need and helping them direct to the right information they require. For instance, if the patient describes severe manifestations, the assistant can suggest contacting a healthcare provider, using telemedicine, or going to the hospital.

Personalized Interaction: NLP helps chatbots and virtual assistants to personalize users' experience and their communication with them based on the patients' characteristics and needs. Such a model helps to create a more compelling and enjoyable atmosphere for a patient, thus contributing to better satisfaction rates and overall health outcomes.

15.4.6 Clinical Trials and Research

NLP can be used to find the patients for the clinical trials through comparison between their medical records and the parameters for the trials. It can also be helpful in studies for finding articles, data extraction, and synthesis of the studies for literature review. Natural language processing and its complexities figure in clinical trials and research throughout, from recruitment to analyzing results.

Patient Recruitment: They can scan patient information from EHRs, clinician's notes, and other clinical documents to identify which patients are eligible for clinical trials. When used to match trial parameters such as demographic data, medical history, symptoms, and lab results among others NLP is very effective since it isolates such information. Thus, the described means enable the process of recruiting patients to be sped up, the work load of the trial organizers to be diminished, and the selectivity of the participants to be improved.

Literature Review: NLP assists researchers in achieving full literature searches when identifying research articles, scientific papers, and clinical guidelines, NLP also assist in extracting and summarizing important information from a pool of numerous documents. Notably, NLP can identify exploitable patterns and extract valuable data through probing of a text's substantive content, specific approach, findings, and conclusion to support independent synthesis of evidence and alignment of research goals.

Data Extraction and Synthesis: There are advantages in using NLP to structure those data from clinical notes, pathology reports, and imaging investigations. Such information can be other characteristics of the patient, features of the disease, treatment effectiveness, and any observed side effects. Such structured documents can be analyzed with NLP algorithms or other translators, which are capable of analyzing texts, parsing meaningful information from the documents and outputting in the desired format. This is convenient for researchers as it eliminates time figuring out the correct tools and methods, freeing up time for data analysis and hypothesis testing.

Clinical Trial Monitoring: Specifically, NLP can monitor and assess quantitative data coming from the clinical practice setting from adverse events to patient reported outcomes and treatment effectiveness data captured during clinical trials. NLP can reveal emergent patterns, identify risk factors or adverse effects, and offer preliminary findings about the effectiveness of investigational treatments based on the analysis of textual information from sources which can be e-patients' diaries or social media.

Protocol Optimization: NLP can also take advantage of trial data and factitious facts to develop and enhance quotidian clinical trial protocols. NLP also helps researchers to achieve clearer aims and objectives as well as revisit protocol design and sample sizes for treatment and correspondence pathways as well as patient outcomes, making for more precision and impactful studies.

Post-Study Analysis and Reporting: In the case of clinical research, NLP can assist in compiling and digesting a study to submit it, for example. By employing NLP tools, realistic findings can be displayed, results summarized, and clear reports generated on trials which would be instrumental in presenting trial findings to stakeholders such as regulatory bodies, care givers, and fellow scientists.

Sentiment Analysis: NLP can also extract insight from feedback/reviews and sentiments made by the patient on social media to assess their degree of satisfaction and the level of public satisfaction with the healthcare services. It offers useful information on patient's response on blogs/forum and health social networks, which will assist healthcare practitioners to quantify and understand patients' perception, satisfaction, and aspects surrounding healthcare delivery systems.

Patient Input Analysis: It is through a way of asking questions to the various patients by using surveys, portals and feedback forms that are provided to the various healthcare institutions. The feedback from patients can then be applied in the NLP tools to find a pattern when patients are happy or when they are not happy. Among the techniques applied to analyze the input, sentiment analysis, which aims to categorize the input as positive, negative, and neutral, helps healthcare providers understand the overall patient satisfaction and pinpoint certain issues or strengths.

Review Analysis: Most of the available data about the interactions between patients and healthcare providers, clinics and hospitals is contained in YELP, Google Reviews, or Healthgrades. Also, some of the information that can be derived from these evaluations include sentiments that indicate the level of satisfaction that the patients have which can be obtained through application of NLP algorithms in extracting reoccurring themes and aspects that are important for the evaluation of the happiness of the patients. The results of this study could be beneficial for healthcare institutions as a guide to addressing individual grievances and complaints, addressing shared concerns, and managing an organization's online reputation.

Social Media Monitoring: Publics also engage with social media particularly in writing lingering experiences on appointment with healthcare providers on sites like X (formerly Twitter), Facebook, and Instagram. NLP can help healthcare practitioners to track social media conversations in real time for their organization, their services or particular healthcare topics, themes, or hashtag. Through sentiment analysis of such messages, healthcare businesses are therefore able to have an insight into people's opinions, addressing some of the issues and needs they may have or serving their needs through some of the messages they post. To effectively respond, healthcare firms use sentiment research to gauge the negativity or positivity shifts occurring during time. Therefore, through the analysis of changes in the sentiment, healthcare practitioners can identify the degree of impact that various programs, campaigns and/or events have to patients. Appreciable patterns of feeling positive might indicate which type of intervention is applicable or alteration is desired, while negative slopes are indicative of issues that have to be fixed or managed.

Identifying Areas for Improvement: This approach can uncover pieces of the healthcare service that are favorable or unfavorable to the patient's sentiment. For instance, the use of negative words will bring out issues like longer patient waiting time, poor communication, or problems with the bills. Therefore, critical aspects such as these, when resolved, can lead to happier and loyal patients by healthcare practitioners.

Benchmarking and Competitive Analysis: The four building blocks of measures of competitive advantage include benchmarking, which is made possible through sentiment analysis in healthcare businesses. By comparing the trend of sentiment scores with similar organizations, the healthcare providers will be in a position to tell where they excel, and where they are lacking, hence development of keyed improvement plans.

Real-time sentiment analysis helps the healthcare professional analyze the negative sentiment or possible problems that may need an intervention at an early stage. For instance, if some negative trend is found in the patients' feedback or social media, healthcare institutions can eliminate the causes of such a decline and show their sincere desire to satisfy patients.

15.4.8 Population Health Management

NLP can work on a large volume of patient information in order to discover high-risk patient groups, forecast disease outbreaks, and design proactive steps for preventive healthcare and population health management. Population health management involves the systematic assessment and monitoring of population health to improve health status of those in a given population. In this discipline, the methodology of NLP is used to assess considerable volumes of patient data to facilitate early detection of vulnerable groups, forecast disease incidence, and develop effective preventative care measures.

Risk Stratification: NLP can analyze EHR consisting of clinical notes, findings, and demographic data to assess the risk level of patients for certain health disorders. NLP algorithms can predict who is more prone to various illnesses, such as cancer, cardiovascular diseases or diabetes by searching for patterns and risk factors in the data.

Predictive Analytics: One benefit of applying NLP is to predict disease outbreaks and epidemics based on a patient's prior medical history. NLP helps recognize infectious diseases or public health emergencies at an early stage by monitoring symptoms, diagnosis, and regions. It helps the healthcare organization and the public health agencies to intervene proactively and prevent the spread of diseases in the population, such as vaccination.

Disease Surveillance: Healthcare data from sources such as EHRs, insurance claims, pharmacy records, and social media can be captured by NLP-powered systems, and can help to assess the disease/health condition incidence in a population. Based on symptoms, treatment records, and other signifiers, NLP can identify disease hotspots, monitor diseases in a population over time, and determine the healthcare needs of a population.

Identifying Social Determinants of Health: NLP may search through text messages that involve social media, online communities, or news websites to identify SDOH that might affect the population's health status. The discussed determinants may concern such factors as socioeconomic status, healthcare utilization, housing and environment. It is by comprehending these characteristics that healthcare institutions can devise specific strategies that focus on altering such social factors to enhance health equality.

Personalized Interventions: NLP can be particularly used in the delivery of personalized prevention and early interventions to high-risk groups according to the patients' risk factors and health threats. Through the analysis of factors, such as medical history, behaviors, and preferences of the patient, NLP can adapt interventions like diet, exercise, improvement of compliance with the screening tests, and care management to each patient.

Quality Improvement Initiatives: Using NLP tools, patient comments and providers' notes and other textual data can be analyzed to find out more about relevant opportunities to improve healthcare. Finally, by comprehending or gathering more information regarding the organizational patient population's experiences and perceptions, it is possible to carry out patient-centered intercessions to enhance patient care coordination, interaction as well as satisfaction.

Resource Allocation: This shall prove to be helpful to healthcare organizations mainly through an effective resource allocation whereby NLP analysis helps to determine individuals and places that need most vigilance and programs that should be put in place to prevent the spread of the disease. This practice is important since this way restrictive funding is directed towards the most productive activity and increase in health standards among the population can be achieved.

15.5 CHALLENGES OF USING NLP IN HEALTHCARE

It was established that NLP in healthcare has the potential of dramatically changing the ways that patients are treated, how decisions are made by clinicians, and how overall healthcare is being delivered and managed. Nevertheless, for these advantages to be attained, they come equipped with several challenges that need to be addressed carefully to preserve the privacy, security, and appropriate use of patients' data besides observing legal requirements like the HIPAA and FDA laws.

Privacy and Security: Consumer health information is perhaps one of the most vital and delicate to protect from third parties since it contains PHI. A lot of unstructured data is often generated as NLP systems work with it, common inputs including clinical notes, test results, and imaging reports. It is thus important to ensure that such data is appropriately protected to reduce on any form of cross-sectional access, data invasion, and misuse. To mitigate the risks of patient's data leakage, identity theft, or data loss, effective encryption mechanisms and access control measures have to be employed for patient data throughout their life cycle.

Ethical Considerations: Several issues have to be considered in ethical NLP, such as patient consent, data confidentiality as well as the possibility of bias. Patients' data can and should be used in NLP applications but patients should be informed how the data will be used and whether they want to participate. Healthcare providers also need to ensure patients' identification is not revealed in every stage of processing data starting from the time it is collected from the patient to the time it was analyzed. In addition, the realities are that NLP algorithms used in AI have to be developed and tested to protect against bias that could lead to prejudice including, but not limited to, diagnostic and treatment advice.

Regulatory Compliance: While using NLP systems, the healthcare firms ought to consider compliance with standards like HIPAA and FDA. HIPAA encompasses strict standards for safety and confidentiality of patient's medical information, application of sufficient measures, restrictions concerning access to information, and reporting cases of violation. NLP applications that perform diagnostic or therapeutic recommendations are also likely to need FDA's sanction to affirm safety and reliability.

Data Quality and Accuracy: The appropriateness of the data used in NLP applications in the support of the heath-care decision making is of great importance in order to obtain reliable outcomes. The documentation that is frequently used in clinical practice may also include mistakes, disparities, and uncertainty, which can affect the functioning of NLP algorithms. As a remedy, input data fed into healthcare businesses have to undergo system validation and this calls for quality checks to be done to enable better performance in NLP systems.

Interoperability and Integration: This integration is challenging since most modern healthcare facilities have complicated IT structures, and the NLP systems themselves are multiformat and multilingual, posing interoperability issues. Thus, for facilitating data exchange and integration of the NLP's working process with clinicians' workflow, these platforms should support the existing electronic systems, including electronic health record systems (EHRS), laboratory information systems (LIS), etc. In this regard, one finds that disciplines with a standardized data format or general interoperability standards can provide help.

To overcome these issues, stakeholders involve healthcare providers, technology suppliers, regulating authorities and other stakeholders who need to develop robust solutions that focus on patients' privacy and security of their data besides ethical applications of NLP technology. Mitigating these challenges will help healthcare organizations achieve the intended gains of NLP so as to enhance efficiency delivery services in healthcare organizations.

15.6 CONCLUSION

NLP is transforming healthcare by providing a myriad of approaches that enhance patient experience, physicians' efficiency and diagnosis, and treatment outcomes, as well as medical advanced research. Cohort construction can be achieved using natural language processing for mining text data from clinical sources such as electronic health records, physicians' notes, literature, etc. Such data can be further applied to optimize clinical documentation, code some of the tasks, develop clinical decision support systems, and personalize communications with patients. NLP is also helpful in population health by using big data for analyzing high-risk representatives, potential epidemics, and possibilities of intervention. According to the present trends in the development of the NLP technology, it was suggested that this technology was going to expand even more extensively in the future in the field of healthcare and will help to develop, reform, and bring more efficiency and equal opportunity to the side of healthcare.

Globally, researches have incorporated NLP into the implementation of healthcare systems. In this pertinent section, we have described how NLP models function in healthcare and several uses of NLP in the healthcare arena. Further, we also pointed out the weaknesses and difficulties related to the application of NLP in the sphere of healthcare. This chapter can be of immense help for researchers looking to venture into the crossroads of NLP and healthcare. Education on the working of NLP models in the healthcare and understanding of the diverse area of application helps the researcher to know how NLP can be harnessed to enhance patient care, client's decision-making, and management of the healthcare.

Furthermore, the recognition of the problems and limitations of the NLP application in healthcare entails the researchers' ability to dedicate their efforts to designing solutions to mitigate these issues and promote the efficient and appropriate implementation of the NLP technology in healthcare.

REFERENCES

Abualigah, L., Alfar, H., Shehab, M., & Hussein, A. M. A. (2019). Sentiment analysis in healthcare: A brief review. In Mohamed Abd Elaziz, Mohammed A. A. Al-qaness, Ahmed A. Ewees, & Abdelghani Dahou (Eds.), *Studies in computational intelligence* (pp. 129–141). Springer, Cham. https://doi.org/10.1007/978-3-030-34614-0_7

Ahmed, U., Iqbal, K., & Aoun, M. (2023). Natural Language Processing for Clinical Decision Support Systems: A Review of Recent Advances in Healthcare. *Journal of Intelligent Connectivity and Emerging Technologies*, *8*(2), 1–16.

Al-Garadi, M. A., Yang, Y., & Sarker, A. (2022). The Role of Natural Language Processing during the COVID-19 Pandemic: Health Applications, Opportunities, and Challenges. *Healthcare*, *10*(11), 2270. https://doi.org/10.3390/healthcare10112270

Attar, R. K., & Komal. (2022). The emergence of Natural Language Processing (NLP) techniques in healthcare AI. In Shabir Ahmad Parah, Mamoon Rashid, & Vijayakumar Varadarajan (Eds.), *Springer eBooks* (pp. 285–307). Springer, Cham. https://doi.org/10.1007/978-3-030-96569-3_14

Basyal, G. P., Rimal, B. P., & Zeng, D. (2020). A Systematic Review of Natural Language Processing for Knowledge Management in Healthcare. *arXiv*. https://doi.org/10.48550/arXiv.2007.09134

Friedman, C., & Elhadad, N. (2013). Natural language processing in health care and biomedicine. In Edward H. Shortliffe & James J. Cimino (Eds.), *Springer eBooks* (pp. 255–284). Springer, London. https://doi.org/10.1007/978-1-4471-4474-8_8

Garg, R., & Gupta, A. (2024). A Systematic review of NLP applications in clinical healthcare: Advancement and challenges. In Swagatam Das, Snehanshu Saha, Carlos A. Coello Coello, & Jagdish C. Bansal (Eds.), *Lecture notes in networks and systems* (pp. 31–44). Springer, Singapore. https://doi.org/10.1007/978-981-99-9521-9_3

Grosz, B. J. (1982). Natural Language Processing. *Artificial Intelligence*, *19*(2), 131–136. https://doi.org/10.1016/0004-3702(82)90032-7

Kumar, A., & Gond, A. (2023). Natural Language Processing: Healthcare Achieving Benefits Via Nlp. *ScienceOpen*. https://doi.org/10.14293/pr2199.000280.v1

Kuwaiti, A. A., Nazer, K., Alreedy, A., AlShehri, S. D., Almuhanna, A., Subbarayalu, A. V., Muhanna, D. A., & Al-Muhanna, F. A. (2023). A Review of the Role of Artificial Intelligence in Healthcare. *Journal of Personalized Medicine*, *13*(6), 951. https://doi.org/10.3390/jpm13060951

Locke, S., Bashall, A., Al-Adely, S., Moore, J. A., Wilson, A. J., & Kitchen, G. (2021). Natural Language Processing in Medicine: A Review. *Trends in Anaesthesia and Critical Care*, *38*, 4–9. https://doi.org/10.1016/j.tacc.2021.02.007

Nadkarni, P. M., Ohno-Machado, L., & Chapman, W. W. (2011). Natural Language Processing: An Introduction. *Journal of the American Medical Informatics Association*, *18*(5), 544–551. https://doi.org/10.1136/amiajnl-2011-000464

Nawab, K., Ramsey, G., & Schreiber, R. (2020). Natural Language Processing to Extract Meaningful Information from Patient Experience Feedback. *Applied Clinical Informatics*, *11*(02), 242–252. https://doi.org/10.1055/s-0040-1708049

Poniszewska-Marańda, A., Vynogradnyk, E., & Marańda, W. (2023). Medical Data Transformations in Healthcare Systems with the Use of Natural Language Processing Algorithms. *Applied Sciences*, *13*(2), 682. https://doi.org/10.3390/app13020682

Tyagi, N., & Bhushan, B. (2023). Natural Language Processing (NLP) based innovations for smart healthcare applications in healthcare 4.0. In Mohd Abdul Ahad, Gabriella Casalino, & Bharat Bhushan (Eds.), *Enabling technologies for effective planning and management in sustainable smart cities*. Springer, Cham. https://doi.org/10.1007/978-3-031-22922-0_5

16 Speech Emotion Recognition for Dialog Systems

M. Soundarya, R. Nancy Deborah, G. Sivakarthi and A. Vinora

16.1 INTRODUCTION TO AMBIENT ASSISTED LIVING

Nowadays, a large number of older persons need ongoing help to do everyday tasks and to meet their medical needs. The development and implementation of effective and economical strategies and systems to offer accessible healthcare and monitoring services, focusing on the aging population, is becoming more widely recognized. This is known as ambient assisted living. Encouraging senior citizens to live as independently as possible in their homes as they age is crucial for their well-being and the long-term viability of public healthcare systems. In 2018, the United Nations released its "World Population Prospects 2019: Highlights," which showed that, for the first time in recorded human history, the number of adults 65 years (Mulam, Navale, Pawar, & Deshpande, 2020) of age or older globally outnumbered that of children under five. Technologies for assisted living can be quite helpful in caring for the elderly. AAL systems use various technologies, including communication tools, smart home appliances, and sensors, to create an environment that adjusts to the user's demands. For instance, it could examine a person's everyday activities and identify any action that deviates from typical activity patterns using ambient or wearable sensors. In the upcoming sections, let us discuss ambient assisted living in more detail.

16.1.1 Role of Technology in AAL

AAL utilizes various technologies to improve the independence, health, and standard of living of the aged and disabled people. Technologies used in AAL are the following:

Smart Home Technologies: Smart home (SH) technology has advanced from research to commercialization in the last ten years. Initially, energy-saving, entertainment, security and surveillance, and other areas made extensive use of SH technologies. Artificial intelligence (AI), the Internet of Things (IoT) (Sanchez-Comas, Synnes, & Hallberg, 2018), and computing methods have contributed to the development of the areas. As a result, it is now easier to focus research and development efforts on things like improving the independence and quality of life for aged and disabled people. When a smart home can sense, anticipate, and react to occupants'

DOI: 10.1201/9781003520184-20

daily activities, it can enhance their lives by providing timely and socially acceptable assistance. It consists of an Internet connection, a smart home gateway, and various devices connected as nodes in the system, such as sensors and actuators with wired or wireless connectivity. With SH technologies, a great deal of systems were created. For instance, climate control, heating, and lighting can be adjusted by user preferences and presence with the help of automated lighting and climate control. Smart appliances, such as the connected kitchen and other home appliances with remote control or programming capabilities, have become more prevalent.

Mobility and Accessibility Aids: To enable daily chores, mobility, and accessibility so that individuals may live more freely and safely in their homes and communities, mobility aids encompass a wide range of devices and technologies. The smart wheel chair is a popular mobility aid that consists of a mobile robot base with a seat attached, or it can be a standard motorized chair with additional sensors and a computer. Intelligent wheelchairs are designed to provide navigation support in several ways, including ensuring accident-free mobility, helping with specific tasks (such as opening doors), and providing autonomous transportation between locations. Electric wheelchairs use smart mobile localization and a mapping system (Cavanini et al., 2014). A wheelchair with electric capabilities was employed to assess the technology in different scenarios. Using sensors and GPS it identifies the best paths and avoids obstacles by navigating through both indoor and outdoor areas. These wheelchairs can alert the users or caretakers of health issues by monitoring vital indications like blood pressure and heart rate. Another helpful concept is mobility scooters, which were developed to improve the flexibility and level of living for the aged and disabled people. For people who need help going around but do not need a wheelchair, these scooters provide the best alternative.

Health Monitoring and Management: In AAL, health monitoring and management plays an essential part in supporting the independence and well-being of the elderly and people with long-term medical issues. In AAL, modern technology improves user's quality of life by enabling immediate action, regular health monitoring, and personalized therapy. The technologies include wearable health devices like fitness trackers and smartwatches, and remote patient monitoring systems, like Teladoc and Amwell, are used to electronically transmit patient health and medical data from one location to another so that medical professionals can assess and provide recommendations. In addition to tracking sleep quality, sensors integrated into chairs, mattresses, and toilets can monitor weight and other health metrics.

16.1.2 Overview of Dialog Systems in Assisted Living

A dialog system, referred to as a conversational system, enables natural language communication between a human and a computer. In ambient assisted living (AAL), dialog systems, also known as conversational agents are essential because they enable communication between residents and their smart home settings. By understanding and responding to human language, it uses AI, ML, and NLP to offer support, companionship, and access to information and services. An interface that allows for somewhat natural interaction between the user and a computer-based application is provided by the conversation system (Arora, Batra & Singh). The system may have several models, a CUI, GUI, or VUI, among others. It applies to web browsers, PDA systems, automobiles, robot systems, and phones. A spoken natural language interface is a key component of spoken conversation systems, which are computer systems with which humans communicate on a turn-by-turn basis.

Types of Dialog Systems: These systems can be classified into various types based on functionality, interaction mode, and underlying technology. Here is an overview of the primary types of dialog systems: Table 16.1 describes different dialog systems, their uses, functionalities, how they interact with each other and its underlying technology.

Importance of Dialog Systems: As a fundamental element of AAL, dialog systems are essential for promoting safety, well-being, and self-reliance. By supporting everyday tasks and routines through natural language contact, enables people in AAL situations to preserve their independence. Users' security and safety are greatly improved. Voice commands, embedded sensors, and conversational bots can identify situations and immediately notify caregivers or emergency services. Fall detection

TABLE 16.1
Dialog System Types

Type	Description
Task-Oriented Dialog Systems	The system is designed to help customers accomplish particular tasks, such as placing restaurant orders, making reservations, or buying tickets. These systems have a laser-like focus on achieving specific objectives. It guides users through controlled interactions to help them complete certain objectives, such as Siri and Google Assistant.
Open Domain Conversational Agents	The system is intended to hold casual discussions about a variety of subjects. These systems can talk about a wide range of topics and are not restricted to any one task. Technologies such as reinforcement learning, deep learning, and generative models such as Open AI's Chat GPT were used.
Hybrid Dialog Systems	Task-oriented and open-domain system characteristics are combined in hybrid conversation systems. They can converse generally and manage particular activities. It offers support for specific tasks as well as general conversational functions. Multi-agent frameworks were utilized, along with the integration of rule-based and machine-learning techniques. Example: Amazon Alexa.
Menu-Based Dialog Systems	Dialog systems that are menu-based direct users through interactions by providing pre-made menus or options. These systems restrict user input to choosing from pre-existing variants. It uses menus and options to provide an organized flow of interaction. NLP and rule-based systems such as bank chatbots and interactive voice response (IVR) systems were applied.

devices and advanced dialog systems can cooperate to deliver emergency aid and alert emergency contacts. Individuals with impairments and the elderly are frequently plagued by social isolation. By promoting camaraderie and communication, dialog systems can lessen this. It promotes learning and the cognitive environment, which aids individuals in continuing their education throughout their lives and preserving their mental sharpness. They can provide games, riddles, and brainteasers that are meant to improve cognitive performance.

16.2 FUNDAMENTALS OF SPEECH EMOTION RECOGNITION

Humans use speech as a form of communication. Speech is a crucial communication medium that consists of a series of words in a predetermined language. A computing technology also known as speech technology enables an electronic device to detect, process, and comprehend spoken words or audio. Studies have been conducted for many years to understand the components of the human brain that make up intelligence. The goal of artificial intelligence is to build systems that are intelligent and capable of developing ideas and behaviors similar to those of humans. Automatic speech recognition (ASR) is one of the key areas of AI and machine-learning research (Darshan & Veerappa, 2020), which seeks to create robots capable of speaking to humans and engaging in speech-based communication. The systems must comprehend the emotions expressed in speech to interact with humans effectively. For machines to communicate clearly and effectively with humans, it is necessary to design machines that can identify paralinguistic information, such as emotion. Emotion is a significant piece of paralinguistic information that is sent together with speech.

16.2.1 Key Features of Speech Emotion Recognition

The primary categories into which the characteristics of SER can be divided are acoustic, linguistic, prosodic, and contextual aspects. Figure 16.1 depicts the features

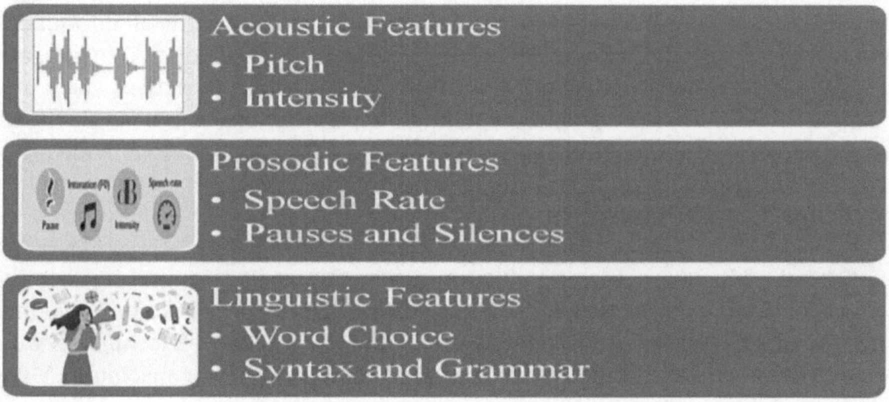

FIGURE 16.1 Features of SER.

of speech emotion recognition systems. To accurately identify the emotions in spoken language these characteristics were needed.

Acoustic Features: The raw audio stream is used to extract acoustic elements, which are crucial for identifying the speaker's emotional state. Pitch and energy are included in it. Pitch variation frequently conveys a range of emotions. Anger, for instance, could have a higher pitch, but melancholy might have a lower pitch. Emotional indicators can be inferred from speech patterns such as volume or intensity. Elevated energy levels may signify agitation or fury, while decreased energy levels may suggest melancholy or indifference.

Prosodic Features: Prosodic characteristics include speech's intonation, rhythm, and stress. These characteristics are important for expressing feelings. Speech rate, pauses, and silences are all included. Speech rate, or a person's rate of speech, might reveal their emotional condition. Another way to express emotions in speech is through the timing and presence of pauses or silences.

Linguistic Features: Analyzing spoken language's content and structure is one of the linguistic features. These characteristics aid in deciphering the emotional meaning behind the words. Emotions can be strongly indicated by certain words or phrases. For example, the terms "happy," "joyful," and "excited" all clearly convey positive feelings. Sentence structure including the use of complicated sentences, exclamations, and questions can provide information about a person's emotional state.

16.2.2 Key Techniques and Methods in SER

SER employs several methodologies and approaches to precisely identify and construe spoken language emotions. Figure 16.2 shows the techniques used in SER. These methods can be broadly divided into three categories: hybrid models, deep learning techniques, and classic machine-learning approaches.

Feature Extraction Methods: One of the most important steps in speech recognition (SER) is feature extraction, which is finding and extracting pertinent information from the speech signal. It consists of prosodic features, linear predictive coding, and mel-frequency cepstral coefficients. One of the most popular aspects of voice processing is MFCC. They are good at capturing the phonetic characteristics of speech and depict the short-term power spectrum of sound. LPC is utilized to provide information on the geometry of the vocal tract by representing the spectral envelope of a compressed digital speech stream.

Traditional Machine-Learning Techniques: Conventional machine-learning methods entail training classifiers that can differentiate between various emotions using features that have been retrieved. Among the often employed techniques were hidden Markov models, K-nearest neighbors, and support vector machines. Many tasks, including text classification, image classification, and speech recognition, can be accomplished with SVMs. KNN is a straightforward, non-parametric technique

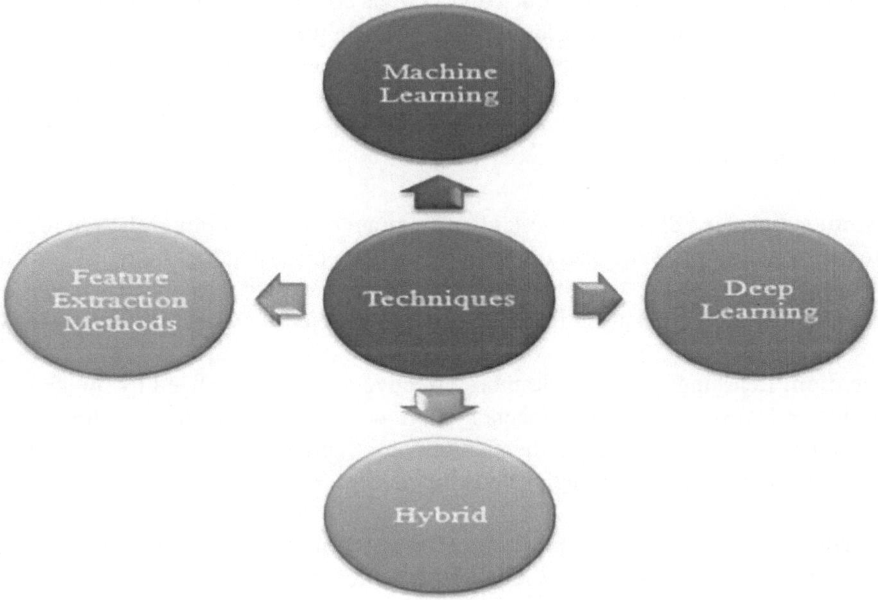

FIGURE 16.2 Techniques in SER.

that compares the attributes of the training and test samples to perform classification. Human-machine models, or HMMs, have proven effective in simulating temporal sequences and capturing the dynamics of speech signals throughout time.

Deep-Learning Techniques: Since deep-learning algorithms can handle enormous datasets and automatically learn features from raw data, they have become more and more popular in the SER. Among the most widely used deep-learning approaches were auto encoders, RNN, and CNN. CNNs are useful for SER tasks because they are good at identifying local patterns and structures in speech spectrograms. RNNs use long short-term memory (LSTM) networks to capture temporal dependencies in voice signals and sequence data. When auto encoders are used for unsupervised feature learning and dimensionality reduction, emotion recognition systems can function more effectively.

Hybrid Techniques: This technique combines deep learning and conventional machine learning to gain the benefits of both. Ensemble models, CNN-RNN hybrid models, and feature fusion are some examples of hybrid techniques.

16.2.3 Applications of Speech Emotion Recognition in Various Domains

The ability of SER technology to identify and react to human emotions from speech has a wide range of applications across many fields. Some of the main areas where SER has a significant impact are mentioned as follows:

Healthcare: SER can be very helpful to the medical community in terms of treatments, patient care, and mental health monitoring. It is a useful tool for identifying signs of depression, anxiety, and other mental health conditions by monitoring the changes in a patient's speech patterns and emotional tone over time. Virtual therapists can interact therapeutically with patients so that they offer more emotional support and real-time attention to their needs.

Customer Service: SER can assess client interactions to determine the emotional state of the client to assist customer service workers in responding more effectively and sympathetically. By knowing the emotional context of a customer's usage of SER, chatbots and virtual assistance can answer customer requests more intelligently.

Education: Learning can be made more effective and individualized by integrating SER into e-learning platforms. Teachers can spot when a student is distracted or confused by keeping an eye on their emotional reactions. This allows for prompt interventions to increase knowledge and engagement.

Entertainment: Games incorporating SER technology react to the feelings of their users by changing the challenge and gameplay to suit, making the game feel more immersive. By allowing systems to respond to users' emotional states, SER can improve VR and AR experiences by enhancing natural and immersive interactions.

16.3 INTEGRATION OF SER IN DIALOG SYSTEMS

The initial part of the system is called automatic speech recognition; here, user speech is used as input, and spoken language is translated into text. It also fixes spelling, punctuation, and case issues in the input text, cleaning and normalizing it. The system's second part, a natural language interpreter, determines the purpose of the user's input. Semantics, syntax, and morphology are used in this component. The dialog manager receives it when the keywords have been determined and a meaning has been formed. The dialog state tracker, which is the third component, keeps track of prior exchanges to control the coherence of the dialog. Policy management comes next, which chooses the subsequent course of action based on the present situation and user input. Rules may be used, or machine-learning models, such as reinforcement learning may be used. Typically, the dialog manager must communicate with another piece of software, like an expert system or database. As a result, the query or plans must be transformed from the conversation manager's internal representation to the external domain-specific system's format (such as SQL). Domain-specific components handle this interaction. Dialog response selection, the fourth component, chooses the response for the input that is provided. Based on its prior knowledge, it selects the answer. Natural language generation, which builds the system answer in natural language, is the fifth component. Language models can be used to produce this or predefine it. Its main purpose is to translate the internal representations and judgments of the system into logical, appropriate-for-context, and naturally sounding text answers. This element is essential to making sure that user-dialog

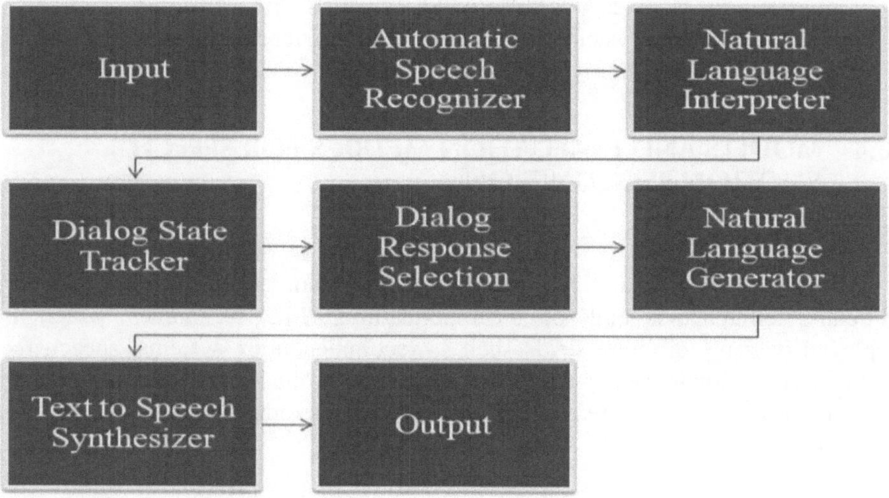

FIGURE 16.3 Architecture of SER.

system interactions are interesting and feel natural. Figure 16.3 shows the architecture of speech emotion recognition. For voice-based systems, the final component, output processing, transforms the generated written response into spoken words. Additionally, it guarantees that, in text-based systems, the response is presented accurately and formatted correctly. Speech conversation systems require databases that hold the information needed to react to users' input.

16.3.1 Role of SER in Enhanced Dialog Systems

Speech emotion detection is essential to dialog systems because it enables them to comprehend user emotions and react appropriately. The effectiveness of the system and user experience was enhanced by this connection.

- The dialog system listens to the user's voice and recognizes emotions like happiness, sadness, rage, or irritation. This enhances the user experience overall by enabling the system to react sympathetically.
- It also offers contextual understanding, which helps the system comprehend the user's intents more effectively. By identifying the user's emotional state, the system may adjust its replies to be more appropriate and tailored, making the interaction feel more human-like.
- It is flexible; for example, if a person becomes agitated while conversing, it can change to a simpler or more encouraging way of communication to stop things from getting worse.
- It gives priority to pressing problems. For example, in customer service applications, identifying negative emotions might assist in prioritizing critical issues so that unhappy or disturbed clients get assistance right away. Continuous

improvement is made possible by SER, which offers insights from users' perceptions of the system's reactions. Emotional feedback, whether favorable or negative, helps improve dialog techniques and replies.

16.4 MODELS AND EVALUATION METRICS FOR SPEECH EMOTION RECOGNITION

16.4.1 Machine-Learning Models for SER

A machine can automatically get better by learning from its historical data. Modern artificial intelligence is built on machine-learning (ML) techniques, which are employed in many different fields such as recommendation systems, speech recognition, etc., support vector machines, naive Bayes classifiers, decision-making, random forests, k-mean clustering, etc., these are a few examples of machine-learning algorithms.

Using Support Vector Machines: A system to identify and categorize speech emotions from three languages databases—the Berlin, Japanese, and Thai emotion databases—was created by Thapanee Seehapoch and Sartra Wongthanavasu. They have extracted features such as fundamental frequency (F0), energy, zero crossing rate (ZCR), linear predictive coding (LPC), and mel frequency cepstral coefficient (MFCC). The support vector machine is used for categorization. It is a non-linear classifier that converts the input feature vectors into a feature space that is typically higher dimensional. The separation plane's ideal location between the borders of two classes yields maximum discrimination. There is a decrease in references since the support vectors cross the plane. Typical kernel functions include the polynomial kernel, radial basis function kernel, and linear kernel (Seehapoch & Wongthanavasu, 2013). For the Berlin, Japanese, and Thai emotion databases, it yields classification accuracy of 89.80%, 93.57%, and 98.00%, respectively.

Using Random Forest: The random forest algorithm is used as a classifier in a speech emotion recognition system created by Susu Yan et al. (2020). Double randomness is the primary feature. The selection of the sample is random, which is the initial randomness. The random selection of features used to train each decision tree model constitutes the second randomness. The double randomness property allows the classification method to perform better against noise in addition to preventing over-fitting. Based on a random forest classifier, we developed a speech emotion identification system for WeChat. To start, the system pre-processes the voice signals it has gathered to cut down on noise. Secondly, the pre-processed speech signals are used to extract 16 acoustic features. By using 12 statistical functions on the initial acoustic characteristics, the system extracts the emotional aspects of speech. The OpenSmile program was utilized by them to extract features. RF and SVM are two classifiers used in the Berlin Speech Emotion Database's emotional classification. The SVM classifier's recognition accuracy is 83%. The random forest classifier (Yan et al., 2020) has an 89% accuracy rate. Ultimately, the voice emotion identification system is constructed using the random forest classifier.

16.4.2 DEEP-LEARNING TECHNIQUES FOR SER

Deep-learning algorithms can recognize complex patterns in photos, text, sounds, and other sorts of data to produce accurate insights and projections. For the SER problem, several deep-learning architectures have been used. The feed-forward and recurrent neural network architectures are two of the most widely used.

Using Deep Neural Network: Architectures for feed-forward networks (Pandey, Shekhawat, & Prasanna, 2019) are composed of several layers of affine transformation, which are followed by sequentially executed non-linear functions. The term "hidden layers" typically refers to the layers that lie between the input and output layers. The softmax layer, the final layer in the network, provides the class probabilities for each of the several classes.

Using Convolution Neural Network: Convolutional neural networks (CNNs) are used to recognize emotions in speech. It has been demonstrated that CNNs can infer a hierarchical feature representation to more accurately classify voice signals based on their local emotional qualities. To cluster the acoustic feature vectors and use the K-means algorithm to create an audio codebook, the training step applies vector quantization. Taking into account the relationships between the audio words in the training database, Word2vec is used to extract the word vector for each audio word. To extract speech features, each input speech signal's acoustic features are first extracted frame by frame. The input word vector matrix is obtained for emotion recognition throughout the generation process. The word vector matrix was then subjected to filtering. To obtain a feature map, convolution is used. After using maximum pooling (Huang et al., 2018), the fully connected layer eventually outputs the scores as the likelihood of each emotion.

Using long short-term memory networks: An optimization method called long short-term memory is used to measure the concentration of emotions across several blocks. Modifying the traditional forgetting gate reduces computing costs. To extract task-related information, an attention mechanism is applied to both the time and feature dimensions in the final output of the LSTM (Leelavathi, Deepthi, & Aruna, 2022). Machine-learning models need numerical values as input. We convert our data into arrays before extracting features from them. The retrieved values are fed into an LSTM model that has been created to exploit these features and forecast the final emotion. This model yielded an overall accuracy of 78.2%.

16.4.3 EVALUATION METRICS FOR SPEECH EMOTION RECOGNITION SYSTEMS

To accurately evaluate the performance of SER systems, a thorough set of measures is needed. The following are the main performance indicators for SER systems:

Accuracy: Ratio of the number of correct predictions to the total number of predictions.

$$\text{Accuracy} = (\text{TP} + \text{TN})/(\text{TP} + \text{TN} + \text{FP} + \text{FN})$$

Precision: Ratio of true positives to the total of true positives and false positives.

$$\text{Precision} = \text{TP}/(\text{TP} + \text{FP})$$

Recall: Ratio of true positives to the summation of true positives and false negatives.

$$\text{Recall} = \text{TP}/(\text{TP} + \text{FN})$$

F1 Score: The harmonic mean of recall and precision is the F1 score. It has been observed that in the accuracy-recall trade-off, recall falls when precision rises and vice versa. The F1 score aims to balance recall and precision.

$$\text{F1 Score} = (2 \times \text{Precision} \times \text{Recall})/(\text{Precision}/\text{Recall})$$

16.5 CHALLENGES IN SPEECH EMOTION RECOGNITION

Due to methodological and technical difficulties, as well as the complexity and diversity of human emotions, SER faces various challenges, which are listed below:

16.5.1 Variability in Emotional Expression

The challenge of accurately characterizing the meaning of emotions is one of the primary problems. Typically, emotions are mingled and difficult to understand (Wani et al., 2021). It is among the most significant difficulties in recognizing emotions in speech. Speech's emotional content can be impacted by regional and linguistic differences in tone and pronunciation. Different vocal traits are frequently displayed by men and women, which results in variations in how emotions are expressed. Emotional expression and interpretation are influenced by cultural context. For example, certain cultures value more restrained expressions while others may encourage strong shows of emotion. Language-specific emotional expressions could have an impact on the way emotions are expressed through linguistic traits. The communication's goal (informing, persuading, entertaining, etc.,) may influence how emotions are expressed. These are a few of the factors that can vary while identifying emotional expressions.

16.5.2 Noise and Environmental Factors

SER systems face substantial obstacles from ambient conditions and noise. These elements may deteriorate the audio signal's quality, confuse emotional cues, and add variability, all of which might make it more challenging for models to recognize emotions correctly. Different sounds like office talk, music, or traffic may mask or misinterpret the emotional content of speech. Similarly, some recording environments (large or small rooms) may add echo and reverberation, which reduces the signal's clarity. The poor microphones can cause additional noise and distortions.

Severe environmental circumstances may affect the quality of the speaker's voice as well as the functionality of the recording equipment.

16.5.3 Culture and Linguistic Differences

Different cultures express their emotions in various ways. For instance, expressing rage may be socially acceptable in some cultures but unacceptable in others. This has an impact on the way emotions come across in speaking. Different cultures can interpret non-verbal cues like tone, pitch, and rhythm differently. In one culture, pitch pattern is regarded as a sign of enjoyment may be interpreted differently in another. Prosody and intonation are used in many languages in different ways to express meaning and emotion. In many languages, the same intonation pattern may convey distinct moods. It is difficult to construct universal models because sounds that are used to indicate emotion in one language may not exist in another.

16.6 APPLICATIONS IN AMBIENT ASSISTED LIVING

By supporting independent living, AAL leverages technology to improve the quality of life for the elderly and those with impairments. Figure 16.4 lists the domain where AAL plays a vital role. Emotionally intelligent assistive technology is essential since it provides individualized and flexible support.

Healthcare and Therapy: Ambient assist systems can track emotional states over time using physiological signals, voice, and facial expressions. It recognizes symptoms of loneliness, anxiety, or despair so that it can set off treatments, such as alerting caregivers or making interesting activity suggestions. Wearable sensors can identify physiological markers of stress or anxiety and trigger relaxation methods, such as guided breathing exercises, or modify the surroundings (music, lighting, etc.) to produce a soothing atmosphere. Vital sign measurements, such as blood pressure (Estudillo-Valderrama et al., 2010) pulsioximeter readings or ECGs for diabetic

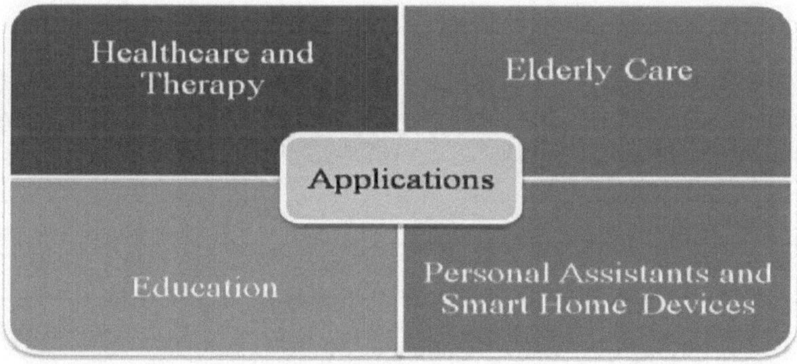

FIGURE 16.4 Applications of AAL.

patient and blood glucose for those with diabetes are the most common medical uses for these devices.

Elderly Care: Using data from heterogeneous sensors, AAL systems continuously monitor the health state of elder people (Mainetti et al., 2016). When a robot is emotionally sensitive, it can identify when an old person is lonely or upset and provide them with company or alert caregivers in a comforting way. When these gadgets detect agitation or disorientation, they can provide appropriate instructions or soothing interactions to help manage illnesses such as dementia.

Education: Learning resources and approaches can be modified by emotionally intelligent educational technologies in response to students' emotional states, resulting in a more successful and individualized learning process. These tools can assist teachers in identifying signs of dissatisfaction or misunderstanding in their pupils with learning difficulties and modifying their teaching methods accordingly.

Personal Assistants and Smart Home Devices: Alexa and Google Assistant are examples of virtual assistants that can learn to be more sympathetic and responsive by tailoring their responses to emotions. To provide a more comfortable living environment, smart home systems can change the lighting, music, or other environmental elements based on the user's mood.

16.7 ETHICAL AND PRIVACY CONSIDERATIONS

When asking questions about moral challenges that may occur while deciding whether technology is suitable for a particular person or group of people with particular traits is an important part of good ethical practice, miniaturization and concealment of these technologies have led to a limited awareness of their presence, which is intimately linked to ethical and privacy-related issues with current ICT (Van Hoof et al., 2007). Figure 16.5 shows the ethical considerations to be followed in ambient assisted living systems.

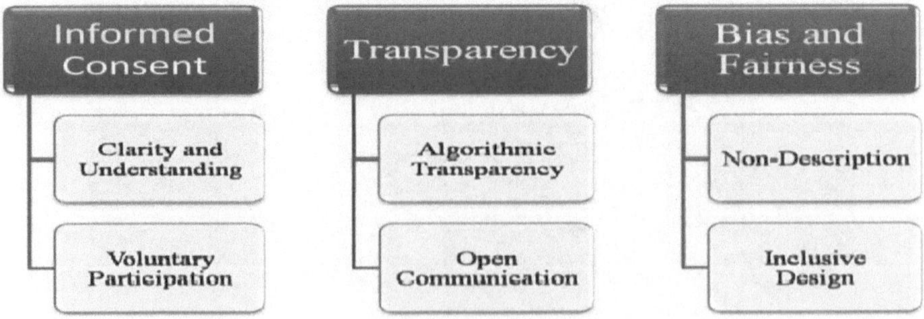

FIGURE 16.5 Ethical considerations.

Informed Consent: Users need to know how their data is gathered, utilized, and distributed. This involves providing a clear explanation for the reason of data collection, the categories of data that will be gathered, and how the data will be utilized. Users should be free to choose whether or not to participate in data gathering and the usage of assistive technologies, and doing so should not have any negative effects.

Transparency: It should be clear how algorithms, especially those that recognize and make decisions based on emotions, operate. The methods used to arrive at findings should be clear to users and caregivers. Setting reasonable expectations requires open communication about the capabilities and constraints of the technology.

Bias and Fairness: Age, gender, ethnicity, and cultural background biases must be eliminated from emotion recognition and other algorithms. Preventing discriminatory outcomes requires ongoing monitoring and a variety of training datasets. All possible users should be able to use devices, and its design should be taken into consideration to meet their varied needs and preferences.

Data Collection and Use: To reduce privacy invasion, only necessary data should be gathered. Over-collection of data may put users' privacy at greater risk. Only the precise uses for which data was gathered should be made of it. Any secondary use should require explicit user consent.

Data Security: To safeguard data from cyber attacks, unauthorized access, and breaches, we need good security measures. To maintain confidentiality and security, data should be encrypted when it is in transfer state and at rest state.

16.8 FUTURE DIRECTIONS AND RESEARCH OPPORTUNITIES

16.8.1 Potential for Personalized Assistance

AAL systems can offer customized support that caters to the individual requirements and preferences of every user by utilizing cutting-edge technologies. Facilitating human–machine interaction is SER's main goal (Harar, Burget, & Dutta, 2017). Chronic condition-specific health markers, such as those related to diabetes, hypertension, or heart disease, can be continuously monitored with personalized help. Based on the patient's prescribed regimen, they can offer tailored medication reminders, promoting adherence and lowering the possibility of side effects. It assists users in organizing their daily schedules, which are customized to their habits and interests, from getting up to going to bed. Depending on the interests and psychological level of the user, customized recreational activities and psychological training can be created to preserve and enhance cognitive functioning. AAL systems can follow customized protocols in an emergency that consider the user's unique medical conditions and preferred methods of communication with family members and emergency responders.

16.8.2 Future Directions

Below is a detailed overview of the various future directions and research opportunities in speech emotion recognition for dialog systems:

- Developments in emotion recognition algorithms like extraction of context and long-term dependencies from voice data by using transformer-based models like BERT and GPT.
- Develop models to identify emotions by combining audio with other techniques like facial expressions and physiological indicators. It should be more reliable.
- Gather information from real-time interactions to improve the applicability of SER systems outside of controlled situations.
- Develop models that take dialog context, previous interactions, and user history into consideration, so that they can give high accuracy.

16.9 CONCLUSION

SER for dialog systems is a developing area that holds great potential to improve human–computer interactions. Its sophisticated machine-learning methods, including CNNs, RNNs, LSTMs, and transformers, are used to identify intricate speech patterns and long-term dependencies. The signal processing was improved by using advanced prosodic and spectral characteristics in addition to standard features (MFCCs) for a complete characterization of emotions. To boost robustness, real-world interaction data is used. With the rapid advancement of SER for dialog systems, more emotionally intelligent and sensitive human–computer interactions could be possible. As ethical and practical issues are resolved, more research and development in this area promises to improve the user experience across wide range of applications.

REFERENCES

Arora, S., Batra, K., & Singh, S. (n.d.). Dialogue system: A brief review. https://doi.org/10.48550/arXiv.1306.4134

Cavanini, L., Benetazzo, F., Freddi, A., Longhi, S., & Monteriu, A. (2014). SLAM-based autonomous wheelchair navigation system for AAL scenarios. In IEEE/ASME 10th *International Conference on Mechatronic and Embedded Systems and Applications (MESA)* (pp. 1–6). https://doi.org/10.1109/MESA.2014.6935628

Darshan, K. A., & Veerappa, B. N. (2020). Speech emotion recognition. *International Research Journal of Engineering and Technology (IRJET),* 7(9), 938–941.

Estudillo-Valderrama, M. A., Roa, L. M., Reina-Tosina, J., & Román-Martínez, I. (2010). Ambient assisted living: A methodological approach. In *2010 Annual International Conference of the IEEE Engineering in Medicine and Biology Society* (pp. 1–4). https://doi.org/10.1109/IEMBS.2010.5626628

Harar, P., Burget, R., & Dutta, M. K. (2017). Speech emotion recognition with deep learning. In *2017 4th International Conference on Signal Processing and Integrated Networks (SPIN)* (pp. 1–5). https://doi.org/10.1109/SPIN.2017.8049931

Huang, K. Y., Wu, C. H., Hong, Q. B., Su, M. H., & Zeng, Y. R. (2018). Speech emotion recognition using a convolutional neural network with audio word-based embedding. In *2018*

11th International Symposium on Chinese Spoken Language Processing (ISCSLP) (pp. 1–5). https://doi.org/10.1109/ISCSLP.2018.8706610

Leelavathi, R., Deepthi, S. A., & Aruna, V. (2022). Speech emotion recognition using LSTM. *International Research Journal of Engineering and Technology (IRJET),* 9(1), 586–594.

Mainetti, L., Manco, L., Patrono, L., Secco, A., Sergi, I., & Vergallo, R. (2016). An ambient assisted living system for elderly assistance applications. In *2016 IEEE 27th Annual International Symposium on Personal, Indoor, and Mobile Radio Communications (PIMRC)* (pp. 1–6). https://doi.org/10.1109/PIMRC.2016.7794963

Mulam, S., Navale, S., Pawar, U., & Deshpande, S. (2020). Video monitoring system for identifying the well-being of elders at home: A survey. *International Research Journal of Engineering and Technology (IRJET)*, 7(12), 1024–1027.

Pandey, S. K., Shekhawat, H. S., & Prasanna, S. R. M. (2019). Deep learning techniques for speech emotion recognition: A review. In *2019 29th International Conference Radioelektronika* (pp. 1–6). https://doi.org/10.1109/radioelek.2019.8733432

Sanchez-Comas, A., Synnes, K., & Hallberg, J. (2018). Hardware for recognition of human activities: A review of smart home and AAL related technologies. *Sensors*, 20(15), 4227.

Seehapoch, T., & Wongthanavasu, S. (2013). Speech emotion recognition using support vector machines. *5th International Conference on Knowledge and Smart Technology (KST)* (pp. 1–6).

Van Hoof, J., Kort, H. S. M., Markopoulos, P., & Soede, M. (2007). Ambient intelligence, ethics and privacy. *Gerontechnology*, 6(3), 155–163.

Wani, T. M., Gunawan, T. S., Qadri, S. A. A., Kartiwi, M., & Ambikairajah, E. (2021). A comprehensive review of speech emotion recognition systems. *IEEE Access*, 9, 47795–47814. https://doi.org/10.1109/ACCESS.2021.3068045

Yan, S., Ye, L., Han, S., Han, T., Li, Y., & Alasaarela, E. (2020). Speech interactive emotion recognition system based on random forest. In *2020 IEEE* (pp. 1–6).

17 Text Analytics for Health Records and Documentations

N. Sharmila Banu and K. Deepa

17.1 INTRODUCTION

The healthcare sector encounters several complications in maintaining reliability and organizing the data. Owing to the large quantity of data that accumulates every day associated with healthcare procedures, general practitioners and healthcare administrators have to dedicate a significant portion of their day to reviewing and organizing healthcare records. The unstructured data contains numerous figures, facts, and statistical data that are not properly organized. It can also be clinical procedures, medical records, medical publications, and many others. Due to disorganized data, it is very critical to access, explore, evaluate, and extract the information.

Text mining is the procedure of transforming unlabeled text into labeled text for easy analysis. Text analytics can be used to improve the speed and efficiency of all functions within the healthcare sector. This allows both patients and healthcare professionals to enjoy simpler and more pleasant healthcare services. The exact information can be obtained with the help of the text analysis procedure. The progression is fully programmed and reliable, which shows actionable data. Text analysis is very effective in categorizing and exploring healthcare records.

The use of data analytics as a tool to exploit healthcare data for competitive improvement is becoming more and more common. Text analytics plays a significant role in describing, encapsulating, and gaining knowledge by providing essential composite information in an exclusive manner by utilizing a range of machine learning methods. A number of clinical and practical domains, such as analysis, physical condition, evaluation, medical management, hospital administration, and healthcare service administration, can benefit from such insights.

The approaches utilized to extract the appropriate and valuable information from the textual data are normally referred to as text analytics or text mining (Meystre et al., 2008). Text analytics is commonly used today to retrieve information from unstructured textual data that may assist in constructing and exploring essential details (Hearst, 1999). NLP in the healthcare sector is growing very rapidly because of its recognized potential by the health sector to explore, examine, and understand numerous amounts of patient datasets. NLP approaches have the power to exploit the appropriate information and the clinical reports that were formerly precise by the

DOI: 10.1201/9781003520184-21

healthcare sector but obscured in textual data. It provides an accurate result from the unstructured data by accepting excellence and effective approaches. Natural language processing tools for healthcare can retrieve key insights from clinical records, like drugs or risk factors that may be related to a particular patient's physical condition, and provide desirable treatments or medications with better precision than manual data processing. NLP in healthcare is capable of recognizing the context within which words are used, permitting us to exactly understand patient discussions and capture the delicate health condition of a person. This assists healthcare experts to supervise data about treatments and investigate actions. The healthcare industry will use its experts to further process patients' data for the betterment of their outcomes.

Natural language processing is utilized to explain any languages used by human beings to discriminate them from programming languages and data demonstration languages used by systems and depicted as artificial. Information extraction is one of the significant fields in healthcare, and name entity recognition (NER) is a subset of data extraction capable of identifying entities like patient names, dosages, and syndromes in the textual data. Machine-learning techniques can effectively extract named entities but involve great annotated training collections. Machine-learning techniques do not utilize human perception and can be reconsidered without retraining in any field. The progress of establishing and attaining insights from the unstructured textual data is said to be text mining (Hearst, 1999).

Data recovery (utilized to gather the applicable texts), data extraction (categorize the associations among the particular types of information), and text mining (analysis of particular types of data from the given texts). The electronic healthcare record (EHR) is a longitudinal compilation of healthcare statistics about a particular patient and many others (Miriovsky et al., 2012). It is mainly utilized for recording health data. The health record may include a group of valuable information that is very significant and essential in many ways, like medical documentation, treatments, and clinical records that improve the quality of the concern (Kruse et al., 2016). The information can be easily retrieved from the structured data with the help of machine-learning approaches because the structured data contains information like age, height, weight, and gender. But in the case of unstructured information, it is very complicated to retrieve the data as it contains discharge summaries, a brief description of the patient's health, which is very hard to extract since it is linked to different backgrounds and the unpredictability of medical records. The textual data that contains spelling errors, uncertainties, acronyms, and grammatical mistakes is very complicated to process and analyze. Natural language processing plays a vital role in showing the exactness of textual data from unstructured information.

17.2 TEXT MINING TECHNIQUES AND APPLICATIONS IN HEALTHCARE

Text mining is the procedure to seek for numerous amounts of records in order to discover knowledgeable information or to show results based on the specific queries. The primary steps involved in text mining are as follows:

(1) Collecting unstructured textual data from various data resources like web, mails, social media, and PDF files.

(2) Identify and eliminate the abnormalities from the acquired data performing preprocessing and refinement process. The refinement process extracts the relevant information hidden within the data source and assists to identify the exactness from the initial stage, with the help of text mining software and techniques this process is possible.
(3) Transform all the textual data extracted from unstructured form into structured form. Further examine the pattern of the textual data through the management information systems.
(4) The extracted relevant data is finally stored in the database to further process and improve the quality of healthcare service.

Text Mining Techniques: The process of extracting textual data and establishing insights from the source is considered text mining. The text mining approaches require data mining tools and applications for the proper execution of results.
The following are the techniques utilized in text mining:

Data Extraction: This technique is utilized to extract the most valuable and relevant information, or textual data, from any kind of data source. The intention of the text mining technique is to identify entities, characteristics, and their correlations from the unstructured textual data. The valuable information is stored in the database for future reference and recovery. The effectiveness and reliability of the results are examined and finally assessed by performing the exactness procedures.

Data Recovery: It is defined as the process of retrieving the significant and related model based on a particular collection of phrases. This technique utilizes many methods to follow and observe the pattern and manage the information accordingly.

Classification: It is considered to be one of the forms of supervised learning that is different from normal language texts, which are allotted to a predetermined group of information from the acquired context. Classification, or relatively natural language processing (NLP), is utilized to collect the textual records and extract relevant synonyms and abbreviations from the textual data.

Clustering: It is a significant and essential progress to formulate a meaningful group of information or clusters from the unstructured data without considering the preceding data. The text mining tools assist in guiding the preprocessing and detection methods.

Summarization: Text summarization is exploited to automatically promote a compressed edition of a precise text that influences valuable information for the individual. This technique gathers the information through several textual data sources and summarizes the text without affecting the originality of the patient's record. It involves various techniques, like bio-inspired algorithms, neural networks, and regression models, to ensure the reliability of the documents. Table 17.1 depicts the techniques, characteristics, and tools of text mining.

Text mining is categorized into two different stages. Initially, the textual data refinement process is performed, which converts the free text records into intermediate

TABLE 17.1
Techniques, Characteristics, and Tools of Text Mining

Techniques	Characteristics	Tools
Extraction	Extracts valuable information from the labeled data.	Clear Forest Text and Text Finder
Recovery	Retrieves valuable information from labeled data.	Intelligent Miner and Text Analyst
Classification	Categorizing the records.	Intelligent Miner
Clustering	Gathering the collection of specific records.	Carrot, Rapid Miner
Summarization	Maintaining the originality of the records by providing the main points.	Sentence Ext Tool, Tropic Tracking Tool

types. Then the information is extracted from the intermediate one (Tan, 2011). This approach may be very useful for retrieving valuable information and maintaining records for future reference. To attain the automatic extraction of keys from the large collection of queries attached to the online healthcare system (Xiaojun, 2011). The aim of this system is to extract related questions from a large set of healthcare sectors (Han et al., 2015).

Natural language processing approaches are implemented using the NLTK library (Cohen & Hersh, 2005). This approach is capable of identifying the medical experts like neuro and cardio disorders and supports provided by governments and industrial sectors. This opportunity is provided by IBM Watson API to support the healthcare industries. Similarly, retrieving significant information based on the health applications on the internet is suggested (Paglialonga et al., 2017). A number of studies used text mining to retrieve significant and valuable information from the insights provided on the web or based on the discussions. The healthcare-linked information is taken from the content generated by the end users on social media with the help of text mining applications. A cancer-associated dataset was considered and specific information like drug names, treatments, and their consequences was extracted (Sutar, 2017). Both unstructured and structured textual data are considered for the extraction of relevant information.

Martínez et al. (2016) described using text mining transforming health-related online content into practical information. In order to recover and transform information derived from real-time streaming social media, an NLP approach was utilized. In addition to extracting the syndromes and their prescriptions, the method was also able to discover relevant connections between prescriptions, discrepancies, and side effects. James et al. (2017) investigated the unstructured feedback provided by the general practitioner. Their intention was to gather responses and focus on the quality services associated with healthcare. The latent Dirichlet allocation (LDA) model was utilized to analyze victims opinions from over 20,000 physicians. Moreover, a dictionary-based textual examination was utilized to recognize the key terms in the general practitioner assessments. The potential of technology to keep patients informed and involved in their healthcare journey has been demonstrated by studies on the function of mobile applications in empowering consumers and strengthening patient control over their health (Alhomod & Alzahrani, 2019).

Elbattah et al. (2021) investigated the possibilities of text mining in automatic clinical analysis. The bag-of-words concept was implemented to represent the medical records. The bag-of-words model generates a word histogram in order to detail the text representation, with each word count being observed as an attribute. Since, every record may be developed as a simple "bag of words", regardless of its grammatical order and progression, In spite of considering a partial dataset, the research proves talented outcomes. In recent times, van Dijk et al. (2021) examined text mining in electronic healthcare records to authenticate the screening acceptability of test patients. The research was based on multi-center and multi-EHR systems. The exactness of the text-mining method was evaluated according to the regular procedure developed by researchers. The precision of the spontaneously recovered information was about 88 percent. To improve healthcare information sharing systems, a multi-method approach that incorporates empirical data and text analysis is absolutely necessary. Text analysis methods that can be used to glean insightful information from user-generated medical content include sentiment analysis, content analysis, and topic modeling (Malhan et al., 2024). By redefining medical documentation through a variety of applications like natural language processing, predictive analytics, and clinical decision support systems, artificial intelligence (AI) is modernizing the health care industry. Large-scale patient data analysis is made possible by AI-powered technologies, allowing for more accurate diagnosis, individualized treatment regimens, and early disease identification (Bongurala et al., 2024). Healthcare organizations confront a variety of issues in the COVID-19 era, but these can be successfully managed by integrating text analytics, data integration, and well-informed decision-making. Text analytics is essential for gleaning insightful information from massive data sets, which helps to clarify patient experiences and hospital workloads and pave the way for implementable solutions. In order to address the complexity of healthcare, a comprehensive database system that supports a range of analytical techniques must be created, and data integration is crucial to this process (Shujana, 2024).

17.3 TEXT ANALYTICS FOR CLINICAL DECISION SUPPORT

Text analytics refers to the computational procedure of segregating the unlabeled textual records, including articles, reviews, and feedbacks, which assist the examinations in the future. Text analytics for healthcare can receive unlabeled text in English, German, French, Italian, Spanish, Portuguese, and Hebrew. There exist seven computational steps in performing unlabeled text records for further study. They are as follows:

Language Identification: Each and every language has its own grammatical rules and regulations. Initially, it should be recognized to verify the textual data from the source for further processing.

Tokenization: Tokenization is the process of separating a phrase into its integral parts. They are generally either words or numbers. Based on the kind of unlabeled textual data an individual is processing, it may be a punctuation mark, links, or notations.

Sentence Breaking: Lengthy records need sentence breakage to segregate every distinct statement. Each and every sentence is divided by a punctuation mark. It is not the same in all situations. It may differ in some cases where sentences containing punctuation marks at times do not refer to the end of the statement.

Part of Speech Tagging: Part of speech tagging is the method of resolving the part of speech of each and every token in a record and designating it by definition. There are some principal rules and patterns that can be authored into a basic part of the speech tagger, which is pursued by most of the languages. When a textual record is displayed, the tagger manages to make out if the token depicts a proper noun, a common noun, or a verb and also represents an adjective or absolutely other commodity. An authentic factor of speech tagging is particular for definite opinion mining. By determining the adjective noun, the affiliations and opinion mining scheme acquires an intimation that it is surveying at a convict bearing expressions.

Chunking: It refers to a sentence breakage system that splits a sentence into its elemental group phrases. It helps to retrieve the significant words alone from longer documents. It plays a vital role in grouping only the necessary phrases, exclusive of all the modifiers, which are not mandatory.

Syntax Parsing: It is the opinion of how a sentence or phrase is structured. It is a demanding preliminary step in sentimental study and natural language processing characteristics. It also holds the procedure of examining grammatical errors, word ranging, and comprehensive recognition associated with words to see if they make sense.

Sentence Chaining: Finally, in developing the unlabeled textual data for further study in sentence chaining, it uses approaches like lexical chaining to correlate separate sentences based on their connection to a lengthy subject (Carchiolo et al., 2019) suggested a method for the spontaneous categorization of clinical documentation (permitted or not permitted) via the text-analytics approach. The text data was first inspected from the instructed medical records. Based on information regarding symptoms, pathology, diagnosis, recommended therapies, and personal medical records for the patient and the doctor, they could generate a professional classifier. According to their perception, only 5% of the instructions were not automatically categorized. Text analytics was utilized in the healthcare sector for analyzing the textual dataset from a wide range of data sources. The dataset can be medical records, descriptive text, predictable electronic healthcare records, content generated by end users on social media, and publications. Text analytics was employed for substantial problems, including extracting evidence-based care interventions and patient's results. Consequently, natural language processing has been developed effectively for dealing with a wide range of text processing tasks. Despite these difficulties, the qualitative analysis showed that physicians noticed the potential advantages of electronic records, such as increased accessibility, readability, and ease of information sharing across healthcare professionals (Ho, 2006).

TABLE 17.2
Recent Studies in Health Records and Documentation

Approaches	Recent Studies and Benefits
Machine Learning	This novel method not only simplifies the data entry and retrieval procedure but also creates opportunities for individualized healthcare interventions based on the needs of each individual patient and real-time monitoring. The capacity to predict probable health issues and take prior actions to remedy them by the medical experts in advance (Czypionka & Drexler, 2022).
	Using deep-learning techniques, meaningful insights are extracted from unstructured EHR data in biomedical NLP that could lead to more accurate and efficient clinical decision-making procedures. By utilizing the enormous amount of data found in electronic health records, this strategy has demonstrated considerable promise for enhancing patient outcomes and expediting the delivery of healthcare (Rostamzadeh et al., 2022).
	Automatic text classification is becoming gradually critical due to the availability of massive corpora. There are two methods for automatically classifying texts: rule-based and data-driven. A rule-based approach divides text into several groups depending on predetermined criteria and subject expertise. A data-driven strategy based on data observations is used to structure the text. The intrinsic relationship between text and its labels can be found using machine-learning or deep-learning algorithms based on data observation (Asudani et al., 2023).
Natural Language Processing	Building flexible models for electronic health record (EHR) texts has become more popular in biomedical natural language processing research. This is done by using domain adaptation strategies and pre-trained transformers to improve the model's performance in clinical NLP tasks and prediction based on the previous reports (Pine & Bossen, 2020).
Big Data	Utilizing big data in healthcare has many important advantages. The most significant advantage is better patient outcomes. Healthcare providers can spot patterns and trends in patient care and regulate treatment plans by gathering and analyzing massive volumes of patient data. Better treatment outcomes, more precise diagnoses, and more patient satisfaction are possible outcomes (Ahmed et al., 2023).

Around the world, medical data processing is extensively automated through the use of technologies like machine learning. A few recent studies in health records and documentation are illustrated in Table 17.2.

17.4 NATURAL LANGUAGE PROCESSING FOR HEALTHCARE

Natural language processing illustrates the rule-based system in which artificial intelligence strategies associate and review unlabeled textual data from the language of individuals to extract indications, obtain significance, and provide responses. This serves the medical management sector to maintain the greatest use of unlabeled textual data. This expertise assists the end user in automating the decision-making task, taking extra care of patients by paying more attention, and enhancing the patient's understanding ability using real-world data. NLP has experienced extraordinary progressions that are extensively considered in the medical management industry, mostly in the area of clinical decision support systems (CDSS). By exploiting natural language processing approaches, the clinical decision support system has obtained the capability to retrieve significant data from a range of clinical textual data sources, consisting of electronic healthcare records (EHRs), clinical documentation, and additional healthcare information. This recovered data has the power to transform clinical decision-making, promote patient results, and simply streamline healthcare procedures.

CDSSs have observed significant advancements by incorporation of NLP, permitting the improvement of complicated structure have the ability to inspect clinical textual data and provide appropriate suggestions to healthcare sources. Holding the potential of natural language processing, these CDSSs acquire the knowledge to extensively examine patient indications, medical summaries, and other related information to produce valuable perceptions and recommendations for healthcare experts. By systematically inspecting the variations of medical textual data, NLP correlated with CDSS can propose effective determination, suggested modified treatment procedures, and affordable medication that assist the individual to improve their health conditions. The suggestions were provided from the information retrieved through the most powerful and effective technique called NLP. These systems are capable of efficiently sorting through the large volume of clinical textual data, discovering prototypes, relationships, and important insights. With the help of this thorough study, CDSS is capable of producing perceptive suggestions that permit healthcare retailers to upgrade their opinions and provide a quality service to the healthcare sector. NLP is a tool that CDSS can use to assist and improve the difficulties related to unlabeled medical textual data. NLP approaches are highly skilled at interpreting the particulars present in clinical summaries, accumulating relevant data, and converting it into practical suggestions. It is a major advancement when clinical text can be comprehended and interpreted by CDSS. The medical narratives and the accuracy of the healthcare records can be upgraded (Reinecke, 1985; Wagholikar et al., 2012).

Natural language processing integrated with the clinical decision support system not only examines individual patient data but also involves a large body of medical knowledge. By utilizing NLP approaches to extract and corporate information from wide-ranging clinical records and clinical procedures, CDSS can endure with the most recent study and optimal procedures (Shortliffe & Cimino, 2014). This combination of NLP and CDSS certifies that healthcare sectors have approaches to retrieving the most relevant and recent data's permitting them to confirm and enhance the quality of patient care in the healthcare sector. It shows the advancements in the medical decision making system and provides a potential tool to traverse the complications of medical records. By appropriate NLP strategies, the large volume of patient data may be explored by CDSS, which assist the recovery of important indications and provide precise and pertinent suggestions (Reyes-Ortiz et al., 2016; Wagholikar et al., 2012). Natural language processing pipelines have been effectively evolved for a range

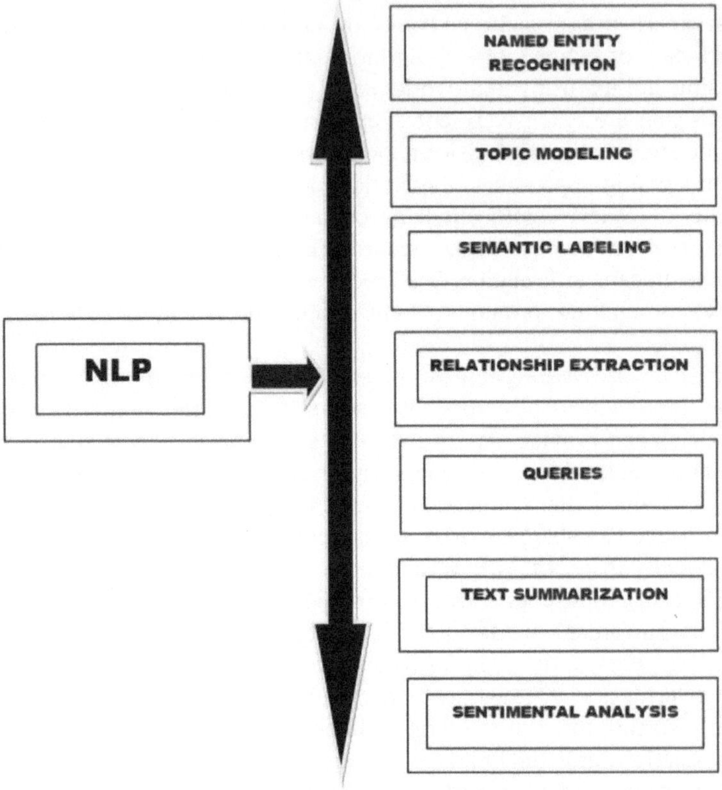

FIGURE 17.1 Leveraging natural processing for healthcare.

of textual processing functions like entity recognition, topic modeling, semantic labeling, affiliation extraction, queries, textual summarization, and emotional analysis. Leveraging natural processing for healthcare is depicted in Figure 17.1.

The availability of high-quality data is a major obstacle to developing reliable natural language processing and machine-learning approaches. Furthermore, the fundamental textual data variations raise a number of ethical questions about the use of NLP models. The literature has lately addressed these ethical concerns (Tayefi et al., 2021; Shortliffe & Cimino, 2014).

17.5 CONCLUSION

Text analytics should be crucial in converting unstructured textual data into applicable perceptions. It is evident that unstructured textual data must be leveraged to hold the process of healthcare in many prospects. A significant amount of clinical data is inevitably accumulated in unstructured documents. Information extraction from user-generated content, medical records, discharge narratives, scientific journals, and free-text data kept in EHR databases. Vector-based representations to convert textual data into a format that machine learning can understand on a range of clinical documents. Sequence-based modeling is used for tasks including sentiment analysis, online forum comments, and notes from clinical reports. The use of NLP has significantly advanced the healthcare industry, especially in CDSS. Through the use of NLP techniques, CDSS is able to extract useful data from a range of medical sources, such as medical literature, electronic health records, and other papers pertaining to healthcare. The information that has been retrieved can be a valuable tool for optimizing clinical judgment, enhancing patient outcomes, and streamlining medical procedures.

REFERENCES

Ahmed, A., Xi, R., Hou, M., Shah, S. A., & Hameed, S. (2023). Harnessing big data analytics for healthcare: A comprehensive review of frameworks, implications, applications, and impacts. *IEEE Access*, *11*(October), 112891–112928. https://doi.org/10.1109/ACCESS.2023.3323574

Alhomod, A. S., & Alzahrani, S. (2019). Patient empowerment via mobile personal health records and mobile health applications: A review of the current use. PICMET 2019 – Portland International Conference on Management of Engineering and Technology: Technology Management in the World of Intelligent Systems, Proceedings, 1–4. https://doi.org/10.23919/PICMET.2019.8893847

Asudani, D. S., Nagwani, N. K., & Singh, P. (2023). Impact of word embedding models on text analytics in deep learning environment: A review. In *Artificial Intelligence Review* (Vol. 56, Issue 9). Springer Netherlands. https://doi.org/10.1007/s10462-023-10419-1

Bongurala, A. R., Save, D., Virmani, A., & Kashyap, R. (2024). Transforming health care with artificial intelligence (AI): Redefining medical documentation. *Mayo Clinic Proceedings: Digital Health*, *2*(3), 342–347. https://doi.org/10.1016/j.mcpdig.2024.05.006

Carchiolo, V., Longheu, A., Reitano, G., & Zagarella, L. (2019). Medical prescription classification: A NLP-based approach. *Proceedings of the 2019 Federated Conference on Computer Science and Information Systems, FedCSIS 2019*, *18*, 605–609. https://doi.org/10.15439/2019F197

Cohen, A. M., & Hersh, W. R. (2005). A survey of current work in biomedical text mining. *Briefings in Bioinformatics*, *6*(1), 57–71. https://doi.org/10.1093/bib/6.1.57

Czypionka, T., & Drexler, S. (2022). Smart Health. In *The Routledge Handbook of Smart Technologies: An Economic and Social Perspective* (Vol. 11, Issue. 7, pp. 588–607). Routledge. https://doi.org/10.4324/9780429351921-35

Elbattah, M., Arnaud, É., Gignon, M., & Dequen, G. (2021). The role of text analytics in healthcare: A review of recent developments and applications. HEALTHINF 2021 – 14th International Conference on Health Informatics; Part of the 14th International Joint Conference on Biomedical Engineering Systems and Technologies, BIOSTEC 2021, *5*(Biostec), 825–832. https://doi.org/10.5220/0010414508250832

Han, J., Nandan, N., & Sun, A. (2015). "Did You Know?" A rule-based approach to finding similar questions on online health forums. Proceedings – 2015 IEEE International Conference on Healthcare Informatics, ICHI 2015, 513–514. https://doi.org/10.1109/ICHI.2015.94

Hearst, M. A. (1999). The role of text analytics in healthcare: A review of recent developments and applicationUntangling text data mining. Proceedings of the Annual Meeting of the Association for Computational Linguistics, 1999-June, *3–10*. https://doi.org/10.3115/1034678.1034679

Ho, K. (2006). Improving the Quality of the Documentation System in a Health Care Environment. Regis University Student Publication.

James, T. L., Villacis Calderon, E. D., & Cook, D. F. (2017). Exploring patient perceptions of healthcare service quality through analysis of unstructured feedback. *Expert Systems with Applications*, *71*, 479–492. https://doi.org/10.1016/j.eswa.2016.11.004

Kruse, C. S., Kristof, C., Jones, B., Mitchell, E., & Martinez, A. (2016). Barriers to electronic health record adoption: A systematic literature review. *Journal of Medical Systems*, *40*(12). https://doi.org/10.1007/s10916-016-0628-9

Malhan, A., Pavur, R., Pelton, L. E., & Hajian, A. (2024). A multimethod approach for healthcare information sharing systems: Text analysis and empirical data. *Information*, *15*(6), 319. https://doi.org/10.3390/info15060319

Martínez, P., Martínez, J. L., Segura-Bedmar, I., Moreno-Schneider, J., Luna, A., & Revert, R. (2016). Turning user generated health-related content into actionable knowledge through text analytics services. *Computers in Industry*, *78*, 43–56. https://doi.org/10.1016/j.compind.2015.10.006

Meystre, S. M., Savova, G. K., & Hurdle, J. F. (2008). Extracting information from textual documents in the electronic health record: A review of recent research. *Yearbook of Medical Informatics*, *17*, 128–144.

Miriovsky, B. J., Shulman, L. N., & Abernethy, A. P. (2012). Importance of health information technology, electronic health records, and continuously aggregating data to comparative effectiveness research and learning health care. *Journal of Clinical Oncology*, *30*(34), 4243–4248. https://doi.org/10.1200/JCO.2012.42.8011

Paglialonga, A., Pinciroli, F., Tognola, G., Barbieri, R., Caiani, E. G., & Riboldi, M. (2017). E-Health solutions for better care: Characterization of health apps to extract meaningful information and support users' choices. RTSI 2017 – IEEE 3rd International Forum on Research and Technologies for Society and Industry, Conference Proceedings. https://doi.org/10.1109/RTSI.2017.8065915

Pine, K. H., & Bossen, C. (2020). Good organizational reasons for better medical records: The data work of clinical documentation integrity specialists. *Big Data and Society*, *7*(2). https://doi.org/10.1177/2053951720965616

Reinecke, R. (1985). The potential for artificial intelligence in manufacturing. *ORSSA Annual Conference*, *6*(2), 94–98.

Reyes-Ortiz, J. A., Gonzalez-Beltran, B. A., & Gallardo-Lopez, L. (2016). Clinical decision support systems: A survey of NLP-based approaches from unstructured data. Proceedings – International Workshop on Database and Expert Systems Applications, DEXA, 2016-Febru*ary*, 163–167. https://doi.org/10.1109/DEXA.2015.47

Rostamzadeh, N., Mincu, D., Roy, S., Smart, A., Wilcox, L., Pushkarna, M., Schrouff, J., Amironesei, R., Moorosi, N., & Heller, K. (2022). Healthsheet: Development of a transparency artifact for health datasets. *ACM International Conference Proceeding Series*, *37*(4), 1943–1961. https://doi.org/10.1145/3531146.3533239

Shortliffe, E. H., & Cimino, J. J. (2014). Biomedical Informatics: Computer Applications in Health Care and Biomedicine: Fourth Edition, 1–965. Springer. https://doi.org/10.1007/978-1-4471-4474-8

Shujana, M. (2024). Navigating healthcare challenges text analytics, data integration, and decision-making in the COVID-19 era. *International Journal of Information Technology and Computer Science Applications*, *2*(1), 54–62. https://doi.org/10.58776/ijitcsa.v2i1.123

Sutar, S. G. (2017). Intelligent data mining technique of social media for improving health care. Proceedings of the 2017 International Conference on Intelligent Computing and Control Systems, ICICCS 2017, 2018-Janu*ary*, 1356–1360. https://doi.org/10.1109/ICCONS.2017.8250690

Tan, A. (2011). Text Mining: The state of the art and the challenges Concept-based. Proceedings of the PAKDD 1999 Workshop On, January, 65–70. www.mendeley.com/research/text-mining-state-art-challenges-3/

Tayefi, M., Ngo, P., Chomutare, T., Dalianis, H., Salvi, E., Budrionis, A., & Godtliebsen, F. (2021). Challenges and opportunities beyond structured data in analysis of electronic health records. *Wiley Interdisciplinary Reviews: Computational Statistics*, *13*(6), 1–19. https://doi.org/10.1002/wics.1549

van Dijk, W. B., Fiolet, A. T. L., Schuit, E., Sammani, A., Groenhof, T. K. J., van der Graaf, R., de Vries, M. C., Alings, M., Schaap, J., Asselbergs, F. W., Grobbee, D. E., Groenwold, R. H. H., & Mosterd, A. (2021). Text-mining in electronic healthcare records can be used as efficient tool for screening and data collection in cardiovascular trials: A multicenter validation study. *Journal of Clinical Epidemiology*, *132*, 97–105. https://doi.org/10.1016/j.jclinepi.2020.11.014

Wagholikar, K. B., MacLaughlin, K. L., Henry, M. R., Greenes, R. A., Hankey, R. A., Liu, H., & Chaudhry, R. C. (2012). Clinical decision support with automated text processing for cervical cancer screening. *Journal of the American Medical Informatics Association*, *19*(5), 833–839. https://doi.org/10.1136/amiajnl-2012-000820

Wagholikar, K., Sohn, S., Wu, S., Kaggal, V., Buehler, S., Greenes, R., Wu, T. T., Larson, D., Liu, H., Chaudhry, R., & Boardman, L. (2012). Clinical decision support for colonoscopy surveillance using natural language processing. Proceedings – 2012 IEEE 2nd Conference on Healthcare Informatics, Imaging and Systems Biology, HISB 2012, 12–21. https://doi.org/10.1109/HISB.2012.11

Xiaojun, W. Berry, Z. M., & Kogan, J. (eds.) (2011). Text mining: applications and theory. *Inf Retrieval*, *14*, 208–211. https://doi.org/10.1007/s10791-010-9153-5

Index

B

C

D

E

F

L

M

N

S

T

U

V

W

Y

Z